To my students, who expected me to write this book.

Primary Health Care

THEORY AND PRACTICE

Trisha Greenhalgh

Department of Primary Care and Population Sciences
University College London
UK

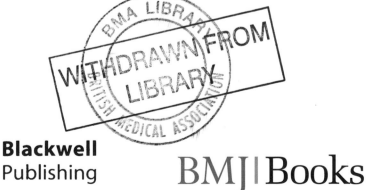
Blackwell Publishing

BMJ|Books

© 2007 Trisha Greenhalgh
Published by Blackwell Publishing
BMJ Books is an imprint of the BMJ Publishing Group Limited, used under licence

Blackwell Publishing, Inc., 350 Main Street, Malden, Massachusetts 02148-5020, USA
Blackwell Publishing Ltd, 9600 Garsington Road, Oxford OX4 2DQ, UK
Blackwell Publishing Asia Pty Ltd, 550 Swanston Street, Carlton, Victoria 3053, Australia

The right of the Author to be identified as the Author of this Work has been asserted in
accordance with the Copyright, Designs and Patents Act 1988.

First published 2007

1   2007

Library of Congress Cataloging-in-Publication Data

Greenhalgh, Trisha.
   Primary health care : from academic foundations to contemporary
practice / Trisha Greenhalgh.
      p. ; cm.
   "BMJ books."
   Includes bibliographical references and index.
   ISBN 978-0-7279-1785-0 (pbk. : alk. paper)
   1. Primary care (Medicine)   I. Title.
   [DNLM: 1. Primary Health Care.   2. Health Services Research. W 84.6
   G813p 2007]

   RA427.9.G74 2007
   362.1–dc22

                                                    2007003618
ISBN: 978-0-7279-1785-0

A catalogue record for this title is available from the British Library

Set in 9.5/12pt Palatino by Aptara Inc., New Delhi, India
Printed and bound in Malaysia by Vivar Printing Sdn. Bhd.

Commissioning Editor: Mary Banks
Editorial Assistant: Victoria Pittman
Development Editor: Lauren Brindley
Production Controller: Rachel Edwards

For further information on Blackwell Publishing, visit our website:
http://www.blackwellpublishing.com

The publisher's policy is to use permanent paper from mills that operate a sustainable forestry
policy, and which has been manufactured from pulp processed using acid-free and elementary
chlorine-free practices. Furthermore, the publisher ensures that the text paper and cover board
used have met acceptable environmental accreditation standards.

Contents

Acknowledgements

This book is my own work, and I alone take responsibility for errors and omissions. It would not have been possible for me to tackle the vast field of primary health care without inspiration, insights and contributions from dozens if not hundreds of academic and clinical colleagues. Many of these people are mentioned by name in the sections of this book where their input has been direct, explicit and auditable. But I am also indebted to the numerous colleagues and students who have provided more subtle, indirect and diffuse input to my knowledge and understanding of primary health care over the years. They are, quite literally, too numerous to list in full. I hesitate to single out any individual or group for special mention because my debt to the academic community is so extensive, but I must acknowledge in particular my outstanding team of tutors on the online MSc in International Primary Health Care at University College London, with whom it is a privilege and a joy to work.

Thanks also to Mary Banks and her team at Blackwell Publishing for the unrivalled quality of their support in taking this book from an idea on the back of an envelope to the finished product. They have seen the work go through many metamorphoses. And finally, to my long-suffering husband Fraser Macfarlane and sons Rob and Al for their forbearance, patience and support as the magnum opus slowly took shape.

Preface

In 1999, the editor of the *Lancet*, Dr Richard Horton, threw down this gauntlet:

> '*Primary care is the subject of more charters, declarations, manifestos, and principles than any other medical discipline, except perhaps its similarly plagued cousin, public health. Yet this efflux of ruminations from worthy experts and respected bureaucracies has contributed hardly anything to the daily practice of family medicine*'.[1]

Horton's words were met with outrage from primary care academics world-wide, and I certainly shared that outrage. But his editorial revealed two important things. First, that the academic foundations of primary care, if not weakly developed in themselves (and perhaps they were), had been poorly articulated by academics within our discipline. Second, that these foundations were, as a result, widely and profoundly misunderstood by people in powerful positions in academia and medical publishing. It was Horton's shot across the bows that prompted me to take on the task of producing a completely new, single-author textbook on the academic basis of primary health care.

The case for such a book was not difficult to make. Remarkably few academic textbooks in this field have ever been written – and to my knowledge, no new first editions have been published in the past 15 years. The giants on whose shoulders I stand include Britain's William Pickles (*Epidemiology in Country Practice*, originally published in 1939[2]) and Julian Tudor Hart (*A New Kind of Doctor*, 1988[3]); Hungary's émigré to Britain Michael Balint (*The Doctor, His Patient and the Illness*, 1956[4]); America's Barbara Starfield (*Primary Care*, 1992[5]) and Robert Rakel (*Textbook of Family Medicine*, 1973[6]) and Canada's Ian McWhinney (*A Textbook of Family Medicine*, 1986[7]).* I have also been inspired by Gillian Hampson's excellent textbook for nurses, *Practice Nurse Handbook*, first published as Bolden and Tackle's Handbook in 1980.[9]

Apart from more up-to-date reference lists, what does this book offer that goes beyond what the greats of a generation ago came up with? First and

---

*I should also mention John Noble and team's *Primary Care Medicine*, the leading US textbook, which is an excellent overview of the clinical problems seen in primary care practice, along with a guide to evidence-based decision making.[8] This is an outstanding reference tome for doctors in clinical practice, but does not attempt to cover the breadth of interdisciplinary territory addressed here. Another comprehensive textbook written for a US audience is Rakel's *Textbook of Family Medicine*, first published in 1973 and now in its 7th edition.[6] While mainly centring on clinical problems, it includes sections on evidence-based medicine and also covers the important work of McWhinney.

foremost, I have deliberately devoted a large section of the book to disentangling the diverse disciplinary roots of primary health care. Pickles, Fry and Starfield took an almost exclusively epidemiological perspective and showed how such a perspective could both emerge from and serve to inform the work of the primary care team. Balint focused on the psychodynamic perspective and showed how this could illuminate the study of the doctor–patient relationship. Tudor Hart linked epidemiology with political science and drew links between social inequalities and health outcomes. McWhinney, to whom I owe a particular intellectual debt,[†] drew on a range of disciplines including epidemiology, psychology and moral philosophy, but did so in a way that produced a unified, multi-level theory (patient-centred medicine; see Section 5.4) rather than – as I have chosen to do – setting out a menu of different disciplinary and theoretical perspectives as possible 'options' for cutting the cake of primary care. It is on McWhinney's important early work, and with the advantage of the last decade in which primary care has matured considerably as an academic field in its own right, that I seek to build.

I have called Chapter 2 'The "ologies" of Primary Health Care' because I believe that no single 'ology' (be it basic biomedical science, epidemiology, psychology, sociology, anthropology or philosophy) can alone underpin either practice or research in primary care. What is needed is not a single, 'minestrone' discipline that primary care can call its own, but a greater recognition by practitioners and researchers that different primary disciplines provide different theoretical lenses through which the complex and multifaceted problems of primary care can be studied. As I explain in Chapter 2, identifying the right 'ology' for a particular primary care problem is one of the key skills of the academic practitioner.

The second unique feature of this book is that it is (to my knowledge) the first general, single-author academic textbook to take an explicitly multi-professional perspective on primary health care (as opposed to general practice or family medicine). The shift from uniprofessional to multi-professional focus reflects changes in the organisation of primary care over the past 20 years and in the diverse roles associated with its delivery – particularly the growth of primary care nursing. It also reflects, I guess, the increasing role of the person who is ill in his or her own care, since the 'expert patient' (see Section 4.4) is also a member of the multi-professional team. Only around half the students on my MSc course in International Primary Health Care (www.internationalprimaryhealthcare.org) are medically qualified; the remainder have backgrounds in nursing, health policy, pharmacy, social work, physiotherapy and management. As I emphasise in Chapter 10, illness in the

---

[†] That is not to say that I regard the contribution of the other authors listed here as less intellectually significant, but that my own take on academic primary care aligns most closely to that of McWhinney and his team.

twenty-first century is characterised by complexity, comorbidity and the need for coordination. In this context, textbooks aimed exclusively at a single professional group are increasingly anachronistic.

The third unique selling point of this book is that every word has been written by a single author. There is a touch of irony here. If primary care is so intellectually diverse, so clinically and organisationally complex and its practice necessarily multi-professional, surely it would be better to include an appropriate range of individuals as chapter authors, each of whom would cover a particular area of expertise. There are certainly some advantages to such an approach – for one thing, the subject matter would be covered more evenly and comprehensively. As it is, this textbook is biased towards my own areas of interest and expertise (sociological aspects of illness and healthcare, ethnic health, electronic records) and somewhat superficial on other areas (such as epidemiological databases). But the upside is – I hope – that this book offers a holistic overview of the field along with consistency of style that simply cannot be achieved in a multi-author textbook. Incidentally, a massive, multi-author reference textbook on primary health care has recently been published in the UK,[10] and an equally weighty *European Textbook of Family Medicine* has recently rolled off the press. I do not seek to compete directly with these tomes, but to supplement them with one woman's take on the parameters of our discipline.

Having said that, I make no claim to comprehensiveness. In a field as diverse and rapidly changing as primary health care, any attempt at encyclopaedic coverage of its multitudinous themes in a single volume is doomed to failure, and in any case the academic journals make a much better job of covering all the latest topics. Like McWhinney before me, I have sought to produce a 'territory map' of academic primary care along with some illustrative examples of how theory and method may be applied to the huge range of potential research topics. Though necessarily incomplete and distorted by my personal interests and prejudices, I hope this map will prove sufficiently coherent to convey the breadth of what counts as the 'normal science' of academic primary health care and sufficiently flexible to accommodate perspectives and theories that I have missed (or which are yet to emerge).

What, then, is my intended audience for this book? To paraphrase John Van Maanen, any book that aspires to the status of academic work has three potential audiences:[11]

1 Scholars in the field. This book is written primarily for people who are already working as academics in primary health care or who aspire to enter the field as researchers or teachers. These are the people who, by and large, see the subject matter of primary health care through similar eyes to mine, who already know (or are learning) the jargon, who share (or are coming to share) the assumptions and are familiar with the main theories and methods used in primary care research. Included in this group are students (PhD, MSc and ambitious undergraduates) who seek to define, with a view to extending, the margins of knowledge in primary care.

2 Thinking practitioners. This book is also intended for general practitioners, practice and community nurses, and other primary care professionals who wish – for personal fulfilment or career progression – to go beyond the multitude of books on the shelves that promise 'ten tips for better consulting' or 'how to organise your practice.' The examination for the Membership of the Royal College of General Practitioners (www.rcgp.org) now includes an understanding of research and the academic basis of general practice in its syllabus. But be warned: I did not set out to write a textbook for the Membership of the Royal College of General Practitioners, nor have I consulted or collaborated with its Board of Examiners, so do not take my word for what will come up in the exam or what the 'right' answers will be deemed to be.

3 General readers. Finally, this book is intended for people – especially in other academic disciplines – who have not the faintest idea what primary health care is and have even less clue about its academic basis. Primary health care is (like education, human resource management and in-flight catering) an applied field of study. Its main subject matter is not a unique set of abstract premises and theories nor a set of observations made in the pure environment of the laboratory, but the messy reality of the real world with all its complexity and situational contingencies. As the opening quote of this Preface illustrates, the academic basis for applied fields is harder for outsiders to grasp, not least because so many practitioners within those fields are unclear about the concepts and theories that inform (often implicitly) the work that they do. It follows that those of us who hold tenured professorships in applied fields must spend at least some of our Sunday afternoons setting out our stall in a way that academics from the traditional 'ologies' can begin to take this seriously. I hope that, in this book, I have begun to address that task.

One final comment about the intended audience for this book: I live and work in the UK, and many (though by no means all) of my examples are taken from my own direct experience. This means that this book will perhaps be more meaningful to readers who are based in the UK. But this book is also intended as the course textbook in an international Masters course that takes students from (so far) four continents and 17 different countries. Whilst I use local examples at both micro level (e.g. the primary care consultation as it generally happens in the UK) and macro level (UK health policy or funding arrangements), I have presented these *as examples,* and have deliberately tried to select ones that provide transferable insights for students from other countries. I hope, therefore, that this book will prove useful to an international audience, and I would be especially keen to receive suggestions for meeting the needs of this wider audience should the book run (dare I say it) to a second edition.

Trisha Greenhalgh OBE
University College London
March 2007

References

1 Horton R. Evidence and primary care. Lancet 1999;353:609–610.
2 Pickles W. *Epidemiology in Country Practice*. Bristol: John Wright; 1939.
3 Hart JT. *A New Kind of Doctor*. London: Merlin Press; 1988.
4 Balint M. *The Doctor, His Patient and the Illness*. London: Routledge; 1956.
5 Starfield B. *Primary Care: Balancing Health Needs, Services and Technology*. New York: Oxford University Press; 1992.
6 Rakel R. *Textbook of Family Medicine*. 1st edn. New York: Elsevir; 1973.
7 McWhinney IR. *A Textbook of Family Medicine*. 1st edn. Oxford: Oxford University Press; 1986.
8 Noble JH, Greene HL, Levinson W, et al. *Textbook of Primary Care Medicine*. 3rd edn. New York: Mosby; 2000.
9 Hampson G. *Practice Nurse Handbook*. 5th edn. Oxford: Blackwell; 2006.
10 Jones R, Grol R, Britten N, et al. *Oxford Textbook of Primary Medical Care*. Oxford: Oxford University Press; 2004.
11 Van Maanen J. *Tales of the Field: On Writing Ethnography*. Chicago, IL: University of Chicago Press; 1986.

Foreword

In 1974, as a working GP in what was then still a functioning colliery village, I was invited to lecture on primary care at Johns Hopkins University Hospital in Baltimore. This was an awesome responsibility. Johns Hopkins was the place where Sir William Osler and William Henry Welch added Rockefeller's oil fortune to German laboratory science, thus realising in practice Abraham Flexner's dream of medical education founded on hospital specialism and scientific evidence.[1] This set a world gold standard pattern for medical education which even today remains largely intact.

True, I was only invited by the Department of Public Health, which, though distinguished in its own right, was still considered by all other faculties as only a minor adjunct to clinical medicine and surgery. And of course there was no department at all for general practice, family medicine, or any other concept of primary health care. However, the phrase "primary care" itself had suddenly become fashionable. Kerr L. White, then at Chapel Hill, North Carolina, had shown that in one average month, out of 1000 adult US citizens at risk, 750 had some sort of illness, 250 consulted any sort of doctor, 9 were admitted to any sort of hospital, and only 1 actually reached a teaching hospital to provide case-material for learning. He originally got this idea from John and Elizabeth Horder's referral data, from the James Wigg practice in Kentish Town.[2] Consultants in teaching hospitals ignored at their peril mounting evidence that existence of cost-effective generalists was a precondition for their own survival as real specialists, rather than "specialoids" – doctors claiming specialist fees but without effective hospital support. That useful term was coined by John Fry[3], one of the first to recognise this truth. It was confirmed by a report from the American College of Cardiology, which found that though in Boston, Miami and New York there were more than 10 cardiologists per 100,000 population, 70% of these had office-based rather than hospital-based practices, and half were not specialist Board-certified.[4] In a market economy, health workers closest to technology make the most money, and nobody wants either to be a generalist, or to provide continuing care.

So before my lecture I was shown around Johns Hopkins Hospital. Like most large hospitals, its ground floor was built around an exhausting and apparently endless corridor, with a network of pipes and cables running along its ceiling. As we approached somewhere about halfway along this corridor I saw a roughly cut cardboard sign hanging from bits of string looped around the pipes. And this is what it said:

DEPARTMENT OF PRIMARY CARE →

My guide was intrigued – he had never noticed it before. We followed the arrow, and found ourselves in the Emergency Room. It was heaving with the sort of events one sees on television doctordramas – children with acute severe asthma whose parents had never been told the difference between a 'preventer' and 'reliever'; diabetic patients in ketoacidosis whose medication had not been reviewed for years; overweight men rigid with low back pain who had never received advice or physiotherapy; elderly people whose undetected hypertension had led to a massive stroke; and smokers whose unchecked habit had finally caused them to cough up blood. These everyday 'emergencies' would occur very rarely in a country with a developed primary care system accessible to the whole population. The barbarism of the scene was confirmed by the presence of several heavily armed policemen. The doctors and nurses confirmed that their work had indeed just been renamed, in tune with fashion. New words, unchanged resources.

I tell this story first to establish two points, and then to draw an important conclusion for the many thousands of students who will use this book, in this first edition and the many others which surely will follow.

First, even in the USA, things have moved on since then, as is the nature of market economies. Specialoids have not been eliminated, but they have been pushed back – by the mighty force of corporate investors in health care, whose profits depend on rationalising the processes of commodity production, and have no interest in maximising doctors' incomes. So *things* get rapidly better, and even if *people* get worse, more and more *things* can be done to repair them. In Britain, where until 1979 the National Health Service, and the medical schools producing its doctors, all operated as a gift economy outside and above the market, both *things* (medical and nursing knowledge and resources) and *people* (staff and patients) steadily improved, even though both service and teaching functions were always grossly under-resourced. In USA in the early 1980s, one single department of family medicine in Worcester, Massachusetts, employed more staff than all the UK departments of primary care and general practice put together. Our health professionals learned how to listen and talk to patients as if they were friends, neither customers to be flattered nor sheep to be herded. Among their most impressive teachers was Trish Greenhalgh, in her frequent columns in the *British Medical Journal*. More than any other medical journalist, she spoke to her fellow GPs in the language of experience, but never without linking this to our expanding knowledge from the whole of human science.

When I compare the outlines of primary care so lucidly presented in this wonderful book, obviously derived from rich experience of real teaching and learning, with the *grand guignol* theatre of London medical schools when I was a student 1947–52, the advance is stunning. Young health workers today are incomparably better educated than they were in my immediately postwar generation, and from what I see of mature students entering medicine at Swansea Clinical School, they are now moving ahead faster than ever before. They know more of what really matters, the body of knowledge from which they draw is larger, simpler, and much more effective, and their attitudes to patients are hugely more sensitive and better informed.

But here we reach my second point. Students in every advanced economy now face an imminent future in which technology will certainly go on improving, but human relationships are rapidly getting worse. In 1996, even before we got incontrovertible evidence of approaching environmental crisis, the United Nations report on human development showed that the world then contained 358 people with one billion or more US dollars. Their total wealth equalled the combined incomes of the poorest 45% of the world population.[5] Disproportionate wealth on this scale creates equally disproportionate power. Health care systems in almost all countries, whatever their stage in economic development, have been conscripted to a single market-oriented pattern determined by the World Bank, which now has a far bigger health budget than the United Nations' World Health Organization.

Students of anatomy will not find what has become the most potent of all human organs, the wallet. The market decides. Even if all these 358 billionaires were angels, determined to address the needs of all people rather than such wants as are profitable, they must maximise their cash returns on investment. If they do not, their corporations will be devoured by competitors.

So the irresistible force of advancing scientific knowledge collides with the immovable object of a global economy in which meeting global needs is allowed to proceed only as a byproduct of making very rich people richer still.[6] They say our world began with a big bang. Unless your generation recognises the difference between natural laws, which cannot be changed, and human laws (including those of economics) which arise from human decisions and behaviour, that may be how it will end. Students today will have to learn, and later to apply their learning, within contexts of crisis no less profound than that from which my generation only just managed to emerge in 1945. Some of the social relationships already established in the pre-"reform" NHS, which were a precondition for developing the ideas and practice outlined in this book, could still provide foundations for rebirth of the honesty and hope we now desperately need.

Julian Tudor Hart

References

1 Berliner HS. A larger perspective on the Flexner report. Int J Health Serv 1975;5:573–592.
2 White KL, Williams TF, Greenberg BG. The ecology of medical care. N Engl J Med 1961;265:885–892. He acknowledged his debt to the Horders in White KL, Frenk J, Ordoñez C, Paganini JM, Starfield B (eds). *Health Services Research: An Anthology*, Vol. 534. Pan American Health Organization Scientific Publication; 1992:217–226.
3 Fry J. *Medicine in Three Societies: A Comparison of Medical Care in the USSR, USA and UK.* Aylesbury, Bucks: MTP; 1969.
4 *Lancet* 1974;i:617.
5 Jolly R (ed.). United Nations Report on Human Development, 1996.
6 Hart JT. *The Political Economy of Health Care: A Clinical Perspective.* Bristol: Policy Press, 2006.

CHAPTER 1

Introduction

Summary points

1 Primary health care has many definitions. Most of them include the following dimensions: first-contact care; undifferentiated by age, gender or disease; continuity over time; coordinated within and across sectors; and with a focus on both the individual and the population/community.

2 In the twenty-first century, traditional academic skills (the ability to think logically, argue coherently, judge dispassionately and solve problems creatively) must be supplemented by contemporary academic skills (communication, interdisciplinary teamwork, knowledge management and adaptability to change).

3 Primary care is an applied (secondary) discipline and its study is problem-oriented. It does not have a discrete scientific paradigm to call its own. Rather, it draws eclectically on a range of underpinning primary disciplines (which will be discussed further in Chapter 2).

4 Different problems in primary care require different perspectives, based on different conceptual and theoretical models. It will never be possible to come up with a single 'unifying theory' that explains all aspects of primary care. Studying different theories can help illuminate why different people look at (and try to solve) the 'same' primary care problem in different ways.

5 There is a tension between the typical 'textbook definition' of primary care (concerned with a tidy disease taxonomy, evidence-based treatments and a compliant patient in a stable family and social context) and its practical day-to-day reality (fragmented and changing populations, unclassifiable symptoms, absent or ambiguous evidence and mismatch of goals and values between clinician and patient). The academic study of primary care should not focus on the former at the expense of the latter.

1.1 What is primary (health) care?

We hear increasingly of a 'primary care led health service', 'primary care based research', 'capacity building in primary care' and 'primary care focus' for healthcare planning. But when we talk about primary (health) care, what exactly do we mean? Is primary care anything that occurs outside a hospital? What about a hospital-based walk-in service for minor illnesses? Is voluntary sector care (such as that provided by self-help charities) part of primary care? If a general practitioner (GP) or family doctor (or a general internist in the

USA) provides specialist services, does that still count as 'primary' care? And, frankly, does it matter? Instead of chasing a tight definition of primary care and enforcing it across all countries and healthcare systems, would we be better off with flexible parameters that can be applied with judgement in different contexts?

Let's start with a working definition and see how it stands up to closer scrutiny.

> *Primary health care is what happens when someone who is ill (or who thinks he or she is ill or who wants to avoid getting ill) consults a health professional in a community setting for advice, tests, treatment or referral to specialist care.*

An obvious primary care contact is a visit to the general medical practitioner or GP (referred to in some countries as the family practitioner or family doctor),* for example, with an episode of acute illness, for ongoing care of a long-term health problem or for a check-up or screening test. But primary care in the UK – and in many other countries – also includes pharmacy services, community-based nursing services, optometry and dental care. It includes not merely the acute care that sick persons might receive *before* they enter hospital with a serious illness (such as a stroke or diabetic emergency), but also the care they receive *after* discharge – rehabilitation, ongoing education and support, and continuing surveillance of their chronic condition.

Until about 1980, the focus of most writing about primary care was the work of the individual GP in treating and preventing illness. Take, for example the following definition produced by the Leeuwenhorst working party in 1974:

> 'The general practitioner is a licensed medical graduate who gives care to individuals, irrespective of age, sex, and illness. He will attend his patients in his consulting room and in their homes and sometimes in a clinic or hospital. His aim is to make early diagnoses. He will include, and integrate, physical, psychological and social factors in his considerations about health and illness.... Prolonged contact means that he can use repeated opportunities to gather information at a pace appropriate to each patient and build up a relationship of trust which he can use professionally. He will practice in co-operation with other colleagues, medical and non-medical. He will know how and when to intervene through treatment, prevention and education to promote the education of his patients and their families. He will recognize that he also has a responsibility to the community'.[1]

This definition reflects some undoubted strengths of primary care: closeness and continuity of the clinician–patient relationship, broad scope of care and embeddedness within the wider healthcare system. But it still seems old-fashioned

---

*Throughout this book I will use the term 'general practitioner' unless I am specifically drawing a distinction between the subtly different roles represented by these different titles. I will also use the term 'primary care' to mean 'primary health care', though I acknowledge that in other contexts primary care includes social as well as health care.

Box 1.1 Examples of primary health care encounters.

• A 63-year-old woman with a sticky eye asks her high-street pharmacist if there is anything she can buy over the counter for it.
• A dentist finds a suspicious white lesion while doing a routine check-up of a 72-year-old woman smoker and offers to refer her urgently to an oral surgeon.
• A 15-year-old schoolgirl visits an evening family planning clinic for a repeat prescription of the contraceptive pill.
• A mother brings her 3-month-old baby to a community centre to be weighed and immunised.
• A 24-year-old HIV-positive gay man attends for a routine blood test and a repeat prescription for his antiretroviral medication.
• A 78-year-old man with diabetes and leg ulcers receives regular visits from both the district nurse (to bandage the ulcers) and the community diabetes team (to monitor the diabetes).
• A 19-year-old single mother attends the accident and emergency department with a sore throat.
• A community psychiatric nurse visits a 53-year-old woman with schizophrenia every 2 weeks to assess the illness, administer a depot injection of medication and provide support.
• A multi-disciplinary community team including doctors, nurses, social workers and health advocates provides a 'health bus' offering a range of services to refugees and asylum seekers on an inner city estate.
• An 82-year-old woman with fading vision and a strong family history of glaucoma visits an optometrist for a routine check-up.
• A 50-year-old man with migraine that has not responded to medication from his GP attends an alternative health centre for a course of cranial osteopathy and aromatherapy.

---

and stereotypical, not just because it appears to assume that the doctor is male, but also because it places 'him' very centrally in charge of the service and responsible for deciding what is best for the patient.

The list in Box 1.1 shows some examples of primary health care problems. It is taken from a seminar in which some of my postgraduate students (GPs, community nurses, pharmacists and managers) told of the last encounter they had in primary care. It illustrates a number of features of contemporary primary care that challenge the Leeuwenhorst definition.

1 *A multi-professional team.* Most so-called GP surgeries or family practices include several doctors, as well as practice and community nurses, dieticians, physiotherapists and counsellors, and there may be close links with an interpreting or advocacy service for minority ethnic groups. Dentists, high-street optometrists, community pharmacists and sexual health clinicians (e.g. family planning) are part of the primary care service but usually have their own list of patients and keep separate records. Whilst in some countries (e.g. Germany), single-handed GPs ('office-based physicians') remain the norm, in others the primary care organisation is a complex social system in which teamwork and coordination are essential.

2 *Proactive as well as reactive care.* Some primary care contacts are patient-initiated (someone feels unwell or worried, so they seek advice), but an increasing number are initiated by a clinician, perhaps via an automated recall system. Clinician-initiated consultations may be for the care of chronic illness (e.g. diabetes, asthma, arthritis, depression), management of risk factors for future disease (e.g. low bone density), prevention (e.g. immunisation) or screening (e.g. cervical smears). In such circumstances, good care is not so much about making clever diagnoses but about the 'three R's' (registration, recall and regular review), as well as supporting self-care (see Section 4.4). It is also about what Julian Tudor Hart once called 'doing simple things well, for large numbers of people, few of whom feel ill'[2] – a task that depends crucially on both continuity of care and high-quality administrative systems.

3 *Population as well as individual focus.* The primary care practitioner is increasingly seen as responsible for health at a population level. Modern IT systems in primary care enable individual patient data to be aggregated (i.e. anonymised and added together) to produce a picture of the overall health of the practice population that can inform the planning of primary care provision and the commissioning of secondary care services. The adverse health impact of poor environments (damp housing, dangerous streets, junk food outlets, sexually explicit media) and, conversely, the positive health benefits of social support and healthy communities are important contributors to the overall disease burden in primary care.

4 *The social and cultural context of illness.* A major advance in primary care over the past 30 years has been the recognition that biomedical models of diagnosing and treating illness (see Section 2.1) are inadequate. Both the social origins of disease and the cultural dimension of the illness experience and self-management are increasingly taken account of in planning services and the advice offered to patients. GP surgeries in multi-ethnic communities often develop positive links with public, religious and voluntary sector organisations who may be able to address the patient's wider social needs and/or provide 'cultural brokering' for ethnic minorities.

5 *The centrality of the patient in his or her own care.* The days of 'doctor's orders' are long gone. Particularly in chronic illness, it is now seen as essential for the individual to understand the nature of the illness and take an active role in monitoring and treating it – often with lifestyle changes as well as (or instead of) medication. All this needs motivation, skills and practical support. Different people have different personalities, learning styles and support needs. 'Empowerment', 'self-management' and 'shared decision making' are different ways of conceptualising the active involvement of the patient (see Section 4.4).

6 *An advocacy role.* According to one definition, an advocate is 'someone who represents the views of another, without judgement, regarding a situation that affects them, in order to influence others'. This role is of course particularly crucial when the patient is vulnerable or disadvantaged in some way (e.g.

learning difficulties, limited language skills, lacking information or social capital). In healthcare systems that rely heavily on the 'empowered' patient engaged in 'self-care', advocacy is increasingly essential to reduce inequities.

7 *Multiple service models*. The examples in Box 1.1 suggest that there is probably no universal formula for organising primary care. Rather, the service must be responsive to local needs, priorities and ways of working. New models of primary care such as drop-in clinics in high-street locations (such as NHS Walk-in Centres) and telephone advice services (such as NHS Direct in the UK), as well as private GPs, alternative practitioners and the voluntary sector (self-help groups and charities), often make an important contribution to the mixed economy of provision. Imaginative local schemes (e.g. travelling health buses) may be developed to make health care more accessible to hard-to-reach groups. An increasing proportion of hospital attenders in reality belong neither to accident nor emergency cases, but are people seeking advice on illness or perceived illness in areas where the primary care sector is underdeveloped or not trusted; some hospitals employ primary care clinicians to deal with these individuals. All these models increase choice for patients but add to the complexity of the system and the difficulty of studying it systematically.

8 *Multiple interfaces*. As Box 1.1 shows, many primary care problems are mild and self-limiting, while others are long-term and/or potentially serious, and require cross-referral within the primary care team (e.g. to a nurse or counsellor) or external referral (typically to a hospital specialist or perhaps to a social worker). In these days of evidence-based practice (see Section 2.2), many such conditions are managed by protocols and care pathways that incorporate the different input of multiple professionals and that transcend the primary–secondary care interface. Consistency of care wherever care is delivered, and close liaison across interprofessional, interorganisational and intersectoral boundaries, and the effective use of new technologies, is essential for a 'seamless' experience by the patient.

These eight features characterise what might be called 'the new primary health care'. Here are some further definitions of primary care and general practice, which capture this more contemporary perspective:

'Primary care is first-contact care, delivered by generalists, dependent (increasingly) on teamwork, which is accessible (both geographically and culturally), comprehensive (interested in old as well as new problems), co-ordinated, population-based (there is responsibility for 'the list' as well as the individual patient), and activated by patient choice'.[3]

'Primary care is the provision of integrated, accessible health care services by clinicians who are accountable for addressing a large majority of personal health care needs, developing a sustained partnership with patients and participating in the context of family and community'.[4]

'The general practitioner is a specialist trained to work in the front line of a health-care system and to take the initial steps to provide care for any health problem(s) that patients may have. The general practitioner takes care of individuals in a society,

irrespective of the patient's type of disease or other personal and social character-istics, and organises the resources available in the healthcare system to the best advantage of the patients. The general practitioner engages with autonomous in-dividuals across the fields of prevention, diagnosis, cure, care, and palliation, us-ing and integrating the sciences of biomedicine, medical psychology, and medical sociology'.[5]

'General practitioners/family doctors are specialist physicians trained in the principles of the discipline. They are personal doctors, primarily responsible for the provision of comprehensive and continuing care to every individual seeking medical care irrespec-tive of age, sex and illness. They care for individuals in the context of their family, their community, and their culture, always respecting the autonomy of their patients. They recognise they will also have a professional responsibility to their community. In nego-tiating management plans with their patients they integrate physical, psychological, social, cultural and existential factors, utilising the knowledge and trust engendered by repeated contacts. General practitioners/family physicians exercise their professional role by promoting health, preventing disease and providing cure, care, or palliation. This is done either directly or through the services of others according to health needs and the resources available within the community they serve, assisting patients where necessary in accessing these services. They must take the responsibility for developing and maintaining their skills, personal balance and values as a basis for effective and safe patient care'.[6]

I find all these definitions useful to some extent. They are, for the most part, both factually accurate and morally inspiring. They implicitly convey the mul-tiple roles played by today's primary care practitioner – including clinical ex-pert (in the diseases and symptoms seen in the community); professional carer (of individuals with chronic disabling conditions); witness (to the illness nar-rative and the experience of suffering or loss); gatekeeper (and coadministrator of limited resources); member (and perhaps manager) of a multi-professional, interagency team and educator (of colleagues, patients and people at risk).

But I also find the definitions above rather dry. Some of them come from a previous era, written as they were before the major social changes – set out in Box 1.2 – had occurred. In addition, these worthy definitions lack the passion that I feel for my own clinical work in primary care, and some of them seem to skirt round the essence of what primary care actually *is*.

I would like to find a definition of primary care that expresses the pride I felt when, as a newly qualified hospital doctor, a patient first said to me, 'I wish you were *my* doctor' and which encompasses the missing piece of the professional jigsaw that I had found so lacking in the organ-specific hospital specialties I had studied in my youth (see Table 1.2). I want a definition of primary care that incorporates the mixture of elation and terror that I felt when I got my first 'list' (i.e. a list of some 2000 people, most of whom were not currently ill, but for whose care I was now responsible) – and the ethical and legal responsibilities that went with it. And finally, I want a definition

Box 1.2 Social changes that have influenced the scope and direction of primary health care in the past 25 years.

Demographic changes

Globalisation and mass migration, leading to multi-ethnic communities and language/cultural barriers in the consultation (Section 7.1)

Ageing population (Section 7.1)

New family structures, especially growth of single-occupancy households (Section 7.1)

Changes in patterns of poverty and social exclusion (Section 7.4)

Changes in disease patterns and understanding of their aetiology

Increase in chronic incurable illness and comorbidity (Section 10.1)

Increased recognition of the interplay between genetic risk, lifestyle choices and environment in the genesis of chronic illness (Sections 4.3, 7.3 and 8.4)

Increased recognition of the importance of healthy communities (Chapter 9)

Changes in delivery of health care

Emergence of evidence-based medicine, replacement of 'clinical freedom' with standardised guidelines/protocols (Section 5.2)

Shift from treating established disease to early detection (screening) and prevention (Section 8.3)

Shift of place of care from hospital to community for chronic conditions (Section 10.1)

New and diverse roles for nurses and professionals allied to medicine (Section 10.4)

Increase in organisational complexity of care, especially across the primary–secondary care interface (Section 10.2)

Changes in social roles and expectations

Increased emphasis on patient autonomy, dignity, self-determination and in-formed consent; decrease in 'doctor's orders' (Section 4.4)

Decline in traditional sick role and rise in 'self-management' and 'expert patient' (Sections 4.1 and 4.4)

Rising expectation that society should change to accommodate the ill and disabled (Section 4.1)

Changing role of women – decline of the full-time wife and mother (Section 7.2)

Decline in public trust in doctors and nurses (Section 5.6)

New definitions of professionalism (Section 5.6)

Technological changes

Increased dependence on technology for administering and coordinating care (Section 10.3)

Standardisation of clinical categories and terms for electronic coding and record-keeping (Section 10.3)

Capacity to generate powerful, population-wide epidemiological data from aggregation of routinely collected clinical data in primary care (Section 8.1)

Universally available medical information (e.g. via Internet) leading to greater questioning by patients of medical advice (Section 8.2)

Growth in high-technology medicine (but not necessarily in the accessibility of such options to everyone)

Changes in the role of the state

Challenges to professional self-regulation, shift from voluntary 'quality improvement' to compulsory 'quality control' (Sections 11.1 and 11.2)

The 'new public management' – with emphasis on accountability, targets and centralised standards and protocols (Section 11.2)

Social movements

Rise of consumerism, leading to increased expectations of health professionals and decreased tolerance of quality gaps (Chapter 11)

Growth in complementary and alternative medicine and re-emergence of humanism as a reaction to over-rationalist models of care

of primary care that does not merely assert the importance of teamwork but which conveys the impoverished contribution invariably made by those who insist on flying solo.[†]

To get a handle on these intangibles, we need to move from descriptions of what happens in primary care to a consideration of why these things are important – that is, we need to shift our focus from the *structure and process*

[†]That is not to say that being a 'single-handed' practitioner is a bad thing. There is considerable evidence that patients prefer their primary care to be provided on a small scale and that benefits such as 'a personal service' and continuity of care are seen as a worthwhile trade-off for a more limited range of clinics.[7,8] But single-handed practitioners will usually be the first to tell you how much they value and depend on their professional friendship networks, their links with colleagues outside their own small practice and the refreshment they get from regular educational meetings, learning sets and so on. Good single-handed practitioners also tend to be especially adept at working in partnership with nurses, physiotherapists, pharmacists and so on. When I talk about 'the impoverished contribution made by those who insist on flying solo', I am drawing attention to the real dangers of refusing to acknowledge the limitations of one's own past training, present knowledge or professional role and those of failing to draw judiciously and creatively on the skills and expertise of others. As I emphasise in the section *What is academic study?*, 'teamwork' is one of the eight essential skills of the academic primary care practitioner, and Chapter 10 considers how this plays out in the complex health care systems of the twenty-first century.

Box 1.3 Core values of primary care.

Holistic. Primary care embraces the complexities and interactions of bodily systems, mental responses, family, community and sociocultural context. It also seeks continuity of care through time.

Balanced. Primary care seeks a middle ground between breadth and depth of knowledge, between lay and medical models of illness and distress and between active intervention and 'leaving well alone'.

Patient-centred. Primary care sees each patient as an individual and seeks to offer personalised rather than standardised packages of care.

Rigorous. Primary care seeks to draw judiciously on multiple sources of evidence (the patient's unique predicament, the relevant research literature and the wider family and social context) when considering the action to take in relation to a particular problem.

Equitable. Primary care takes responsibility for social justice in the allocation of scarce resources; hence it works proactively with, and plays an advocacy role for, the disempowered, inarticulate and socially excluded. This may include challenging the educated worried well when they seek a disproportionate share of healthcare resources.

Reflective. Primary care is always practised in conditions of ignorance and/or uncertainty. It requires a questioning attitude, willingness to revise provisional diagnoses in the light of emerging findings and the humility to defer to higher authority (the specialist, the parent, the patient) when appropriate.

Developed from various sources.[9,10–15]

---

of primary care to the *core values* of primary care. Values are defined by the Oxford English Dictionary as 'principles, standards or qualities considered worthwhile or desirable'. The core values of primary care are those aspects of our practice which we hold dear, which give us satisfaction, for which we seek to perform especially well and for which we are disappointed if we fail to deliver on. Box 1.3 shows some core values of primary care.

Table 1.1 summarises some important changes in the scope and organisation of primary care in the past 30 years, and Table 1.2 shows the implications of these changes for how illness and its management are approached, using one condition (diabetes) as a worked example. You can see that there has been a fundamental reframing since the 1970s (when diabetes was a relatively rare condition treated in hospital by specialists who focused on lowering the blood glucose level) to the present day (when it is seen as a multifaceted condition affecting both the patient and the wider family and requiring active self-management and a coordinated and individualized package of multi-professional support). Table 1.2 should not be taken to imply that primary

Table 1.1 Trends in the scope and organisation of primary health care.

Feature	Traditional general practice	Modern primary health care
Core business	Diagnosis and treatment of acute illness	Prevention, surveillance and support of chronic illness
Typical encounter	Reactive (patient-initiated)	Increasingly proactive (clinician-initiated)
Focus of care	Uniprofessional (doctor-focused)	Multi-professional (team-focused)
Place of care	Most encounters occur in the GP surgery	Diversity and choice in place of care
Principle of resource allocation	'Health for me': resources allocated by patient demand	'Health for all': resources allocated by population need
Basis of clinical decision making	Clinical freedom (sometimes idiosyncratic)	Evidence-based (often directed by guidelines and protocols)
Nature of clinician–patient relationship	'Doctor's orders': paternalistic advice with limited information	Patient preference: shared decision making based on informed choice
Purpose of record-keeping	Paper-based and constructed as aide-memoire for individual doctors	Electronic and designed to organise the work of multiple professionals around the patient's illness and provide aggregated data for monitoring disease trends

care has driven these changes. Quite the contrary, it was hospital specialists (both diabetologists and diabetes-specialist nurses) who first recognised the need for these changes and worked to achieve them across the primary–secondary care interface.[16] Profound shifts in the attitudes of GPs and practice nurses were needed, as well as education, improved administrative systems and new models of care across the interface (e.g. the introduction of advice hotlines, open-access appointments and 'fast-track' foot clinics). But once the sea change had occurred in how diabetes was conceptualised and managed, it ceased to be a disease that could be comfortably accommodated in a hospital setting.

All this began to happen in the mid 1980s, when I was training to be a diabetologist and undertaking my first research project – into the kinetics of insulin absorption in patients with 'brittle diabetes'. I did not know at the time that my lack of fulfilment from my research project (and the feeling that I wasn't getting anywhere despite collecting vast numbers of blood samples from poorly controlled patients) reflected the exciting paradigm shift shown in Table 1.2, nor that my decision to change career and enter general practice in 1989 marked the imminent shift in the care of a substantial

Table 1.2 An example of primary care principles and values: a new model of diabetes.

	Traditional biomedical model	New model informed by primary care principles and values
Diabetes conceptualised as	Disease of the pancreas (absolute or relative insulin deficiency)	Multifaceted disorder arising from metabolic defect, which leads to imbalance in multiple embedded systems (biochemical, endocrine, physiological, psychological, family/community, society)
Cause seen in terms of	Damage to pancreatic cells and/or cellular resistance to insulin	Complex interaction between nature (genetic risk), nurture (environmental mediators and moderators) and culture (behaviours, norms and expectations of the group)
Management focused on	a Correcting the deficiency with insulin injections or medication b Ensuring compliance	Multiple dimensions and levels of care: a Developing a partnership for care b Drawing up a personal management plan that reflects the patient's goals and priorities c Providing culturally appropriate education and resources for self-care d Supporting positive lifestyle choices e Managing overall cardiovascular risk f Regular structured surveillance ('annual reviews') for early complications g Judicious referral for specialist assessment or management
Main goals of management	Near-normal blood glucose control Avoidance of hypoglycaemia	Understanding, confidence, self-efficacy, well-being Reduction in overall cardiovascular risk Prevention of secondary complications (amputation, blindness) Social integration Personal goals of patient (e.g. pregnancy, marathon run, renewal of driving licence)
Main model of care	Doctor-driven	Self-management supported by multi-professional team
Main indicators of success	Blood or urine testing Patient's HbA1c level	Complex risk profile including HbA1c level Lifestyle choices, e.g. smoking cessation, exercise Well-being
Quality failures detected via	Critical events, e.g. hospital admission, death	Surveillance at patient level Regular, multidimensional audit at system level including process measures (e.g. data capture) and outcome measures (e.g. proportion of patients with blood pressure adequately treated) Structured review of critical and near-miss events

proportion of people with diabetes in the UK from hospital clinics into primary care.

Here is one final definition that reflects not only a description of what happens in primary care, but also the core values listed in Box 1.3. You will see that it is a refinement of the initial back-of-envelope that I proposed on page 2.

Primary health care is what happens when someone who is ill (or who thinks he or she is ill or who wants to avoid getting ill) consults a health professional in a community setting for advice, tests, treatment or referral to specialist care. Such care should be holistic, balanced, personalised, rigorous and equitable, and delivered by reflexive practitioners who recognise their own limitations and draw appropriately on the strengths of others.

Box 1.4 summarises what I personally believe to be the defining characteristics of primary care and what I have called the 'four pillars of professionalism' in this field of practice. Later chapters in this book address these four pillars in more detail.

Box 1.4 Definition and scope of primary health care: a summary.

Primary health care has 10 defining characteristics:
1 It provides the patient's first point of contact with the health care system.
2 It deals with both acute and chronic health problems regardless of age, sex or disease type.
3 It provides person-centred care to the individual, taking account of his or her family and the wider community.
4 It considers health problems in their physical, psychological, social, cultural and existential dimensions.
5 It is ideally delivered via an ongoing clinician–patient relationship, built over time and characterised by high levels of communication and trust.
6 It is proactive as well as reactive, promoting health and well-being by supporting healthy lifestyle choices and offering interventions to manage risk.
7 It takes responsibility for the health of the community as well as of the individual.
8 It has a particular role in the early stages of potentially serious illness when symptoms and signs are mild or non-specific.
9 It assumes an advocacy role for the patient when needed (and/or works flexibly with others who take on this role).
10 It strives to make efficient use of health care resources through coordinating care, working with other professionals and managing the interface with other specialities.

To practice this specialty, the primary care practitioner must be competent in three areas:
- Clinical care
- Communication
- Management

Professionalism in primary care rests on four pillars:
- Ethical: drawing on core values, principles and virtues
- Scientific: adopting a scholarly and reflective approach to practice, including (but not limited to) the use of best up-to-date research evidence in clinical decisions
- Organisational: addressing issues such as access, equity, relevance to social need, efficient use of resources and so on
- Educational: taking ongoing responsibility for continuous professional development of oneself and one's staff

Developed from various sources[6,9,10–15]; see text for further discussion.

1.2   What is academic study?

All the definitions in the previous section point to an important conclusion: primary health care is not itself an academic discipline. In the eyes of the people writing these definitions, primary care is a practice rather than a theory, based on 'doing something' rather than 'thinking in the abstract'. For those with the time and inclination to take an academic perspective, we might say that primary care is a problem-oriented field of study that draws variously on a range of concepts and theories drawn from different disciplines. If you study primary care from such a perspective, you may initially be frustrated at the intellectual fuzziness in this field of study compared to (say) the kind of well-demarcated subject areas that are taught in universities (e.g. biochemistry, mathematics). Before the end of this chapter, I hope to have persuaded you that primary care has (or *could* have) a robust academic basis. But before I take on that argument, I would like to consider in more detail what 'academic study' actually means.

The German academic, philosopher and educationist Friedrich Wilhelm von Humboldt (1767–1835), who founded Berlin's first university and who was once described as 'the last universal scholar in the field of the natural sciences', believed that there are four core skills that the graduate of academic training will display. He or she will be able
1 To think constructively
2 To argue coherently
3 To judge dispassionately
4 To solve problems creatively

As well as these *traditional academic skills*, I would further add four essential skills for the academic scholar in the twenty-first century. I have called these *contemporary academic skills*:

5 To communicate ideas and concepts to the non-expert

6 To work effectively and efficiently[‡] as a member of a multi-disciplinary team

7 To manage knowledge – that is to find, evaluate, summarise, synthesise and share information

8 To adapt appropriately to change

If these eight core skills (four traditional, four contemporary) are taken as the defining features of an *academic* approach, such an approach is entirely congruent with the core business of primary care and with primary care as a fundamentally practical (and inherently fuzzy) field of enquiry.[§] Others might define academic study as to do with abstract thoughts rather than real-world problems or practical action, and I guess those are the people who believe that primary care has no academic basis! I return to contemporary academic skills in Section 5.1 when I consider the nature of generalist knowledge.

In order to unpack academic study further, we need to consider the notion of an academic discipline. If you ask your children what 'discipline' is, they would probably say 'punishment for breaking the rules' or (as self-discipline) 'behaving according to a particular set of rules'. In the world of academia, a discipline is a body of knowledge that has a well-defined set of intellectual conventions and rules.

There are two sorts of academic discipline. The first – primary or theoretical disciplines – comprise the traditional academic 'subjects' that have been offered at universities for decades. Examples of primary disciplines include physiology, immunology, sociology, statistics, philosophy, history, geography and so on. In Chapter 2, I will refer to these as 'the ologies'. Each of these has an agreed body of knowledge (we can generally say that X is or is not part of the discipline), an agreed focus and set of concepts (the 'stuff' that is deemed worthy of study by experts in the discipline), a theoretical model of how these concepts

---

[‡] *Effectiveness* is sometimes defined as 'doing the right thing' and *efficiency* as 'doing things right'. The former is essentially a clinical dimension; the latter is largely an economic one. If I make a tasty and nutritious meal, dirtying only the minimum of pots, for someone who is not hungry, I have done something efficient, but not effective. If I jump into water to rescue a drowning person but ruin my expensive watch in the process, I have been effective but not efficient since I could (perhaps) have achieved the same outcome by removing the watch first.

[§] If you are interested in seeing how these academic skills link to an official policy map of the practical skills and 'know-how' needed for delivering primary care in the twenty-first century, take a look at the 2004 report from the US Society of General Internal Medicine on 'The Future of General Internal Medicine'.[9] As well as expertise in providing comprehensive long-term care to an unselected population, this national task force identified the following skills as essential for the general internist practising in a community setting: effective communication with patients and colleagues, evidence-based practice (including critical thinking and knowledge management), reflection and lifelong learning, leadership and team working, professionalism and adaptability to a changing world.

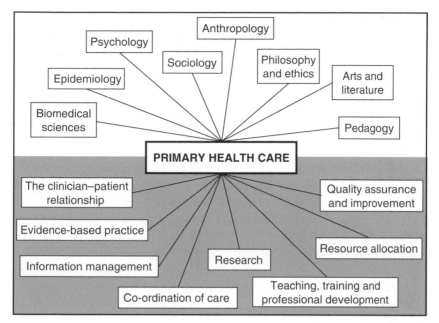

Figure 1.1 Primary health care: underpinning disciplines (upper half) and key themes in contemporary practice (lower half).

fit together (see Section 1.3) and a more or less agreed approach to research design (immunologists, for example, do experiments on rabbits, whereas historians study ancient manuscripts and philosophers discuss premises and what can be deduced from them). Within each theoretical discipline, scholars generally agree about the main research questions and about what counts as good (or poor) research. Until recently – with a few notable exceptions – scholars from different primary disciplines rarely exchanged ideas with one another.‖

The second sorts of discipline – secondary or applied – focus on problems rather than concepts and theories. Scholars in secondary disciplines consider real-world issues from many different angles, drawing eclectically on the different primary disciplines to address different dimensions of the problem. Examples of secondary disciplines include business studies (which draws on economics, marketing, anthropology and organisational theory), education (which draws on learning theory, linguistics and psychology) and primary health care, whose underpinning disciplines are illustrated in Figure 1.1.

‖ Philosopher Thomas Kuhn introduced the concept of a *paradigm* (a particular scientific approach characterised by four things: concepts, theories, methods and instruments).[17] If you are interested in the philosophical basis of different approaches to primary care, I recommend Kuhn's book, which is short, inspiring and easy to follow.

Table 1.3 Primary care: textbook versus gritty reality.

The textbook	The reality
Diagnoses	Non-specific conditions
Families	Unsupported individuals
Housing	Homelessness
Continuity of care	Episodic care
Evidence and guidelines	Pragmatic solutions
Compliance	Compromise
Predictability	Uncertainty
Healthy lifestyle choices by individuals	Structural and practical barriers to healthy choices

Adapted from Murdoch.[18]

Figure 1.1 raises an important question: Given the number of different un-underpinning disciplines relevant to the academic study of primary care, where should one start? The answer is, with a real-life problem. The theoretical literature often only makes sense when *applied to* a practical problem; the different theoretical perspectives represented by the 'ologies' can be thought of as different 'lenses' through which to view real-life problems. Strictly speaking, secondary disciplines such as pedagogy are not 'disciplines' at all but 'applied fields' – since a discipline in the pure sense is a single conceptual framework with its own conventions and rules. But in practice, the word 'discipline' is now used for both theoretical and applied fields of study.

Please do not assume that the only disciplines relevant to primary health care problems are the ones shown in Figure 1.1, nor that all the disciplines shown will be relevant to all primary care problems. Table 1.4 sets out the definition and scope of some key underpinning disciplines of primary care, some of which for clarity, are not shown in Figure 1.1. You might like to modify Figure 1.1 by adding and subtracting different disciplines in a way that allows you to make sense of particular problems in the context of your own work in primary health care. Like the rest of this book, Figure 1.1 is intended to set the scene for further reflection and discussion, not to be memorised as 'fact'.

Traditionalists often bemoan the fact that universities are offering their students an increasing array of secondary disciplines from in-flight catering to Frisbee throwing and (probably rightly) argue that the main task of a university is to introduce its undergraduates to bodies of theoretical knowledge and the rules and conventions of the primary disciplines. It is certainly true that one can (and some universities do) approach practical subjects in a superficial, unrigorous way and that all applied fields of study (including primary care) have a continuing responsibility to demonstrate their academic rigour if they are to be considered credible. Whilst non-academic (e.g. continuing professional development) courses can offer useful tips and tools for the primary care practitioner, the academic study of primary care problems is impossible unless students have a sound theoretical grasp of the main underpinning

Table 1.4 Underpinning academic disciplines for primary health care.

Discipline	Definition	Contribution to the study of primary health care
Primary disciplines		
Anthropology	The study of human cultures and how they have evolved and influenced each other	Culture, values and identities (includes organisational culture, professional culture and so on as well as the ideas and practice of different ethnic groups)
Biomedicine	The study of the structure and function of the human body, its disease processes and treatment	Diseases and how to treat them
Epidemiology	The study of disease patterns in populations	Prevention and management of diseases and risk factors in populations (both infections, e.g. HIV, and non-infectious, e.g. obesity)
Health economics	The study of the production, distribution and consumption of goods and services in health care	Models of payment for primary care. Issues of affordability and access
Law (strictly, jurisprudence)	The study of the body of enacted or customary rules recognised by a community as binding	Legal rights of patients, legal obligations of health professionals. Informs the study of medical ethics
Philosophy	The study of the nature of knowledge (ontology) and how it is used in practice (epistemology). Also, moral philosophy or ethics which concerns what is the right way to live and behave	The nature of knowledge, e.g. differences between scientific knowledge and experiential knowledge or know-how
Psychology	The study of mind and behaviour. Factors that influence human beings to act, particularly cognitive and emotional influences	Motivation, incentives, rewards, emotional needs. Influence (e.g. impact of 'medical advice' vs. 'lay advice' on patients' decisions)
Social psychology	The study of social influences on human behaviour	Interpersonal influence, roles, modelling, norms
Sociology	The study of human society and the relationships between its members, especially the influence of social structures and norms on behaviours and practices. Includes medical sociology (the study of the norms, behaviours and social networks of health professionals)	Organisational, family and peer structures. Group norms and values. Social influences on clinician behaviour (e.g. adoption of guidelines)

(Continued)

Table 1.4 (*Continued*)

Discipline	Definition	Contribution to the study of primary health care
Secondary disciplines		
Pedagogy	The study of learning – in particular, how knowledge can be understood, used and valued	Acquisition and application of knowledge by both patients and professionals
Health promotion	The study of strategies and practices aimed at improving the health and well-being of populations	Disease prevention, healthy lifestyles
Organisational studies	The study of the structure and function of organisations	Organisational factors influencing accessibility, process of care, financial efficiency and health outcomes
Political sciences	The study of government structures and their function in developing and implementing policy	Impact of different political structures on the effectiveness of policymaking (includes 'modernisation' of urban bureaucracies, citizen involvement)

primary disciplines such as the biomedical subject areas (physiology, pharmacology, epidemiology and so on), social sciences (sociology, anthropology) and psychology.

For this reason, I believe that primary care is a particularly difficult subject to study. It should be considered as a postgraduate (advanced) discipline by people who recognise its complex foundations, and not as 'the easy bits' of biomedicine. For this reason also, I believe that the study of primary care is best accomplished through open and pluralist discussion in learning groups that are both *multi-disciplinary* (i.e. comprising individuals who studied different theoretical disciplines as undergraduates) and *multi-professional* (i.e. comprising individuals who have a wide range of roles in their working lives – and hence different perspectives on primary care problems).

Professor J. Campbell Murdoch has drawn attention to the difference between the primary care of most textbooks and the reality with which most of us deal in our daily practice (Table 1.3).[18] As Murdoch pointed out, most of us spend our first few years in clinical primary care 'unlearning' the tidy theories and taxonomies of textbook biomedicine and becoming more or less comfortable with the 'grey zone' of practice we have found ourselves in. We learn, more or less, to manage without the things we expected to find (the left-hand column in Table 1.3) and to cope with what we actually find (the right-hand column). We also learn that the knowledge base of primary care is potentially infinite and that however hard we try, we cannot ever get on top of everything.

Much of primary care is characterised by *untidiness*, *uncertainty* and many different potential approaches to a single problem. The notion of uncertainty, and the gap between theory and reality, will be recurring themes throughout this book. The academic study of primary care includes the theoretical study of 'grey areas' and uncertainty in clinical method. It also includes the use of multiple theoretical perspectives to build up a rich picture of a complex and contested field of study. You can probably begin to see why the contemporary academic skills of teamwork, knowledge management, communication and adaptability to change are going to be particularly critical to the study of primary care.

1.3   What are theories – and why do we need them?

Theories are conceptual models that help us make sense of reality.[19] Look at the example of Dr Begum and her colleagues in Box 1.5. The clash of approaches between these three health professionals results from the fundamental way they conceptualise the problems they deal with in their work. Dr Begum's conceptual model of primary health care is one where patients suffer from diseases, which have causes (and risk factors) and which respond to a greater or lesser extent to specific treatments, which in turn have been tested in randomised controlled trials. In other words, she uses the biomedical model (see Section 2.1) – a rational, scientific model that underpins anatomy, physiology, biochemistry, cardiology, immunology and so on. If Dr Begum were to conduct a research study, it would probably be a randomised controlled trial or a survey of symptomatology in a particular disease.

Box 1.5 Different perspectives on primary care problems.

A young GP, Dr Begum, works in a busy group practice. She is a keen proponent of evidence-based medicine. She considers every problem in terms of 'diagnosis', 'prognosis', 'therapy' and so on. She searches for research evidence on the Internet. She carefully evaluates the research evidence and draws conclusions that she believes are rational and logical. But she cannot understand why the other doctors in her practice (who are older and more experienced) do not share her enthusiasm for exploring the research literature and applying the results in practice. Her practice nurse, Mrs Perkins, suggests, 'The best thing to do is spend a bit of time listening to the patient, and getting to know their family and their situation, so you can view their illness from their point of view and in its proper context'. One of the older doctors, Dr Brown, has a different piece of advice, 'My dear, when you have accumulated as many years of experience as I have, you won't need to rely quite so much on your super-scientific research evidence. You'll be able to improvise like the rest of us. When people come in asking for some new fangled medication, you'll be able to get them out the door believing they never wanted it in the first place'.

Mrs Perkins has a different model – based centrally around the achievement of empathy through shared experience and active listening. The question for her is not 'what is the diagnosis?' but 'who is this patient and what is he or she going through?' Note that Mrs Perkins views her work not as *doing something to* the patient but as *being there for* the patient. Her work is built around a 'care' relationship, not a 'cure' relationship, and the mental model for the former is not a rational (scientific) one but an experiential (phenomenological) one (see Section 11.5).[20] If Mrs Perkins were to do a research study, it might take the form of an in-depth case study, written up as a detailed narrative, of a patient whose illness was an epic struggle for survival or quest for meaning.[21]

Dr Brown's model of primary care problems is different again. Like Dr Begum, he is interested in influencing the course of the illness, but his ideas about treatment are not primarily biomedical. He uses the word 'improvise' – a term more frequently used in relation to jazz music or unscripted theatre. This suggests that his mental model is based on the view of general practice as an art – where the demonstration of a bit of priestly authority and mystical divination might just help the healing process. The conceptual world of artistic improvisation has little place for 'causes' and 'effects', but has much to do with the performative relationship between the 'actor' and his or her 'audience', the roles they assume and the games they play. Dr Brown might even take a psychodynamic model of his work – the notion that in general practice, trivial illness is the vehicle through which painful subconscious (emotional) issues are brought for discussion (the so-called hidden agenda – see Section 6.3).[22] If Dr Brown were to conduct a research study, it might be a series of reflective discussions between him and his fellow GPs, in which they work through a series of challenging patients and how they attempt to use their professional position (what Balint called 'the doctor as the drug' – see Section 6.3) to promote emotional (and thereby symptomatic) healing in their patients.[22]

If you have a conventional hospital-based medical training, you will almost certainly feel most comfortable with the rational, scientific model. If you come from a nursing background, the 'care' model might make more sense to you, because much of your undergraduate training would have been based on it (and because much of your work is to do with caring). However, nursing curricula throughout the world vary considerably, and scientific models are increasingly privileged (perhaps reflecting the emergence of the extended role of the nurse in diagnosis, treatment and so on). If you are a British GP, or come from a comparable health care system (such as the Netherlands or New Zealand), you may well be most comfortable with an 'artistic' model of general practice and/or with models that consider subconscious, as well as conscious, influences on behaviour. Which model is correct? Think about this for a little before you read on.

If you believe that any one model is the 'correct' way to conceptualise every problem you encounter in primary health care, you have probably not seen very many real-life problems or listened to many people from other professional (and lay) backgrounds. You have probably also not understood Section 1.2 about the multiple underpinning disciplines of primary care! But if you are an experienced generalist, and especially if you work a lot in multidisciplinary teams, you will almost certainly know that different conceptual models help us with different sorts of problems – and allow us to have multiple 'takes' on the same problem. A rational, 'evidence-based' model helps us when the problem can be couched in the taxonomy of a specific disease (or a differential diagnosis), whereas the 'improvisation' model might become dominant when the problem is best expressed as 'Mrs Jones making yet another appointment after all those negative tests'.

Different primary disciplines are generally based on different conceptual models, though most of the hospital-based medical disciplines share a common biomedical model (in which problems can be analysed at different levels including the molecule, the cell, the organ and so on). There are many other conceptual models relevant to primary care that I have not yet mentioned. If you work in a managerial or executive role, your mental model of primary care is probably one of a complex organisation and you will see problems in terms of appropriate skill mix, effective teamwork, efficient project management and so on. You will have a natural tendency to analyse problems at the level of the team (e.g. particular project groups). And if you work in social services, you are more likely to view problems in terms of the social structures, norms and relationships that produce particular behaviours – that is, your conceptual model will be the social system and your unit of analysis will be the social group (e.g. teenage mothers).

Take another look at Table 1.4, which illustrates the diversity and scope of academic primary care. You will probably return to it (and perhaps add to it) when you begin to conceptualise and theorise about the primary care problems you meet in your own practice. Once you begin to do that, even if you do not find any easy answers, you can call yourself an academic primary care practitioner.

References

1 Leeuwenhorst Working Party of European General Practitioners. *The General Practitioner in Europe: A Statement by the Working Party Appointed by the European Conference on the Teaching of General Practice.* Leeuwenhorst, Netherlands: WONCA Europe; 1974.

2 Hart JT. *A New Kind of Doctor.* London: Merlin Press; 1988.

3 Gordon P, Plamping D. Primary health care: its characteristics and potential. In: Gordon P, Hadley J, eds. *Extending Primary Care.* Oxford: Radcliffe Medical Press; 1996:1–15.

4 Donaldson M, Yordy K, Vanselow N. *Defining Primary Care: An Interim Report.* Washington, DC: Institute of Medicine; 1994.

5 Olesen F, Dickinson J, Hjortdahl P. General practice – time for a new definition. BMJ 2000;320:354–357.

6 European Academy of Teachers of General Practice. European definition of general practice/family medicine. Available at http://www euract org/html/page03f shtml; 2002.

7 van den Hombergh P., Engels Y., van den Hoogen H., van Doremalen J., van den Bosch W., Grol R. Saying 'goodbye' to single-handed practices; what do patients and staff lose or gain? Fam Pract 2005;22:20–27.

8 Campbell JL, Ramsay J, Green J. Practice size: impact on consultation length, workload, and patient assessment of care. Br J Gen Pract 2001;51:644–650.

9 Larson EB, Fihn SD, Kirk LM, et al. The future of general internal medicine: report and recommendations from the Society of General Internal Medicine (SGIM) Task Force on the domain of general internal medicine. J Gen Intern Med 2004;19:69–77.

10 Toop L. Primary care: core values. Patient centered primary care. BMJ 1998;316:1882–1883.

11 McWhinney IR. Primary care: core values. Core values in a changing world. BMJ 1998;316: 1807–1809.

12 Dixon J, Holland P, Mays N. Primary care: core values. Developing primary care: gate-keeping, commissioning, and managed care. BMJ 1998;317:125–128.

13 Roberts J. Primary care: core values. Primary care in an imperfect market. BMJ 1998;317: 186–189.

14 Neuberger J. Primary care: core values. Patients' priorities. BMJ 1998;317:260–262.

15 Jones R. Core values in primary care. BMJ 1998;317:1394–1396.

16 Greenhalgh T. Shared care for diabetes: A systematic review. Occasional Paper 67. London: Royal College of General Practitioners; 1994.

17 Kuhn TS. *The Structure of Scientific Revolutions*. Chicago: University of Chicago Press; 1962.

18 Murdoch JC. Mackenzie's puzzle – the cornerstone of teaching and research in general practice. Br J Gen Pract 1997;47:656–658.

19 Alderson P. The importance of theories in health care. BMJ 1998;317:1007–1010.

20 McCance TV, McKenna HP, Boore JR. Exploring caring using narrative methodology: an analysis of the approach. J Adv Nurs 2001;33:350–356.

21 Frank A. Just listening: narrative and deep illness. Fam Syst Health 1998;16:197–216.

22 Balint M. *The Doctor, His Patient and the Illness*. London: Routledge; 1956.

CHAPTER 2

The 'ologies' (underpinning academic disciplines) of primary health care

Summary points

1 Two medical disciplines are crucially important to the effective practice of primary health care:

  a Biomedical sciences (anatomy, physiology, pathology, cardiology, pharmacology and so on); and

  b Epidemiology (the study of disease patterns in populations, and interventions to change these). Clinical epidemiology (evidence-based medicine) requires judicious application of the findings of rigorously conducted epidemiological research to individual clinical decisions.

2 However, focusing exclusively on these medical sciences would give us a narrow and incomplete view of primary care. This chapter covers six additional disciplines that underpin an academic perspective on primary care:

  c Psychology (the study of mind and behaviour);

  d Sociology (the study of human society and the relationships between its members);

  e Anthropology (especially cultural anthropology – the study of the ways of life and meaning-systems of groups and societies);

  f Literary theory (the study of the human condition as presented in stories, poetry and drama);

  g Philosophy, including epistemology (the study of how we know things) and ethics (the study of what we should do); and

  h Pedagogy (theories of learning).

3 Each of these disciplines contains a number of key concepts and theories that can serve as a conceptual 'lens' through which to make observations and design interventions. An academic approach to primary health care requires these concepts and theories to be made explicit, for the methodological approach and level of analysis to be appropriate to the chosen theory and for the unit of analysis to be clearly and consistently defined.

4 Multi-level theories, though conceptually complex and challenging to investigate, can provide rich insights into primary care issues, but should not be equated with 'anything goes' methodologically or analytically.

2.1 Biomedical sciences

It is beyond the scope of this book to give even the briefest outline of the biomedical basis of primary health care. Even if you are not medically qualified, you will know that a good deal of the work of doctors* requires a sophisticated understanding of anatomy (the structure of the human body at the level of organs, tissues and cells), physiology (the study of how the body works), biochemistry (the study of the chemical reactions, especially enzyme pathways, that are crucial to bodily function at microcellular level), pathology (the study of what goes wrong when people get ill, including a classification of different diseases and what they do to you), immunology (the study of the immune system and how it both fights disease and mediates allergy – which is strictly a branch of pathology but likes to have its own identity), therapeutics (the study of things that help people get better) and pharmacology (the study of the chemical structure and biochemical impact of drugs – a branch of therapeutics of course).

The reason why I am not going to cover these subjects here is that there are already some excellent textbooks that set out the principles and practice of these important sciences. Some of these books are oriented to a particular organ system (such as 'cardiology'), disease entity (such as 'diabetes') or patient group ('paediatrics'), and cover all the biomedical sciences relevant to the chosen territory. In relation to the clinical side of general practice, I can recommend John Fry's *Common Diseases*[1] as a collector's classic from the early sixties (but updated many times since) that includes chapters such as 'the catarrhal child'. The modern day equivalent is the splendid tome from John Noble's team *Textbook of Primary Care Medicine*[2] or the weighty Volume 2 of the *Oxford Textbook of Primary Medical Care*,[3] both of which cover every disease you are ever likely to see in primary care and many others besides, from an evidence-based perspective.†

For the purposes of this book, I want to position all the biomedical sciences as coming from essentially the same stable and to highlight the conceptual and theoretical assumptions implicit in all of them.

Biomedical sciences share three key concepts:
• *The body is a physical system* that obeys the laws of science. In other words, the body is composed of substances that behave in a way previously described by physicists and chemists in relation to the physical world. Hence, bodily

---

*The same can generally be said of the work of physiotherapists, pharmacists, osteopaths and nurses (depending on how the country and healthcare system defines the role of each of these professions).

†If you want a short book of 'what to do' advice with a bendy cover and thumbable index that will fit in your back pocket, try the *Oxford Handbook of General Practice*[4] or Bob Mash's *Textbook of Family Medicine*.[5] Numerous pocket paperbacks aimed at undergraduate medical students such as Anne Stephenson's classic[6] are also useful general introductions for a wider readership.

substance and processes can be broken down into the behaviour of molecules, compounds, fluids, and gases (mostly dissolved ones, and some attached to transfer proteins). And whilst the molecules, compounds, mixtures and processes that make up the living world tend to be more complex than those of the non-living world, the same fundamental physical principles apply.

• *The logical and causal nature of ill health.* When I was a medical student, I spent my life learning lists: the 20 causes of chest pain; the 20 causes of an old person going 'off legs'; the 20 causes of fever in a person recently returned from a trip to Africa. The small print of these lists was (sometimes implicitly, though you never knew when you might have to set it out in full in an exam answer) a particular sequence of causation such as 'mosquito bites man → malaria parasite enters bloodstream as sporozoite → sporozoite takes up residence in man's liver → dormant period ensues while sporozoite reproduces asexually → sporozoites are periodically released from liver and enter red blood cells → dying red blood cells produce chemical with pyrogenic properties[‡] → man's homeostatic thermostat is shifted up two degrees every few days → man gets periodic fever' – and thus, the disease and its symptoms could (or should) be explicable entirely in terms of what had 'gone wrong' with the body, in what order.

• *The logical and causal nature of therapeutic interventions.* It follows from the previous two concepts that the treatment of ill health is about correcting the physical abnormality that set the undesired causal sequence in motion. Correcting pathological processes at the molecular level is, of course, the raison d'etre of the pharmaceutical industry. Millions of people worldwide owe their lives to anti-malarial drugs that were developed by the logical analysis of the disease sequence outlined briefly above.

As Table 1.2 in the previous chapter shows, the biomedical model of diabetes is not 'incorrect' in any simple sense. Diabetes is indeed the product of a pancreas that makes too little of the hormone insulin and/or the result of cells becoming resistant to its effect (so that more is needed to do the job). But I hope you can see that this is only one 'framing' of the problem of diabetes – and it is a framing that drives us down a very particular approach to managing the problem of diabetes. Patients will be put on medication to boost their insulin levels (or improve their sensitivity to insulin); they will need to have this medication prescribed by a doctor and 'comply' with instructions on how to take it; and they will need to attend for regular blood tests to check-up on how the biological repair work is going. The right-hand column in Table 1.2 illustrates how going beyond the biomedical model can open up new framings of what diabetes is and new opportunities for how it is managed. Sections 2.3–2.8 of this

---

[‡] You may have spotted the tautological (circular) nature of this explanation. A 'pyrogen' is something that causes a fever. The man gets a fever because he produced a pyrogen – which hasn't said much except to imply that there *must* be a pyrogen since a fever has to have a cause. Such reasoning is, sadly, very common in biomedical textbooks.

chapter offer the principles and theoretical basis of some (though not all) of the disciplines that underpin this right-hand column, and Section 2.9 introduces the notion of multi-level theories. You might like to draw a comparable table suggesting how the study of malaria (or indeed, drug dependency, anorexia nervosa, peptic ulcer or any other illness you care to name) could be framed differently, opening up new avenues for its prevention or treatment.

It is worth noting here that patients can often receive excellent primary health care for their problem when doctors and nurses behave *as if* the biomedical model explained everything, even when it doesn't. But in many situations, the biomedical model can dangerously limit the clinician's insight into the problem and the options he or she considers feasible – sometimes to the detriment of the patient. A sizeable branch of mainstream psychiatry (the study of mental illness and its treatment), for example, works on the assumption that mental illness is the result of a deficiency in a neurotransmitter in the brain, and that the treatment of everything from depression to schizophrenia will come in the form of a pharmacological 'magic bullet' designed to restore that deficiency. As we shall see later in this book, other models of mental illness often prove more illuminating for the clinician and more helpful for the patient.

2.2 Epidemiology

Epidemiology is the study of disease patterns in populations. We usually think of an *epidemic* as a disease that spreads rapidly by contagious transmission (SARS, influenza, cholera and so on), but as non-infectious diseases contribute increasingly to the overall burden of disease, we often talk about 'the epidemic of obesity in affluent countries' or 'the emerging epidemic of lung cancer in the developing world'. We are using the term 'epidemic' here not to imply contagion but to denote a problem that demands to be looked at the level of the population. We must consider its causes and management at environmental and policy level as well as at the level of the individual patient. Chapter 8 discusses some examples of population level questions in primary care, and shows how epidemiology (among other 'ologies') contributes to addressing these.

Clinical epidemiology is the application of research conducted on population samples to inform individual health care decisions. Box 2.1 gives some examples. Clinical epidemiology was once a somewhat marginal branch of medicine, but was rebranded a few years ago with the catchy title 'evidence-based medicine' (EBM).[7] It has since become a 'must-do' discipline for both undergraduate and postgraduate students of health sciences.[§]

[§] EBM is sometimes referred to as 'evidence-based health care' (EBHC) or 'evidence-based practice' (EBP) so as to avoid the implication that it is only for doctors. In this book I use the term EBM throughout for consistency, but many of my examples are drawn from studies conducted by (and highly relevant to) nurses, psychologists, physiotherapists and alternative practitioners.

> **Box 2.1 Examples of how epidemiology can help in the clinical encounter.**
>
> • A 24-year-old woman with a history of epilepsy is surprised to be expecting her first child, and asks her GP whether she should stop her tablets (or change to a different medication) to reduce the risk of drug-related damage to her unborn baby. The GP contacts the pharmaceutical company's medical adviser, who consults their international database of post-marketing surveillance data on the safety of the drug in pregnancy.
>
> • A 39-year-old woman seeking family planning advice asks the nurse 'is the oral contraceptive pill safe for me?'. The nurse consults a set of risk tables based on large population cohorts which take account of age, smoking status, blood pressure and other risk factors, before advising the patient on her chance of developing side effects.
>
> • A 76-year-old man who lives an active and independent life has a mild stroke and is found to have an irregular heartbeat (atrial fibrillation). His physician recommends that he take warfarin to 'thin the blood', thereby preventing further strokes. But the man is reluctant to have the weekly blood tests required for warfarin therapy and asks just how much his risk of stroke is going to change if he takes the drug. His GP consults the Cochrane database for evidence from randomised controlled trials and is able to provide the necessary information for the man to make an informed choice about whether the blood tests are worth the inconvenience.

I do not plan in this book to give a comprehensive overview of either general epidemiology or clinical epidemiology (EBM). Rather, this section will highlight the key theoretical concepts that underpin these disciplines. For general epidemiology, Geoffrey Rose's *Epidemiology for the Uninitiated* (now revised by Coggon)[8] offers an accessible introduction to the basics; and Barbara Starfield's *Primary Health Care* provides a weighty application of these principles to the specific disease patterns relevant to the primary care clinician.[9] For a basic introduction to clinical epidemiology, you might try my own book *How to Read a Paper – the Basics of Evidence Based Medicine*[10]; for a more detailed introduction I recommend Fletcher et al.'s *Clinical Epidemiology – the Essentials*; and for those after a 'black belt' in EBM, Sackett and colleagues' big red book *Clinical Epidemiology*[11] is still unparalleled. Mark Gabbay's *Evidence Based Primary Care Handbook* repackages the concepts of EBM focusing specifically on primary care examples.[12]

Let us briefly consider the key concepts and theoretical framework within which epidemiology (and therefore evidence-based medicine) makes sense. The first thing to say is that EBM is predicated very strongly on the biomedical model described in the previous section. The second concept to highlight is the role of mathematics (especially probability theory) in informing decision making. Dave Sackett, who I believe deserves more credit than anyone else for popularising EBM, produced what is probably the most widely quoted sentence ever printed in the British Medical Journal when he said *'Evidence based medicine is the conscientious, judicious and explicit use of current best evidence when making decisions about the care of individual patients'.*[7] This definition (which, you will note, welds EBM inextricably to the professional virtues of integrity, commitment and wisdom) has taken on an almost religious significance within the EBM movement while producing nothing but controversy outside it. The problem in my view is that apart from his cheeky claim to the high moral ground of professional practice, Sackett didn't define tightly enough what 'current best evidence' meant. I prefer a different definition of EBM which I developed with Anna Donald:

> *'Evidence based medicine is the use of mathematical estimates of the risk of bene-fit and harm, derived from high-quality research on population samples, to inform clinical decision-making in the diagnosis, investigation or management of individual patients'.*[13]

EBM helps to establish both the *size* of effect expected from a certain course of action, as well as the *likelihood* of its occurring, such as the likelihood that the measles, mumps and rubella (MMR) vaccine causes autism (see Section 8.1). Typically, EBM helps to answer questions of the general form 'What is the chance that outcome X will result from course of action Y in population Z?' For example, 'What is the chance that topical anti-inflammatory cream will cure tennis elbow?' or 'What is the chance that the combined MMR vaccine is just as safe and just as effective as individual vaccines in children aged 2–6 months?' Such questions (sometimes referred to as the 'four-part clinical question' as shown in Table 2.1) must be answered with quantitative research, which gives answers in the form of probability estimates, such as 'one half', or '70% as likely'

Table 2.1 The four-part clinical question, which forms the basis of much of evidence-based medicine.

	Element	Suggestions to help	Example
1	Patient or problem	'How would I succinctly describe a group of patients similar to this one?'	In children under 12 years with eczema ...
2a	Intervention (i.e. test, treatment, process of care)	'What is the main action I am considering?'	would adding tiger balm ointment to their existing therapy of 1% hydrocortisone cream ...
2b	Comparison (where relevant)	'What are the alternative option(s)?'	... compared to continuing with hydrocortisone cream alone ...
3	Outcome	'What do I/the patient want to happen/not happen?'	... improve symptom control without increasing the risk of adverse events ...
4	Time	'Over what period of time should the outcomes be evaluated?'	... over the subsequent three months?

or '2% more likely'. The research that produces these numerical estimates is covered briefly in Sections 3.3 and 8.1–8.4, and in more detail in the specialist textbooks listed on the previous page.

I have my differences with Dave Sackett about what EBM is, how it should be promoted and where its limitations lie, but it's worth acknowledging that the idea of combining the most elegant and abstracted science – mathematics – with the one closest to our own vulnerable humanity – biomedicine – was nothing short of brilliant. Doctors have known for centuries that the 'causes' of a particular disease do not *necessarily* produce that disease (take smoking and lung cancer for example) nor does a single 'abnormal' diagnostic test mean that a patient has actually got a particular disease (take a suspicious breast lump detected on a mammogram for example – which means either genuine breast cancer or a 'false positive' with all the attendant anxiety and unnecessary tests). I explain all this in more detail in Section 8.3, but for now, I just want to convey the idea that numbers (if they are numbers we can trust) can improve the quality of information and advice we offer our patients. Before EBM, all we could say to a woman with an abnormal mammogram was 'You've got a suspicious lump; it might be cancer but it might be just a lumpy breast'. Using research studies from epidemiology, we can now say that the overall chance (based on the entire population of women who have had mammograms) of an abnormal lump detected on mammography being cancerous is around 1 in 10. But based on a stratified (i.e. divided up by age) analysis of the same dataset, we can say that if the woman is 35, the chance of her lump being cancer is approximately 1 in 35; if she is 55 the chance is 1 in 11; and if she is 75 the chance is 1 in 5 (Figure 2.1).[14] This information is considerably more helpful to the

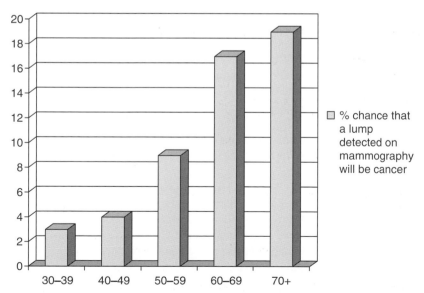

Figure 2.1 Positive predictive value of screening mammography at different ages[14] (see Section 8.3 for an explanation of the term 'positive predictive value').

patient than 'it might be cancer and it might not'! In Section 5.2, I describe a more complex example, but based on the same fundamental principle, about how to estimate a patient's chance of having conjunctivitis given certain combinations of physical signs, and in Section 8.3, I talk about screening for Down syndrome using similar principles.

A word of caution. Epidemiology might appear very scientific and precise (since it involves a lot of numbers), but as Chapter 3 will emphasise, any epidemiological estimate is only as sound as the representativeness of the samples, the validity of particular measurements (e.g. does a particular 'quality of life' questionnaire really measure the quality of someone's life?) and the thoroughness and transparency of the data collection process (can all the researchers and data entry clerks be trusted not to invent results to fill gaps, for example?). If we make our measurements in a group of individuals who differ systematically from the population we are interested in and if we use the wrong instruments or poorly trained or motivated staff, our figures will be not merely useless but positively misleading.

So, for example, the statement 'One man in ten is homosexual' (which as you will learn in Section 3.3 is an estimate of *prevalence*, except that homosexuality isn't a disease!) *sounds* like science, but a critical epidemiologist will want to know where that figure has come from – and, indeed, why the question was asked in the first place. What sort of men were in the sample? Old? Young? Army recruits? Actors? People who agreed to answer a market research survey in the street? What proportion of these was telling the truth? How was 'homosexual' defined? One experience ever? A regular same-sex partner? Fantasies? In any case, why did the researchers want to know? And surely, a tick-box questionnaire with 'homosexual' and 'heterosexual' as the two categorical (mutually exclusive) responses fails to represent the fluid, context-dependent and complex nature of sexual orientation. And so on. We begin to mistrust the 'hard' figure of 10%. This fictitious example shows that although the results of epidemiological surveys are generally quantitative (numerical) in nature, the questions we ask about *where the numbers have come from* tend to be qualitative (i.e. relating to context, meaning and experience). This example also raises epistemological questions (i.e questions about the nature of knowledge). Primary care knowledge is *inherently* ambiguous and uncertain, as Section 1.1 illustrated, so it's not simply a question about working harder to 'fill the evidence gap'. More on epistemology in Section 2.7.

In Section 1.3 (Box 1.4) I described the example of Dr Begum, the young EBM enthusiast who considered every problem in terms of 'diagnosis', 'prognosis', 'therapy' and so on. She searched for research evidence on the Internet, evaluated it carefully and drew conclusions that she believed were rational and logical, and she then applied them in practice. In Dr Begum's version of primary care, patients suffer from diseases that are attributable to specific causes (and risk factors), and which respond to a greater or lesser extent to the treatments that have been tested in randomised controlled trials. It is worth summarising here the principles (and assumptions) on which Dr Begum's view is based:

• *The logical and causal nature of disease and its treatment.* As with biomedical theories, EBM assumes a rational and predictable universe in which the findings of research in one group of people can be used to inform the management of a different group.

• *The availability (and the accuracy and precision) of mathematical estimates of benefit and harm.* The EBM model breaks down where the mathematical estimates on which decisions are supposed to be based is absent, flawed, imprecise, conflicting, ambiguous, contested or relating to a group of patients that differs in important characteristics from the one you happen to be treating. The reality of primary health care (see Section 1.1, especially the right-hand column of Table 1.2) is that research evidence on much of its subject matter does not (and never will) exist in the form that EBM requires.

• *Both clinician and patient operate as rational decision makers.* As Section 5.3 shows, neither patients nor clinicians always make decisions by weighing up the pros and cons of different options in an essentially 'mathematical' way. Many years ago, my father (an intelligent enough man) was advised to take tablets for a chronic condition. He refused, because he didn't like taking tablets – a decision that eventually killed him. Not taking tablets is a common choice made by patients the world over, perhaps because their identity (see Section 2.4.3) is strongly linked to not being a 'tablet-taker'. Competent care for such people is about understanding the motives of such patients and reaching the best compromise – an approach that needs a different theoretical lens from that of EBM.

• *Evidence-based decision making is feasible in the clinical encounter.* In the world of contemporary primary health care, busy clinicians see patients at intervals of a few minutes, and much needs to be achieved within the encounter. Achieving evidence-based care at the front line of primary care rests heavily on accessible summaries of the best evidence (see, e.g., www.clinicalevidence.com) being available on the GP's desktop (and perhaps tied into his or her computer system). The challenges of evidence-based decision support are covered in Section 5.2.

In summary, the main point to grasp about epidemiology is that it is a numbers game whose primary purpose is estimating how many people in a population have a particular disease or complication. Clinical epidemiology (EBM) can be thought of as a tool that provides numerical estimates of benefit and harm that clinicians and patients can draw on to inform health care decisions. But the numbers used in 'evidence-based' decision making often raise important qualitative questions about their trustworthiness, generalisability or precision. I will discuss the different types of epidemiological research in Section 3.3, and Sections 5.2, 5.3, 10.2 and 11.2 all give examples of the practical and philosophical challenges of delivering the so-called gold standard of 'evidence-based' primary care.

2.3   Psychology

2.3.1   Overview

There are many definitions of psychology and a host of branches to this vast discipline.[||] Psychology extends from the observation of animal behaviour ('rats in mazes') to the interpretation of unconscious desires (psychoanalysis). A typical psychology textbook might include the following chapter headings: psychobiological processes; sensation and perception; consciousness; learning; memory; thinking and language; intelligence; motivation; emotion; development; personality; psychological disorders; psychotherapy; psychology and health; social cognition; social influence. Some (but not all) of these topics feature in the different applications of psychology to primary care problems covered in Chapters 4 through 11.

The most common definition of psychology is 'the scientific study of mind and behaviour'. But this definition is hotly contested, especially by psychologists who are less interested in a narrowly 'scientific' perspective (observing, and trying to influence, human behaviour) than in exploring the meaning that individuals and society give to that behaviour.[#] In other words, much of psychology sits more comfortably in an interpretive, humanistic paradigm than in an experimental and narrowly scientific one. The research methods of psychology are equally diverse. Some psychologists use methods based on the natural sciences – observation and experiment – to study human (and animal) behaviour. Much of their research comprises either laboratory experiments or questionnaire studies (see Section 3.4) – typically using undergraduate psychology students as their 'subjects'! Psychologists who take a more interpretive stance generally use qualitative methods such as semi-structured interviews (see Section 3.2) in which they ask participants[**] to describe the world as they perceive it. Common to all branches of psychology is the attempt to make sense of how people see the world and how they behave within it.

Given the broad scope of knowledge that is encompassed under the heading 'psychology', it is not surprising that a number of more or less circumscribed subdisciplines have arisen within it. For example:
• *Behavioural psychologists* study the conditions under which a behaviour can be learned and the situations (incentives, rewards, punishments) that make that behaviour more or less likely to occur;

[||] I am grateful to Dr Petra Boynton for illuminating this discipline for me. Petra is the psychologist on my own team and has written a very accessible textbook on research methods called *The Research Companion*.[15]

[#] The best book I have ever read that explains what the study of meaning adds to psychology is Jerome Bruner's *Acts of Meaning*.[16]

[**] People who volunteer to take part in experiments are often called 'subjects'. But 'subject' is a rather old-fashioned and (arguably) politically incorrect term, since it implies a passive individual who does not understand what is being done and has no power to influence what goes on – a situation at odds with the principles of research ethics described in Section 3.1. I will use the term 'participant' throughout this book to refer to people who take part in research studies.

• *Cognitive psychologists* investigate memory, thought, problem solving and how these factors influence learning and behaviour. Because of the close links between cognitive and behavioural approaches, in practice they are usually combined as cognitive-behavioural psychology;

• *Social psychologists* are concerned with the effects of social situations on human behaviour;

• *Personality theorists* study how attitudes, motives and behaviour differ between individuals (and why they are often relatively constant within individuals);

• *Developmental psychologists* study the principles and processes responsible for changes in cognition and behaviour throughout life – but particularly during childhood;

• *Physiological psychologists* are concerned with the biological bases of behaviour (of which a subset, neuropsychologists, are particularly interested in neurotransmitters and other biochemical influences on the brain);

• *Psychodynamic psychologists* (including psychoanalysts) study the impact of unconscious and irrational forces on human motivation, attitudes and behaviour.

These different subdisciplines (divisions of psychology as a science) underpin a number of different vocations (divisions of psychology as a profession). A person might study a number of the above subdisciplines as part of a psychology degree, and then choose to train in one of the following as a profession:

• *Educational psychologists* apply a range of psychological theories (especially cognitive-behavioural theory, motivation theories, social learning theories and theories of identity) to improve understanding of how new behaviours are learned and maintained and how a child's learning and development might be supported;

• *Industrial or organisational psychologists* apply a similar range of psychological theories to improve understanding of how the physical and social aspects of work environments affect the activity and output of individuals at work (and advise on how these can be improved);

• *Sports psychologists* apply the principles of motivation and cognitive psychology to the coaching and support of athletes;

• *Community psychologists* apply the principles of social psychology to attempt to solve social problems in communities;

• *Clinical psychologists* apply a wide range of psychological theories (about the biological, social, cognitive and affective bases of behaviour) to the assessment, prevention, treatment and rehabilitation of psychological disability, dysfunctional behaviour and risky lifestyles, and to the enhancement of psychological and physical well-being;

• *Psychotherapists* apply selected theories of mind and behaviour (either cognitive or psychodynamic) in an effort to relieve psychological distress;

• *Critical psychologists* question the discipline of psychology itself by challenging the questions it deems important and the methods it uses to explore those questions. Within this group are feminist psychologists (who evaluate how psychology has marginalised and perhaps harmed women) and Marxist psychologists (who consider how bourgeois ideology has distorted the research agenda).

The branch of psychology most familiar to primary care professionals is clinical psychology, since clinical psychologists may be part of the primary health care team or a secondary care service to which patients are referred. Clinical psychology includes both scientific research (laboratory-based or community-based studies that seek to add to the knowledge base) and clinical service (patient-oriented work that focuses on the study and care of individuals with psychological needs). An important branch of clinical psychology draws on moral philosophy (see Section 2.7) and is devoted to supporting and monitoring patient welfare and professional conduct – for example, respect for dignity, responsible caring, integrity in relationships and responsibility to society.

Psychological theories generally take the individual as the unit of analysis (see Section 3.9) and offer explanations in terms of rewards and punishments, attitudes and motivation, identity (the 'self' and how it is constructed and presented) or unconscious desires. Of the hundreds of psychological theories available in the literature, I have referred to only a few in this book: Prochaska and DiClemente's stages of change theory (also known as the transtheoretical model – Section 4.3), Azjen and Fishbein's theory of reasoned action (Section 4.3), Freud's psychoanalytic theory (see Section 6.3), Bandura's social learning theory (which incorporates self-efficacy theory – see Section 2.8.1), and Vygotsky's social development theory (see Section 2.8.2). I have included these for one or more of the following reasons: (a) they are widely cited in the primary care literature, so you may have heard of them already; (b) they are good examples of how the study of mind and behaviour can be applied to real-life problems in either clinical primary care (explaining and influencing patients' beliefs and actions), professional development (how clinicians learn and reason) or organisational change; or (c) they raise general issues about how we draw on theories to help us develop an academic approach to primary care problems. They are intended to be used as examples, not as an exhaustive selection of the contribution of psychology to the study of primary care.

2.4   Sociology

2.4.1   Overview

Sociology is the study of human society and the relationships between its members, especially the influence of social structures and norms on behaviours and practices. The unit of analysis in sociology is generally the social situation (or, sometimes, the expression of social norms and expectations in individuals' behaviour). The sociologist may look at social situations and relationships at a micro level (e.g. how do individuals locate themselves and behave in their family or friendship group) or at a more macro level (e.g. how does the prevailing social system shape and constrain individuals' views about how they should behave and what they might achieve in life). In other words, the sociologist looks at what we do and the meanings we place on objects, acts and relationships – and asks 'what do these actions and interpretations say about the society we live in?'

The term 'sociology' begs the question of what is 'society'; what are 'social situations' and 'social relationships'; and how might these be studied. Britain's ex-prime minister Margaret Thatcher one infamously said that 'there is no such thing as society'. Most academics would disagree with that statement, but it is certainly true that the norms and relationships that constitute 'society' are elusive, contested and hard to measure. A good definition of a social situation is 'people orienting their actions towards one another' – and this can be measured both quantitatively (who interacts with whom, who is influenced by whom and what is the impact on particular outcomes) and qualitatively (what is the *meaning* of particular acts, and particular interactions, to individuals).

Like anthropologists, sociologists have moved in recent years from analysing the strange and exotic to focusing on familiar experiences and social relationships. Increasingly, therefore, sociology requires the researcher to develop a high degree of self-awareness and critical consciousness. As Peter Berger points out in his classic textbook 'Invitation to Sociology',[17] this 'sociological consciousness' has four defining features:

• *The goal of 'debunking'* – '[Sociology's] built-in procedure of looking for levels of reality other than those given in the official interpretations of society... a logical imperative to unmask the pretensions and the propaganda by which men cloak their actions with each other';

• *Attention to the underclass and the socially excluded* – hence, 'studying the social reality of the community not only from the perspective of city hall, but also from that of the city jail';

• *Relativism* – the notion that today's norms and values are not absolute, but are the product of the historical and social changes that gave rise to them (and hence recognising that tomorrow's norms and values will be different); and

• *Cosmopolitanism* – in Berger's words, 'a taste for other lands, inwardly open to the measureless richness of human possibilities, eager for new horizons and new worlds of human meaning'.

Sociology has many subdivisions (one official library taxonomy lists 342 of them), including, for example, the sociology of education (the study of how social structures and norms influence education systems and the learning that takes place within those systems); organisational sociology (the study of social relationships and work patterns in organisations); and the sociology of information (the study of how information is used, interpreted, transferred and valued in society). My main concern in this book is the sociology of health and illness (known as medical sociology in the USA), which has a number of subdivisions that overlap with other branches of sociology:

• *Social epidemiology* – the study of how a person's experience in society influences the risk and outcome of disease (most notably in relation to health inequalities between socio-economic, ethnic and gender groups);

• *The sick role* – the impact of social norms and expectations on illness and help-seeking behaviour (i.e. how we behave when we are ill);

- *The professional role* – the identities, behaviour patterns, social norms and social networks of doctors and other health professionals;
- *The clinician–patient interaction* – how patient and health professional relate to one another and enact society's expectations in the consultation or other healthcare encounter; and
- *The organisation of clinical work* – how work patterns and routines are developed and enacted in healthcare organisations (including the impact of new technologies on clinical work and its administration).

An important theme in sociology is how a particular society achieves control over its members' behaviour. In different social systems, this may occur predominantly through violence or threat of violence; through economic constraints; or through norms, expected behaviour patterns and social pressure from family or institutions such as schools or workplaces that become internalised and perceived as the individual's free choices. The general theme of social control (and particularly the debate around 'internal norms' versus 'external regulation') informs the study of how we regulate professional behaviour and the incentives and rewards that drive the implementation of health policies.

People who are not familiar with sociology as an academic discipline sometimes confuse it with social work (the practice of helping people, typically disadvantaged ones, in an official capacity) or with social reform. But as Berger suggests, sociological information can be valuable to anyone – and is not equal to humanitarian information.[17] It can be used for fighting crime and (in the wrong hands) for promoting crime! As he says: *'Sociological understanding can be recommended to social workers, but also to salesmen, nurses, evangelists and politicians – in fact, to anyone whose goals involve the manipulation of [people], for whatever purpose and with whatever moral justification'.*

In this book, I will introduce a selection of classic sociological theories, some of which have already featured prominently in primary care research and some of which I feel deserve greater attention: Parsons' theory of the sick role (see Section 4.1); Goffman's theory of stigma, and of the self and its presentation (Sections 4.1 and 4.4); Strauss and Corbin's theory of chronic illness as biography (Section 4.4); Putnam's social capital theory (Section 9.2); Mead's theory of symbolic interactionism (Sections 4.4 and 6.2); Everett Rogers' diffusion of innovation theory (see Section 5.4); sociological theories of professionalism and professional bodies (Creuss et al. – see Section 5.6); the theory of communicative action (Jurgen Habermas – see Section 6.5); structuration theory (Anthony Giddens and others – see Section 9.3) and sociotechnical systems theory (Marc Berg and others – see Section 10.3).

2.5 Anthropology

Anthropology is the 'study of humans' in the broad sense. There are three main subdisciplines of anthropology: (a) cultural anthropology (with which we are mainly concerned here), (b) archaeology and (c) physical (or biological) anthropology, which is mainly concerned with comparing physical measurements between different populations. A fourth, linguistics (pertaining to language), was once a subdiscipline in its own right but seems to have been absorbed by cultural anthropology (and particularly structuralism) in recent years.

Cultural anthropology deals with myriad aspects of human society, culture, behaviour, beliefs, ways of life and so on. Traditionally, it focused on the study of primitive or unusual societies or groups, but increasingly these days it studies more developed societies and familiar groups within those societies (such as professional bodies or organisations). In the past, cultural anthropology suffered from intellectual imperialism (benchmarking 'their' beliefs against 'our' knowledge). These days, the research tools of the anthropologist (mostly in-depth qualitative methods) can be applied to the study of one's own culture through self-awareness and distancing techniques designed to 'make the familiar strange'. Because the study of humans is so relevant to many academic disciplines, cultural anthropology cross-cuts a number of other disciplines traditionally taught in universities – for example, foreign languages, economics, psychology, sociology, political science, ecology, women's studies, history and of course the health sciences.

Medical anthropology is the branch of cultural anthropology that studies the cultural influences, which promote, maintain or contribute to disease or illness, and the strategies and practices that different human communities have developed in order to respond to disease and illness. Exchanges between anthropology and medicine date as back as the end of the nineteenth century, with the pioneering works of Rudolph Virchow, the distinguished nineteenth century pathologist whom doctors may know as the author of the famous 'Virchow's triad' (the three classical signs of thrombosis) but who also emphasised the need to consider the patient's illness in the particular cultural context of his or her society.

Apart from this early influence by Virchow, the roots of medical anthropology can be traced back to the founding fathers (and mothers) of mainstream cultural anthropology, such as WHR Rivers (the anthropologist-psychiatrist who became famous for treating Siegfried Sassoon and Wilfred Owen for battle shock in the First World War), Sir Edward Evans-Pritchard and Margaret Mead (the brilliantly unconventional US anthropologist who shocked the academic community with her graphic description of sexual rituals in Pacific islanders). These and other researchers undertook detailed ethnographic studies (i.e. they donned a pith helmet and moved in with their chosen 'tribe' for several years at a time). Their studies on health beliefs and healing rituals were presented as part of a wider description of the culture and practices of that society. During and immediately after the Second World War, medical anthropology began to arise as a separate subdiscipline – partly as a result of greater political awareness amongst academics and researchers (i.e. the obvious health differentials between different societies became a subject for ideological statements and political action). In the 1950s, many anthropologists began to join with other academics to address problems of international health – and thus began the systematic and proactive study of health and culture in its own right, which in a single generation developed into an extensive literature.

In the subsections that follow, I have deliberately not tried to cover all the main anthropological theories (I have, e.g. omitted functionalist theories which take what I believe to be an overly 'scientific' approach to the study of culture). I have chosen three theories that will recur in later chapters of this book – structuralism (which is closely linked to the work of Claude Lévi-Strauss), what I have called post-structuralism (Pierre Bordieu), and symbolic (or narrative) anthropology (Clifford Geertz and Mary Douglas).

2.5.1 Structuralist anthropology

This theoretical school was established almost single-handedly by the French anthropologist Claude Levi-Strauss. It assumes that cultural forms are based on common properties of the human mind. The goal of structuralism is to discover what universal principles of the human mind underlie each cultural trait and custom.

Structuralist anthropology is derived from structuralist linguistics, a school of thought developed by Ferdinand de Saussure. We all know how to use language, even though we may not be aware of the grammatical and phonetic rules we are applying. Structuralist anthropology holds that there is a comparable 'grammar' of cultures. Just as the linguist's task is to discover the unconscious rules and principles embedded (and expressed) within a language, claimed Lévi-Strauss, the anthropologist's task is to uncover the underlying 'structure' of different cultures.

A key premise of structuralist theory is that human thought processes are the same in all cultures, and that these mental processes exist in the form of binary oppositions. These oppositions include hot–cold, male–female, culture–nature and raw–cooked, and they are reflected in various cultural institutions. Anthropologists may discover underlying thought processes by examining such things as kinship, myth and language. Implicit in structuralist theories of anthropology is the notion of hidden reality or 'deep structure' that exists beneath all cultural expressions.

Another premise of structuralism is that just as the meaning of a word must be interpreted in relation to the meaning of all the words in a language, so elements of culture must be understood in terms of their relationship to the entire cultural system. Thus, elements of culture are not explanatory in and of themselves, but rather form part of a meaningful system.

The main criticism levelled at structuralist theories of anthropology is the possibility that independent structural analyses of the same phenomena could arrive at different conclusions – yet if this 'deep structure' exists, such analyses should always lead to the same conclusions. Structuralism has close links to psychology since (in its basic form) it is primarily concerned with the structure of the human psyche and does not concern itself with historical aspects of culture or changes in culture through time. Others have criticized structuralism for its lack of concern with human individuality. An extreme application of structuralism depicts human thought as uniform and invariable.

Structuralist anthropology is not linked directly to any of the examples in this book, but it has had a powerful indirect influence on medical anthropology since (regrettably in my view) doctors' perceptions of cultural issues are often subconsciously driven by a structuralist world view.

2.5.2   Post-structuralist anthropology

As the name implies, post-structuralist theories in anthropology developed out of structuralism and are closely linked to the work of Pierre Bourdieu.[††] Bourdieu rejected the structuralist notion of a universal set of human thought processes 'hard wired' in the structure of the human mind, and instead proposed that dominant thought processes are a product of society and determine how people act.

One example of socially produced thought processes is Bourdieu's notion of symbolic capital (e.g. prestige, honour, the right to be listened to), which he saw as a crucial source of power. When a holder of symbolic capital uses this power against someone who holds less, seeking thereby to alter their actions, they exercise symbolic violence. A patient, for example, might disclose to her GP that she is thinking of consulting a homeopath. The patient may be met with disapproving looks and gestures, symbols which serve to convey the GP's message that pursuing the homeopathic option is unacceptable, but which never make this coercive fact explicit. People come to experience symbolic power and systems of meaning (culture) as legitimate. Thus, the (less powerful) patient will often feel a duty to 'obey' the (more powerful) GP's unspoken demand to abandon the homeopathic option so as not to jeopardise their relationship. In this way (Bourdieu would argue), the patient has been made to misunderstand or misrecognise the essential nature of the homeopath. Moreover, by perceiving the GP's 'symbolic violence' as legitimate, the patient is complicit in her own subordination.

I draw on post-structuralist anthropological theory and the work of Bourdieu in Section 9.2 when I address social capital theory.

2.5.3   Symbolic anthropology

One of anthropology's all-time great scholars, Clifford Geertz, once defined culture thus: '*Believing, like Max Weber, that man is an animal suspended in webs of significance he himself has spun, I hold culture to be those webs, and the analysis*

[††] Bourdieu was actually a sociologist, but he fits better in the anthropology section as he made such a critical contribution to post-structuralism. He was also a philosopher with Marxist leanings and a passionate campaigner for social justice – but that's a subject for another book.

of it to be therefore not an experimental science in search of law but an interpretive one in search of meaning.[18] These 'webs of significance', Geertz believes, are constructed of religious beliefs and practices, customs, social interactions, attitudes and behaviour – everything that we have constructed as rational, social beings capable of thought and imagination. According to Geertz, the role of the anthropologist is to 'decode' the symbolic meanings of the events, practices, customs and interactions that take place within a specific culture, however insignificant they may seem to the observer.

A perennial controversy within anthropology is whether (and to what extent) it is ever possible to understand a culture that is alien from one's own. Structuralism, which is covered in Section 2.5.1 above, and even more so, functionalism (which is not covered in this book) would hold that a good deal of decoding can be achieved through rigorous empirical and analytic methods. Geertz makes no such claims – indeed, he suggests that anthropological writing is merely a 'thick description', an interpretation of an interpretation. The anthropologist's task is much more humble – first to understand how an event is interpreted by the culture in which it takes place, and then to make an interpretation of that interpretation. Furthermore, the reader of anthropological writing must in turn interpret the anthropologist's interpretations.

There is thus (say the protagonists of symbolic anthropology) nothing absolute, rational or strictly logical about the study of culture – rather, it is akin to literary analysis (see Section 2.6). Cultural anthropology is merely the process of creating various imaginative hypotheses, examining those hypotheses, and then deriving explanations from the best hypotheses. It is difficult (indeed, probably impossible) to derive hard-and-fast factual conclusions from data constructed of so many interpretive layers; thus, the argument goes, anthropological interpretation is no more definitive than a commentary on the meaning of a novel or play.

Another anthropologist who has contributed significantly to this theoretical tradition is Mary Douglas. Her extensive fieldwork has examined how people give meanings to their reality and how this reality is expressed by their cultural symbols – most famously in *Purity and Danger* – her classic study of what is defined as 'dirty' in different societies (*'our idea of dirt is compounded of two things: care for hygiene and respect for conventions'*).[19] By defining what is dirty or polluted, people classify their social life into two opposite categories: what is acceptable and what is unacceptable. This symbolic system gives moral order to societies – but may also produce intractable prejudices (such as those against people with AIDS, for example). Douglas argues that humans actively create meanings in their social lives – particularly through ritual – in order to maintain and sustain their society.

I draw on anthropology in Section 5.4 when I refer to Kleinman's work on patients' models of illness; in Section 6.5 when I consider how to study the complex goings-on in the interpreted consultation; and in Section 7.1 when I discuss changes in family structure and social organisation in recent years. It is also worth pointing out that anthropology and sociology are growing closer together as the latter moves from the study of strange far-flung tribes to 'making the familiar strange'. In Section 10.3, I discuss how the ethnographic observation, which is the traditional hallmark of anthropology, may be applied in the 'sociotechnical' study of the impact of electronic patient records.

2.6 Literary theory

A patient's account of symptoms, and a clinician's account of an aspect of professional practice, is often presented in story form. Stories are a universal form of communication. They are also the unit of clinical memory (we remember cases better than we remember lists) and the form in which informal insights and warnings are transferred between clinicians. Yet despite this acknowledged reliance on the story form, primary health care (and health sciences in general) draws remarkably little on the best established academic approach to analysing stories – literary theory.

The online encyclopaedia Wikipedia (http://en.wikipedia.org) defines literary theory as '*the theory (or the philosophy) of the interpretation of literature and literary criticism. Its history begins with classical Greek poetics and rhetoric and includes, since the 18th century, aesthetics and hermeneutics. In the 20th century, 'theory' has become an umbrella term for a variety of scholarly approaches to reading texts, most of which are informed by various strands of Continental philosophy*'.

The father of literary theory is undoubtedly Aristotle, whose book *Poetics* is still a classic some 2500 years after its publication. In it, Aristotle proposed that a story (narrative) has a number of characteristics, including chronology (the unfolding of events and actions over time); characters (people of greater or lesser virtue who take action and/or respond to the actions of others); context (the local and wider world in which the characters enact their business); emplotment (the rhetorical juxtaposition of events and actions to evoke meaning, motive and causality); and trouble (*peripeteia* – a breach from the expected, as in surprise or 'twist in the plot').[20]

Aristotle gave particular prominence to emplotment as a key component of narrative. Emplotment is the use of literary devices to align events and link them through the purposeful actions of characters, thereby getting the heroes and villains in and out of trouble and to show (at least implicitly) whose fault it all was. Trouble, and the response to it, is conveyed through literary tropes such as repetition, metaphor, irony, surprise, suspense and so on.

The psychologist and narratologist Jerome Bruner has argued that there are two fundamental forms of reasoning – logico-scientific reasoning (based on formal logic) and narrative reasoning (based on an appeal to the emotions about the human condition). In his words, '*A good story and a well-formed argument are different natural kinds. Both can be used as a means for convincing another. Yet what they convince of is fundamentally different: arguments convince of their truth, stories of their lifelikeness. The one verifies by eventual appeal to procedures for establishing formal and empirical truth. The other establishes its truth by verisimilitude*'.[16]

The 'narrative turn' in healthcare studies is the term given to a move away from logico-scientific theories and methods for exploring and managing illness (such as evidence-based medicine – see Section 2.2) and towards narrative-interpretive approaches (as proposed in the various 'talking therapies', including the family therapy practised in primary care[21,22]). I have argued elsewhere that pitting an 'evidence-based' approach against a 'narrative-based' approach to clinical practice is a spurious exercise, since there is no zero-sum relationship between these and each must be approached judiciously and within the parameters of its paradigm.[23]

Literary theory is most obviously relevant to the analysis of individuals' written accounts of illness in novels, personal stories or (increasingly) Internet blogs. But as I have argued elsewhere,[23] it can also inform and enrich the clinician–patient consultation even when there is no obvious 'story' to start with. For example, questions like these (which are, of course, at a different level of abstraction) can augment the usual checklist of questions like 'How long has she had the pain?' and 'What medication is she taking?':
• Who is the narrator?
• Is the narrator reliable?
• From what angle of vision does the narrator tell the story?
• What has been left out of the narrative?
• Whose voice is not being heard and why?
• What kind of language and images does the narrator use?
• What effect does that kind of language have in creating patterns of meaning that emerge from the text?
These 'literary' questions (questions *about* the medical history rather than ones that form part of it) can also be used to interrogate the professional's version of events and compare it with the patient's. As Anne Hudson Jones and others have pointed out, ethical problems in clinical care are always 'framed' by the actors involved in ways that suggest a particular 'plot'. For example, to use an example I raised earlier in this chapter, a cancer patient's choice to take homeopathy rather than undergo chemotherapy might be framed by doctors as non-compliance, denial or confusion, and the patient's character presented as flighty, ignorant or stubborn, though this would not, presumably, be the patient's (or the homeopath's) construction of the story. A crucial contribution of the narrative perspective in medical ethics is in mapping the territory and constructing the description of what is conventionally referred to as 'the case'. As Susan Rubin argues in a paper entitled *Beyond the authoritative voice*, the use of the patient's own narrative as the starting point for ethical analysis precludes the clinician (or ethicist) from using his or her own perspective and values to decide what are and are not important components of the 'case'.[24]

I draw on literary theory in Section 4.2 when I introduce the work of Arthur Frank on illness narrative; in Section 6.4 when I consider how the work of Bakhtin might illuminate the study of the clinician–patient relationship; and again in Section 11.3 when I consider the significant event audit approach to quality improvement.

2.7   Philosophy and ethics

Philosophy is derived from two Greek words: 'philo' meaning love and 'sophia' meaning wisdom. Not wisdom itself, note, but *love of wisdom*. Merely having a certain amount of knowledge doesn't make you a philosopher. A philosopher is someone who hungers for the truth about the world – specifically, the truth about the general principles of how the world works. Many philosophers from Socrates to Sartre have been passionate political activists and social reformers whose philosophical musings were put to immediate practical use. Philosophy can be a remarkably practical tool for 'getting your head round' the challenges of primary care too.

In the summary which follows, I have drawn almost exclusively on secondary sources (modern philosophers who have summarised and in many cases clarified the work of their predecessors), especially Bertrand Russell's *History of Western Philosophy*,[25] Roger Scruton's *Modern Philosophy*[26] and the charmingly illustrated *The Story of Philosophy* by Bryan Magee.[27] I have not referenced the great works of the masters (and mistresses) in this text because I suspect that, like me, you will not have time to study them in-depth. But if after reading this introduction you are keen to access the original sources, note that such classical texts as Plato's *Republic*, Aristotle's *Rhetoric*, Descartes' *Discourse on Method*, Kant's *Critique of Pure Reason*, John Stuart Mill's *Utilitarianism* and Mary Wollstonecraft's *A Vindication of the Rights of Women* are now reproduced in full on the Internet, so just put the titles into Google!

The history of western philosophy is marked by three revolutions (i.e. relatively abrupt changes in direction) of thought, which can be simplified as follows:

• *The rationalist revolution* – the switch from religious or mythical (magical) ways of thinking to a rational (scientific) way of thinking, which occurred in ancient Greece at around the time of Socrates (470–399 BC);

• *The epistemological revolution*, which occurred around the time of the French philosopher Rene Descartes (1596–1650), and he is often credited with starting it. For a long time thinkers had been taking something for granted which they used in all their work – knowledge. They had assumed the reliability of the human mind. It was Descartes who called into question the very foundations of all knowledge by doubting the reliability of knowing. All philosophy since that time has had to deal with this issue (see 'Epistemology' below);

• *The linguistic revolution*, which occurred at the beginning of the twentieth century. In a parallel move to Descartes' attack on the reliability of knowledge, twentieth century philosophers challenged the reliability of another previously taken-for-granted aspect of their work – language. The German philosopher Ludwig Wittgenstein (1889–1951) questioned the very purpose and function of language and its use and misuse in philosophical discussions. Wittgenstein's philosophy is unusual in that his first major work, called the *Tractatus Logico-Philosophicus*, published in 1921, put forward the view that philosophical problems are generally based on a misuse of language, and that a careful logical analysis will clarify the meaning of these issues. But his second book, *Philosophical Investigations*, published in 1953 (two years after his death) was an attack on his previous work and proposed a new type of linguistic analysis, which proposed (in essence) that a sentence is understood not by itself, but only in the context of its use.

Different philosophers divide their discipline differently, but broadly speaking there are six main subdisciplines: epistemology, moral philosophy, argumentation (rhetoric and logic), metaphysics, political philosophy and aesthetics. The first three are considered briefly in turn below; the last three, though interesting, are less relevant to our purposes and is not considered further in this book.

2.7.1 Epistemology

Epistemology is the study of valid forms of knowledge. It comes from the Greek 'episteme' which means knowledge and is sometimes called 'theory of knowledge'. Its roots as a distinct subdiscipline in modern times probably began with Descartes, who raised such questions as: 'Is genuine knowledge attainable at all?' 'Is the skeptic (see below) right?' 'What are the limits of knowledge?' 'From what faculties of the mind does knowledge originate?' 'Which method should be used to obtain valid knowledge?' 'How do you justify *a priori* statements?' 'Where is the boundary between subjective and objective knowledge?' 'What is the nature of truth?'

Some important schools of thought within epistemology are

• *Scepticism* – the view that questions whether valid or reliable knowledge is ever attainable by a human being. An extreme sceptic holds that nothing can ever be known. A less extreme form of scepticism holds that we do not know whether knowledge is possible, so we should suspend judgment on the issue. Descartes (1596–1650) defined scepticism as 'systematic doubt', and using that definition we can see why scepticism built the very foundations of epistemology and the scientific method.

• *Rationalism* – the view that valid knowledge comes only through the mind. Rationalists hold that the mind knows truths that were not placed there by sensory experience. There are innate ideas which you can know independent of what you can see, hear and measure. Mathematics and geometry are examples of abstract truths which are known with certainty, even though the physical illustrations of these truths may vary. The Greek philosopher Plato (427–347 BC) was an early rationalist. He stated that ideas have an existence independent of human minds. These independently existing ideas are the only reality in the universe since they are absolute and unchanging. Valid knowledge comes then when the mind grasps these ideas. More recently, Descartes (1596–1650), who initially went through a period of scepticism, later came to the conclusion that only ideas that are clear and distinct to the mind represent valid knowledge; all else is somehow tainted. Rationalism is somewhat out of favour these days, given the rise of other philosophies of knowledge (see below).

• *Empiricism* – the view that valid knowledge comes only through the five senses, first proposed by Aristotle (384–322 BC) but not widely accepted until after the death of Descartes. John Locke (1632–1714) was an English philosopher and doctor who compared the mind to a blank tablet. When a person is born they know nothing. As they go through life, the experiences they have with their five senses write information on the tablet of their mind. In other words, Locke held a representational view of knowledge. Ideas in our mind are representations of the things in the real world. If they accurately represent these things we can say we have valid knowledge. Locke strongly influenced the British physician Thomas Sydenham (1624–1689) who was the first doctor prospectively to record detailed observations of his patients' diseases and follow their course though time. Later empiricist philosophers included George Berkeley (1685–1753) and David Hume (1711–1776). Whilst empiricism has its critics, the notion that not merely knowledge but *understanding* is grounded in experience is of course a central tenet of adult (experiential) learning. Much of evidence-based medicine (Section 2.2) is built on an empiricist view of knowledge.

• *Objectivism* – the view, put forward by (among others) Ayn Rand, that there is an objective reality independent of the human mind that perceives it and studies it. According to this view, individuals are in contact with reality through sensory perception; they gain objective knowledge from perception by measurement and they develop understanding by forming concepts that correspond to natural categories in the external world.

• *Relativism* – the view that there are no absolute truths, but only relative viewpoints. Extreme relativism (like extreme scepticism) is, according to Scruton, the first refuge of the scoundrel. I can dismiss any statement with the line 'that is merely your opinion' – hence, no view is 'better' than any other. But more moderate forms of relativism allow useful insights into modern science. Thomas Kuhn, for example, in *The Structure of Scientific Revolutions* argued that science progresses dialectically through paradigms and that different paradigms are dominant at different times in history.[28] A paradigm shift in science is the point at which one version of 'truth' (i.e. one conceptual framework within which scientific questions are asked, addressed and findings interpreted) becomes displaced by another – such as, the displacement of Newtonian physics by Einstein's theory of relativity or the rise of the feminist perspective in social science, which allowed both male and female scientists to recognise the distortions that can arise from privileging the measurable over the experiential.[29]

• *Social constructivism* – the view that reality is created by individuals through their thoughts, actions, stories and interpretations. This perspective, originally put forward by Peter Berger and Thoams Luckman in the 1960s,[30] is currently very popular in social science research. In direct contrast with objectivism, a strong social constructivist view holds that there is no objective reality 'out there' waiting to be discovered, but that reality is dynamically created through individuals' thoughts, actions and interactions. Few academics would admit to holding an extreme position but many (myself included) describe themselves as 'weak social constructivists' – i.e. whilst accepting that there is something 'out there', much of the reality we perceive is far from fixed and objective. A *social construct* is an idea, which may appear to be natural and obvious to those who accept it, but in reality is an invention or artifact of a particular culture or society – such as the historical notion that women, ethnic minorities and slaves are not fit to vote in a democracy or that the content of medical records should not be shown to the patient.

• *Phenomenology* – Phenomenology is the study of the mind (especially consciousness) as experienced from the first-person point of view. Literally, phenomenology is the study of phenomena – happenings as perceived by the individual experiencing them.[31] A phenomenologist is interested in the artist rather than the painting he or she produces; the mind of the politician rather than the political process; and the person who is ill rather than the disease as defined by clinical coding systems. Central to phenomenology is the issue of personhood and the structure of personal experience. Experiences are always 'real' in that the person perceives something. Phenomenology is concerned with how meaning is assigned to external events and phenomena as part of perception. The sensations of seeing, hearing and so on are part of mainstream phenomenology, but so are more abstract perceptions that are given meaning in the context of a particular experience, such as humiliation, rejection, empathy and so on. The difference between a phenomenological analysis and (say) the analysis of a tick-box survey is the difference between *living through* a visit to the sexual health clinic and *knowing about* such a visit. In Section 11.5, I suggest that phenomenology might be used to enrich the use of 'mystery shopper' patients in the evaluation of health services.

• *Deconstructionism* – the view that all texts have hidden meaning as well as the overt meaning of the spoken or written words, and that there is no firm, fixed or ultimate meaning in any text. Careful analysis (deconstruction) of texts (including asking questions about what is *not* said) will reveal the unspoken and implicit assumptions, ideas and frameworks that form the basis for thought and belief, and will also shift and complicate the overt (apparent) meaning of the text itself. This perspective is associated with the German philosopher Martin Heidigger (1889–1976), the French philosophers Jacques Derrida (1920–2004) and Jean-Francois Lyotard (1924–1998) and America's Richard Rorty (1931–). Deconstructionism underpins the technique of discourse analysis in which texts (interview transcripts, media articles academic papers, policy documents) are studied with a view to revealing the assumptions and ideologies behind their construction (see Section 6.2 for an example).

One of the major schisms within primary care research is that between researchers who take what might broadly be called the logico-deductive approach (which includes objectivism, realism and logical positivism) and those who adhere to one of a range of approaches that come under the 'interpretive' umbrella (including social constructivism, phenomenology and deconstructionism). Some key differences between these two broad schools are set out in

Table 2.2 Differences between logico-scientific and interpretive approaches to knowledge (adapted from Plummer).[32]

	Logico-scientific approach	Interpretive/humanistic approach
Epistemology	Realism Objectivism	Social constructivism Phenomenology Deconstructionism
Goal	To measure To generate causal explanations	To interpret, appreciate or understand To describe
Reasoning	Deductive	Inductive
Focus	The external world The 'facts' The structure of reality	The inner world The meaning or symbolism of things The person
Main output	Generalisable truths	Local insights
Style	Cold Systematic Reliable 'Objective'	Soft Imaginative Valid 'Real'
Main methods	Quantitative (counting and measuring)	Qualitative (watching, listening and reading)
Values	Ethically and politically neutral	Ethically and politically engaged

Table 2.2. I consider the fundamental schism between interpretive/humanist perspectives on knowledge and objectivist perspectives in a number of places in this book, notably Section 4.4 (where I critique different approaches to research in self-management), Sections 5.2 and 5.3 (where I contrast rationalist and humanist dimensions of clinical method) and Sections 11.2 through 11.6 (where I offer a selection of perspectives on healthcare quality, each based on a different philosophical perspective on what quality is and how to measure it).

2.7.2 Moral philosophy

Moral philosophy (ethics) is the study of the moral value of human behaviour. It is important to distinguish between ethics as a division of philosophy (which uses the tools and techniques of philosophy – rhetoric and reason) and 'ethical' religious doctrines and dogma (which are taken by the faithful as incontestable). The questions of moral philosophy include 'What is good?' 'How should we live?' 'What method should we use to determine moral standards?' 'Why be moral at all?' and so on. Translated into the healthcare arena, these principles often translate into questions such as 'Who should get access to expensive healthcare resources?' and second-order questions such as 'How should we decide who should get access to these resources?'.

Some important schools of thought within moral philosophy are:

• *Consequentialism*. This school holds that the moral goodness or badness of an act or rule is determined by its results or consequences. This theory is sometimes called 'results-based ethics' or 'teleological ethics'. Telling a lie is morally wrong because of the damage this lie will cause both to the liar and to society which depends on honest relationships. A particular example of consequentialist thought is called utilitarianism ('the greatest good for the greatest number'), a movement started by philosopher and social reformer Jeremy Bentham (1748–1832) whose long list of personal achievements included founding University College London.

• *Deontology*. Under this theory, sometimes called 'duty ethics' or 'standards-based ethics', you determine if an act or rule is morally right or wrong if it meets a predefined moral standard. One famous philosopher who developed such a theory was Immanuel Kant (1724–1804). Kant developed a 'universal test' to see if a rule could be a universal standard. If a rule can be made universal without contradiction, then it is morally good; if a rule cannot be made universal without contradiction, then it is morally bad. Not keeping your promise is morally wrong because you cannot make it a universal law that everyone can knowingly make promises with no intention of keeping them.

• *Ethical intuitionism*. This school holds that an act or rule is determined to be right or wrong by an appeal to the common intuition of a person. This intuition is sometimes referred to as your conscience. Anyone with a normal conscience will know that it is wrong, for example, to kill an innocent person. The developments in medical ethics over the past 50 years have shown a move from intuitionism to other (arguably, more defensible) positions such as utilitarianism.

• *Virtue ethics*. This school, whose most famous protagonist was probably Aristotle (384–322 BC) and whose more recent advocates include Alasdair MacIntyre, holds that we will achieve a good society by developing the character traits or 'virtues' in its citizens. Such citizens will do what is morally right because they are inherently virtuous, not because they are obeying rules or principles. Aristotle believed that virtue ethics was the way to attain true happiness. Virtue ethics is particularly relevant to the education and training of health professionals – can we or can't we develop a formula for producing 'virtuous practitioners'?[‡‡] Incidentally, virtue ethics has been linked to literary theory by the feminist philosopher Martha Nussbaum through the argument that actions only make sense in the context of a particular story and that one's

---

[‡‡] My friend Dr Peter Toon inspired my interest in philosophy as applied to primary health care. In his book *The Virtuous Practitioner,* he applies Aristotle's virtue ethics to define the qualities of the ideal general practitioner,[33] and Alan Armstrong has done the same for nurses in an excellent recent paper in *Nursing Philosophy*.[34]

emotional response to a story is not merely an allowable component of the ethical decision but should actively drive that decision.

• *Emotivism.* This theoretical position is based on a study of the type of language used in ethical sentences and discussion. You may have noticed that people get emotional about ethical issues. According to this view, ethical pronouncements are a type of language used by a speaker or writer who has particular emotions about an issue, which attempts to evoke similar emotions in the hearer or reader.

I return to these different perspectives on ethics in Section 5.6 when I consider 'the good clinician'.

2.7.3   Rhetoric and logic

Rhetoric is the study of persuasion. In his classic philosophical text *Rhetoric*, Aristotle defined three dimensions to the scholarly art of persuasion: *logos* (the argument itself), *ethos* (the credibility of the speaker) and *pathos* (the appeal to emotion), all of which he considered worthy of academic study. It is worth noting the difference between ancient Greece, where the ability to 'spin' was seen as a positive attribute of a scholar and modern times where scholars (especially scientific ones) are often taught to strip the *pathos* of an argument so as to gain more clarity.

An argument, seen from the perspective of *logos* (formal logic), is a set of statements in which there is a set of premises and a conclusion and in which (unless the argument is fallacious) the premises support the conclusion. In other words, an argument is a statement along with the evidence that supports it. If we have a rational discussion of different philosophical positions, the discussion must use the rules of logic. An important point to grasp is that logic will not specify what the content of the statements are, but it will tell you how to arrange the statements in a logical fashion. There are three basic kinds of argument:

• *A deductive argument* is one in which the conclusion is certain, based on the premises. In a deductive argument the conclusion is contained in the premises. One of the earliest forms of deductive logic, developed by Aristotle, is categorical syllogism – a deductive argument containing two premises and one conclusion. Each of the three statements is a categorical statement – that is it is either true or not. These statements can be of the form: All S are P, No S are P, Some S are P or Some S are not P. An example of a valid categorical syllogism is All humans are mortal. Socrates is a human. Therefore, Socrates is mortal.

• *An inductive argument* is one in which the conclusion is probable, based on the premises. In an inductive argument the conclusion goes beyond the premises. A common form of inductive argument is the argument by analogy – in which a conclusion is drawn about a situation based on similarities of this situation (analogies) to previous situations. For example, if we predict that since it is Sunday the church bells will ring because in the past when it was Sunday the church bells have rung, we are making a probabilistic argument based on an analogy. Most of evidence-based medicine (see Section 2.2) is based on inductive logic because it uses the language and methods of probabilistic reasoning.

• *Fallacies.* An important contribution of logic is its consideration of *incorrect* ways of reasoning. A fallacy is a set of statements that appears to be an argument, but which on closer analysis is not. One example of this is called a 'circular argument', in which the conclusion is used as the premise. Why is drug dealing illegal? Because it is against the law! Since 'illegal' and 'against the law' are the same concept, nothing has been proven. Another common fallacy in medical research is the ecological fallacy – assuming that A caused B when in fact A and B were both caused by something else (call it C) which we did not measure. Thus, for example, just because a town has a large number of unemployed people and a very high crime rate, it does not necessarily follow that the unemployed are committing the crimes! In fact, both unemployment and high crime rate may well have a different cause (or, more accurately, a determinant) – the state of the national economy.

I draw on these principles of rhetoric and logic in many places throughout this book, especially Section 8.2 when I discuss the notion of causality.

2.8 Pedagogy

Pedagogy (theories of learning and their application) deserves a book all to itself, so crucial is this science to primary health care, since so much learning is involved by both patients and professionals. In this section, I have chosen to cover three theories that have particular relevance either to the materials covered in later chapters or in the planning of your own learning as a student of academic primary health care. They are not the only important theories of learning, and some would say I have omitted others that are more relevant, but if nothing else, they serve as examples of how psychological theories (see Section 2.4) might inform the design of educational materials and experiences.

2.8.1 Experiential learning theory

Experiential learning theory (sometimes known as adult learning theory) goes back over 50 years to the work of child psychologist Jean Piaget, sociologist Kurt Lewin and educationist John Dewey.[35] They all emphasised the role of active experience and reflection in shaping understanding. Lewin believed that the failure to learn effectively was usually attributable to a lack of adequate feedback to feed the process of reflection, resulting in an imbalance between observation and action. His widely cited experiential learning cycle is reproduced in Figure 2.2. Dewey held similar views, but placed more emphasis on *ideas* as an impetus for learning.[36] He depicted a progressive spiral in which judgments based on concrete observations lead the learner, via new ideas, closer to an ultimate purpose or goal. Experiential learning theories accord with what we see as 'common sense' in the early twenty-first century, but at the time of their development some 80 years ago, they were a fundamental challenge

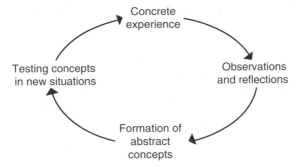

Figure 2.2 The experiential learning cycle (Lewin and Kolb[35]).

to prevailing wisdom, which was based on instructivist theories (which saw learning in terms of the accumulation of facts, like storing money in a bank, and which assumed that learning could be assessed by the reproduction of these facts) and behaviourist theories (which saw learning in terms of performance outputs, like teaching a dog to beg for a reward, and which denied – or at least, refused to analyse – any key role of meaning-making in the learning process).

Experiential learning theories assume that facts are not fixed and immutable elements of thought, but are constantly formed and re-formed through reflection, experience and feedback. Such approaches view learning as a continuous process in which every new experience builds on, and integrates with, the accumulated experiences that have gone before. Thus, says Kolb, no two thoughts are ever the same, since experience always intervenes.[35] I return to experiential learning theory in Section 11.4 when I discuss reflective practice and peer discussion as a tool for quality improvement.

2.8.2 Social learning theory

Social learning theory, developed by the social psychologist Albert Bandura in the 1970s, focuses (as its name implies) on the learning that occurs within a social context.[37] Its main claim is that people learn from one another, and its core concepts are as follows:

• *Observational learning* – people learn by observing the behaviour of others and the outcomes of those behaviours (e.g. they observe that a particular behaviour is socially accepted, experienced as fun or fulfilling or brings a reward);

• *Modelling and imitation* – a key mechanism of learning is observing behaviour in action and imitating it in the same or a similar social context (Bandura emphasised, however, that people can learn by observing *without* directly imitating a behaviour);

• *Direct reinforcement* – people are often rewarded (e.g. by praise, social acceptance or personal satisfaction) when they model the behaviour of others in a social situation, and this increases the likelihood that the behaviour will be sustained and repeated;

- *Vicarious reinforcement* – people who observe someone being rewarded for a particular behaviour are more likely themselves to exhibit the behaviour[§§];
- *The role of cognition* in learning – awareness and expectations of future reinforcements or punishments can have a major effect on the behaviours that people exhibit. But reinforcement will only increase behaviour (and punishment decrease it) if the learner is aware of the link between the behaviour and the reward or punishment;
- *The role of attention* in learning – learning involves cognitive processes, and hence requires attention. The expectation of reinforcement influences the processes that promote learning, and attention in turn influences this expectation.

Whilst social learning theory has many parallels with behaviourist theories (e.g. its emphasis on the role of rewards and punishments in shaping behaviour), Bandura recognised that rewards and punishments have only an indirect effect on learning (humans are not 'rats in mazes'). He also developed a theory of moral thinking and moral behaviour based on the concepts of observation and modelling. Children, he claimed, learn to make moral judgments in part through the modelling of such judgments by their parents and peers.

Bandura believed that four conditions are necessary before an individual can successfully model the behaviour of someone else: (a) attention (the person must first pay attention to the model); (b) retention (the observer must be able to remember the behaviour that has been observed – this may be improved by rehearsal); (c) motor reproduction (the person must be physically able to replicate the behaviour that the model has demonstrated); and (d) motivation (the learner must want to demonstrate what they have learned).

Bandura later extended social learning theory to include a specific emphasis on self-efficacy, which he defined as *'the belief in one's ability to organise and execute the courses of action required to manage prospective situations'*.[38] As well as the previously described concepts of observation, modelling, imitation and motivation, self-efficacy theory includes the additional concepts of confidence and self-belief. People are more likely to engage in behaviours when they believe they are capable of executing those behaviours successfully. Self-efficacy is determined by three things:

- *Personality* – some people have greater confidence and belief in their ability than others;
- *Past successes and failures* – and the rewards, punishments and other feedback received in these experiences. Included in this category is the vicarious learning from seeing others rewarded or punished for their efforts;

[§§]This was shown by the highly controversial 'clown doll' experiments in which Bandura showed two films to groups of children. In one, the child in the film was praised for hitting an inflated doll; in the other, the child was admonished for the same behaviour. Children watching the former film were much more likely to be violent towards the clown doll themselves.[36]

- *Self-regulation* – the individual's ability to, and propensity to, set specific goals, work towards them, evaluate his or her performance and construct personal rewards for achieving particular behaviours.

Self-efficacy in turn influences:
- *Enjoyment* – individuals typically choose activities they feel they will be successful in doing;
- *Effort and persistence* – individuals will tend to put more effort end activities and behaviours they consider to be successful in achieving;
- *Learning and achievement* – individuals with high self-efficacy tend to achieve more (e.g. self-efficacy in students is associated with higher grades).

Promoting self-regulation is an important technique for shaping behaviour. This is usually done by teaching the individual to reward him or herself for particular achievements. For example, a person who seeks to give up smoking might be encouraged to save the money that would have been spent on cigarettes towards a desired (and otherwise unaffordable) treat. Other teaching techniques based on social learning theory are self-instruction (in which the individual is taught to give him or herself specific instruction to guide the desired behaviour) and self-monitoring (in which the individual is taught to measure their own behaviour and reflect on the standard achieved).

In Section 4.4, I apply social learning theory to a contemporary 'hot topic' in primary care: self-management of chronic illness and lay-led programmes to promote and support this.

2.8.3 Social development theory

Lev Vygotsky, born in Russia in 1896, is not nearly as famous as he ought to be. His social development theory of learning was responsible for a sea change in psychological thinking. He proposed not merely that social interaction profoundly influences cognitive development, but that – crucially – social interaction *precedes* cognitive development. Learning is social and cultural before it is cognitive. This approach is best understood when contrasted with the more conventional view of learning and development proposed by the French psychologist Jean Piaget, who saw children as little intellectuals who go through four main periods of cognitive growth: sensorimotor, preoperational, concrete operations and formal operations – each of which adds a 'step' to what is going on inside the child's head and each of which may lead to changes in the externally observed (social) behaviour. Vygotsky, in contrast, believed that development is *primarily* social and cultural and is only later internalised to produce cognitive changes. He also held (again in contrast to Piaget) that development is a lifelong process which can never be said to have been 'completed'.

Vygotsky believed that this lifelong process of development was dependent on social interaction and that social learning is what drives cognitive development. He used a rather strange term for the social interaction that sows the seeds for learning: the Zone of Proximal Development, which he defined as '*the distance between the actual development level as determined by independent*

problem solving and the level of potential development as determined through prob-
lem solving under adult guidance or in collaboration with more capable peers'.[39] In
other words, a student (or indeed a patient) can perform a task under expert
guidance or with peer collaboration that could not be achieved alone. The ZPG
bridges the gap between what is known and what can be known – and it is in
this zone that learning occurs.

The fundamental difference between Piagetian and Vygotskian models of
learning has major implications for the design of educational programmes
for both patients and health professionals. If learning is considered through
a 'Vygotskian' theoretical lens, then the nature of interaction (with whom is
the discussion occurring, in what social context, how often and with what
assumed purpose) is at least as important as the 'content' of the learning (what
is being discussed). If considered through a more conventional Piagetian lens,
learning will occur in pretty much the same way (and in the same sequential
order) whatever the social context.

Both social learning theory and social development theory have huge implications for the education of both patients and professionals (Box 2.2). In
Section 4.5, I speculate about how such theories might enrich research into improving health literacy. In Section 5.5, I draw on these theories to explain the
rather dismal success of efforts to make doctors' practice more evidence-based.
And in Section 11.4, I consider social learning and social development as the

---

**Box 2.2 Implications of social learning theory for education of patients
and health professionals.**

• People often learn a great deal simply by observing other people.
• Describing and discussing the consequences of different behaviours can increase appropriate behaviours and decrease inappropriate ones.
• Modelling is often a more efficient way of shaping behaviour than rewarding
or punishing existing behaviour. To promote effective modelling, a teacher
must make sure that four essential conditions exist; attention, retention, motor
reproduction and motivation.
• Teachers and other opinion leaders must themselves model appropriate behaviours and take care that they do not model inappropriate behaviours.
• Learners must believe that they are capable of accomplishing a particular
desired behaviour. Teachers can promote such self-efficacy by ensuring that
learners receive confidence-building messages, watch others be successful and
experience success on their own.
• Teachers should help students set realistic expectations for their accomplish-
ments so as to avoid the disappointment and disillusionment that leads to a
behaviour being abandoned.
• Goal-setting, self-monitoring and self-regulation techniques can all be effective techniques for changing and sustaining behaviour.

fundamental drivers for quality improvement in the context of peer review and quality circles.

References

1 Fry J, Sandler G. *Common Diseases: Their Nature, Prevalence and Care*. London: Petroc Press; 1993.
2 Noble JH, Greene HL, Levinson W, et al. *Textbook of Primary Care Medicine*. 3rd edn. New York: Mosby; 2000.
3 Jones R, Grol R, Britten N, et al. *Oxford Textbook of Primary Medical Care*. Oxford: Oxford University Press; 2004.
4 Simon C, Everitt H, Kendrick T. *Oxford Handbook of General Practice*. Oxford: Oxford University Press; 2005.
5 Mash B. *Handbook of Family Medicine*. 2nd edn. Cape Town: Oxford University Press; 2006.
6 Stephenson A. *A Textbook of General Practice*. 2nd edn. London: Hodder Arnold; 2004.
7 Sackett DL, Rosenberg WC, Gray JAM. Evidence based medicine: what it is and what it isn't. BMJ 1996;312:71–72.
8 Coggon G, Rose G, Barker DJP. *Epidemiology for the Uninitiated*. 5th ed. London: BMJ Publications; 2003.
9 Starfield B. *Primary Care: Balancing Health Needs, Services and Technology*. New York: Oxford University Press; 1992.
10 Greenhalgh T. *How to Read a Paper: The Basics of Evidence Based Medicine*. 3rd edn. London: BMJ Publications; 2006.
11 Sackett DL, Haynes RB, Guyatt GH, Tugwell P. *Clinical Epidemiology: A Basic Science for Clinical Medicine*. Boston: Little Brown & Company; 1991.
12 Gabbay M. *The Evidence Based Primary Care Handbook*. London: Royal Society of Medicine Press; 1999.
13 Greenhalgh T, Donald A. Evidence based medicine as a tool for quality improvement. In: Jones R, Grol R, Britten N, Culpepper L, Silagy C, Mant D et al., eds. *Oxford Textbook of Primary Medical Care*. Oxford: Oxford University Press; 2002.
14 Kerlikowske K, Grady D, Barclay J, Sickles EA, Eaton A, Ernster V. Positive predictive value of screening mammography by age and family history of breast cancer. JAMA 1993;270:2444–2450.
15 Boynton PM. *The Research Companion: A Practical Guide for the Social and Health Sciences*. London: Psychology Press; 2005.
16 Bruner J. *Acts of Meaning*. Cambridge: Harvard University Press; 1990.
17 Berger P. *Invitation to Sociology*. London: Sage; 1963.
18 Geertz C. *The Interpretation of Cultures*. New York: Basic Books; 1973.
19 Douglas M. *Purity and Danger: An Analysis of Concepts of Pollution and Taboo*. London: Routledge and Kegan Paul; 1966.
20 Aristotle. Poetics. *Translated by Malcolm Heath*. London: Penguin; 1996.
21 Launer J. *Narrative Based Primary Care: A Practical Guide*. Oxford: Radcliffe; 2002.
22 Young V, Tomson D, Tomson P, Asen E. *Ten Minutes for the Family: Systemic Interventions in Primary Care*. London: Routledge; 2003.
23 Greenhalgh T. *"What Seems to be the Trouble?": Stories in Illness and Health Care*. Oxford: Radcliffe; 2006.
24 Rubin SB. Beyond the authoritative voice: casting a wide net in ethics consultation. In: Charon R, Montello M, eds. *Stories Matter: The Role of Narrative in Medical Ethics*. London: Routledge; 2002.

25 Russell B. *History of Western Philosophy*. London: Routledge; 2000.

26 Scruton R. *Modern Philosophy: An Introduction and Survey*. London: Arrow Books; 1997.

27 Magee B. *The Story of Philosophy*. London: Dorling Kindersley; 1998.

28 Kuhn TS. *The Structure of Scientific Revolutions*. Chicago: University of Chicago Press; 1962.

29 Oakley A. *Ways of Knowing: Gender and Method in the Social Sciences*. London: Sage; 2000.

30 Berger P, Luckman T. *The Social Construction of Reality*. London: Penguin; 1966.

31 Merleau-Ponty M. *The Primacy of Perception* (J. Edie, Transl.). Evanston IL: North Western University Press; 1964.

32 Plummer K. *Documents of Life 2: An Invitation to Critical Humanism*. London: Sage; 2001.

33 Toon P. *Towards a Philosophy of General Practice: A Study of the Virtuous Practitioner*. Occasional Paper 79. London: Royal College of General Practitioners; 1999.

34 Armstrong AE. Towards a strong virtue ethics for nursing practice. Nurs Philos 2006;7:110–124.

35 Kolb DA. The process of experiential learning. In: Thorpe M, Edwards R, Hanson A, eds. *Culture and Processes of Adult Learning*. London: Routledge; 1993:138–156.

36 Dewey J. *Experience and Education*. New York: Simon and Schuster; 1938.

37 Bandura A. *Social Foundations of Thought and Action*. Englewood Cliffs, NJ: Prentice-Hall; 1986.

38 Bandura A. *Self-Efficacy in Changing Societies*. New York: Cambridge University Press; 1995.

39 Vygotsky LS. *Mind and Society: The Development of Higher Mental Processes*. Cambridge, MA: Harvard University Press; 1979.

CHAPTER 3

Research methods for primary health care

Summary points

1 Research that informs practice and policymaking in primary care includes a wide range of study designs, methodological approaches and underpinning theories. The 'best' research design and method depend on the nature of the question.

2 Good research in any discipline builds critically and constructively on what has gone before, addresses a clear and relevant question, has specific and measurable objectives, uses appropriate methods and instruments (including methods of analysis), takes account of users' perspectives and priorities and is ethical.

3 Qualitative research addresses questions that begin with 'How...?' 'Why...?' or 'In what way does...?' Qualitative methods include interviews, focus groups, observation and shadowing. They may be used alone or as part of a mixed-method study – for example, to explore the process elements of a clinical trial.

4 Quantitative research addresses the question 'What is the chance that....?' or 'What proportion of....?' It is the cornerstone of epidemiology, in which most research questions consider one of five aspects of a disease or condition: prevalence, incidence, prognosis, harm or therapy.

5 Questionnaire research may include both quantitative (closed-ended) and qualitative (open-ended) questions. Questionnaire studies may use off-the-peg (previously validated) instruments or they may require extensive preliminary work to validate a new instrument. Questionnaire studies may be freestanding or used as part of a wider mixed-method research study.

6 Action research links the search for generalisable truths with efforts to work with local communities to improve their situation and generate tangible benefits for local people. It requires reflexivity and a continuous cycle of learning and change.

7 The analysis phase is often what marks out high-quality research studies from mediocre ones. In general, quantitative data must be analysed by using the appropriate statistical test(s) and qualitative data using a formal interpretive method such as thematic analysis.

(Continued)

(Summary points continued)

> **8** Critical appraisal means systematically studying published research papers with two questions in mind: 'Is this paper relevant to my work?' and 'Can I trust it?' A checklist of around 10 questions allows the reader to address these questions, thereby rejecting papers that are irrelevant to the question or which lack validity.
>
> **9** A systematic review is an overview of a defined topic area in which the author has been systematic about what to include and about how to assess the value and relevance of each study. Different approaches to systematic review reflect different philosophical positions about the nature of knowledge (objectivist or interpretive) and also different goals (to produce generalisable findings or to illuminate an issue with a view to informing local decision making).
>
> **10** Multi-level, mixed-method research has great potential to illuminate the complex and multifaceted problems encountered in primary care. Approaches include the biopsychosocial model, social ecology theory and the stream of causation theory.

3.1   What is good research in primary health care?

It is beyond the scope of this book to explain in any detail how to do research in primary care (see Judith Bell's excellent text on this[1]) or to look critically and systematically at papers describing research done by others (on which I have written a separate book[2]) The goal of this chapter is more modest (but important nonetheless) – to give you a flavour of what research can (and cannot) offer the academic primary care practitioner.

Before you read any further, you might like to try this exercise. Take a blank piece of paper and write down an idea for a research study. Start with a problem based in your own practice (or perhaps from your own experience as a patient or carer), and set out a specific question or questions that you would like the research to answer. Then decide what sort of broad research approach (e.g. qualitative or quantitative) and more specific research design (e.g. a randomised controlled trial for a quantitative study, or interviews or focus groups for a qualitative study) best matches your question. If you do this exercise, you will realise that from every primary care problem there spins off a large number of potential research questions, each of which could be answered in multiple different ways with multiple potential designs. It is often surprisingly hard to decide what a 'good' or 'useful' piece of research might look like in the complex world of primary care.

Figure 3.1 shows some potential spin-off directions from a single primary care problem. You can see that the problem – a high rate of teenage pregnancy and sexually transmitted infections locally – offers countless opportunities for research studies. You will also see that whereas some research questions start with the words 'How many . . . ' or 'What is the chance that . . . ', and hence seek an answer in terms of *numbers* (quantitative research), others begin 'How . . . ' or

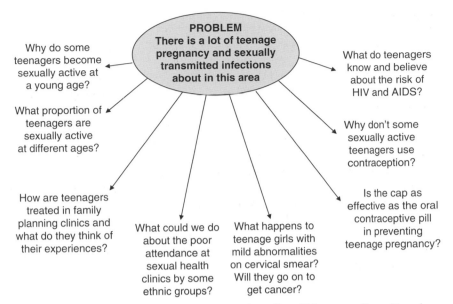

Figure 3.1 One primary care problem, multiple questions. *Note:* All these questions will need focusing further before they become researchable.

'Why . . . ' and seek an answer in terms of *descriptions* or *explanations* (qualitative research). One of the most common errors made by novice researchers is to embark on a quantitative study when a qualitative one is needed or vice versa. Table 3.1 shows examples of both qualitative and quantitative research questions that arise from the same primary care problem. Sections 3.2 (*Qualitative research*), 3.3 (*Quantitative research*), 3.4 (*Questionnaire research*) and 3.5 (*Participatory ('action') research*) set out the principles of each of these basic designs, and the remainder of this book uses examples from the published research literature to illustrate the value of studies from these different genres in primary care decision making. But before we go on to distinguish the different types of research form one another, let's think about research in general and what makes it good (or bad).

A few years ago, a group of tutors and dissertation students on the MSc in International Primary Health Care at University College London considered a selection of research papers that had won the Royal College of General Practitioners' Research Paper of the Year and comparable awards (e.g. from the Royal College of Nursing) over a 10-year period. We asked ourselves 'What is so good about this prize winning paper?' We concluded that:
• Good research starts with (and tries to illuminate or solve) a real clinical or organisational problem via a clear, focused research question;
• Good research builds on, rather than duplicates or ignores, the existing body of knowledge in the field;
• Good research has a firm theoretical basis, which justifies the particular approach, research design and choice of data to collect;

Table 3.1 Examples of quantitative and qualitative research questions.

Clinical field	Example of a quantitative research question	Example of a qualitative research question
Acute myocardial infarction	'What is the chance that prompt thrombolytic therapy improves survival in acute myocardial infarction compared with survival in those not receiving this therapy?'	'Why do some patients delay seeking help when they have acute central chest pain?'[4]
Cervical screening	'What is the chance that a woman with a history of genital warts will have a pre-cancerous cervical smear, compared to the chance in a woman without such a history?'	'When a woman is told her smear is "mildly abnormal," what does she think is happening?'[5]
Smoking cessation	'What is the chance that a smoker will give up when advised to do so by a doctor?'	'What sort of smoker responds to advice to quit, and how to improve the success rate with other smokers?'[6]
Acute febrile illness in young children	'What features of acute febrile illness predict serious disease such as bacterial meningitis?'	'What worries parents when their preschool children are acutely ill, and why?'[3]

• Good research works towards SMART (specific, measurable, achievable, relevant and timely) objectives;
• Good research has a simple and appropriate study design and is practically possible within the timescale and budget of the designated research period;
• Good research uses well-established methods and instruments where possible, but adapts and extends them creatively to produce new empirical techniques;
• Good research is relevant to service users and measures its success in terms of 'patient relevant' outcomes;
• Good research is undertaken according to high standards of ethics and governance (Box 3.1); and
• Good research is value for money in terms of the deliverables on investment.

Note that this list of worthy criteria does not include any prescriptive advice on the 'best' research design for addressing primary care questions. It is often assumed by students with a superficial knowledge of evidence-based medicine (see Section 2.2) that the best design is a randomised trial and that a survey is necessarily a lower form of life. But as Sackett and colleagues made clear a generation ago,[11] the randomised trial is *only* the preferred design if the question concerns the efficacy of a therapeutic intervention (e.g. is anti-inflammatory cream better than placebo cream in treating tennis elbow?). A question about, for example, how teenagers from minority ethnic groups feel about sexual health services is best addressed by a design that collects free-text accounts (e.g. semi-structured interviews or focus groups), and the best

---

Box 3.1 What is research governance?[7–9]

Research governance is the system of administration and supervision through which research is managed, participants and staff are protected and accountability is assured. In the UK, the main reference point is the Research Governance Framework for Health and Social Care,[10] whose stated purpose is to enhance ethical and scientific quality, promote good practice, reduce adverse incidents and ensure lessons are learned. The Framework, which reflects European Union regulations, sets out the responsibilities of the individuals and organisations involved in research, including funders, researchers, organisations employing researchers and health care organisations and goes some way to dispelling the persistent view of research *management* as something separate from the *science* of research.

Research governance includes (but is not restricted to) the ethics of research, which is not restricted to gaining formal approval from a research ethics committee or equivalent overseeing body. In the UK, all research on National Health Service staff and patients must be approved by a Local or Multicentre Research Ethics Committee (LREC or MREC; see www.corec.org.uk), and non-NHS research may require approval from one or more other bodies (e.g. university ethics committee, school governing body, company board and so on). 'Ethical approval' from a formal body does not necessarily make a research study ethical, nor does the refusal of an ethics committee to grant approval necessarily make it unethical (though it may make it illegal to continue with the project).

Active involvement of patients and carers in the management and governance of research projects tends to reduce the chance of unethical practices. For more on such involvement, see www.invo.org.uk

---

design for finding how young children feel about having epilepsy might be one in which the children produce a drawing or painting of what epilepsy means to them![12] The important issue is whether the research design matches the question asked.

The issue of research governance (Box 3.1) and particularly the task of getting 'ethics committee approval' for a piece of research is a bone of contention amongst students, who are often required to plan, execute and write up a small research project within a very limited time span. But scientists have a poor track record of addressing the important tasks of respecting participants' autonomy (including gaining informed consent), protecting them from harm, promoting benefit (including informing participants of the findings after the research is completed) and keeping adequate records. Box 3.2 lists some shameful highlights from the past, which should serve to remind us that the paperwork for ethical approval is not an administrative formality. For further advice on research governance both in the UK and more generally, see the websites in Box 3.1 and a recent series in the *Journal of the Royal Society of Medicine*.[7–9]

Box 3.2 Fraud and misconduct in medical research: disproportionate impact on vulnerable groups.

The strict and bureaucratic regulations for research ethics approval in the UK may seem overassiduous, but scientists have a long and inglorious history of ethical failures, including:

Minority ethnic groups

Between the 1930s and 1960s in Tuskegee in the South of America 400 poor, Black men from rural areas were recruited without their knowledge or consent into a long-term follow-up trial of the prognosis of untreated syphilis; effective treatments were withheld from them for decades. Jews, Gypsies and Slavs were included within human experiments throughout the Holocaust, particularly those relating to warfare such as the testing of effects of gas attacks, battle injury or surviving freezing temperatures subjected to a range of experimentation.

Institutionalised groups

Prisoners and military personnel have not always been given the opportunity to give full-informed consent or opt out of research without changes in their care or status.

Developing countries

Poor communities in developing countries have occasionally been targeted by pharmaceutical companies for trials of medicinal products that would not meet stringent restrictions in the countries where the company is based.

Socially excluded groups

Studies of 'treatments' for homosexuality up to the 1970s can, with the wisdom of hindsight, be classified as ideologically driven research that supported and perpetuated social prejudice and exclusion.

The recently dead

The Alder Hey Hospital scandal highlighted the removal and retention of children's organs and body parts for scientific study without full parental consent or knowledge.

Reproduced with permission from Shaw et al.[7]

One of the most important things to note about research (and primary care research in particular) is that no single study is going to provide all the answers. A research study (which typically takes 2 or 3 years and costs tens if not hundreds of thousands of pounds) generally adds a rather small and humble brick to the 'wall' of knowledge being built about a topic. If you want a different metaphor, a single study alters the colour and tone of the overall picture by a fraction of a shade. A common mistake made by novice academics (such as BSc or MSc students writing their first essay) is to assume that the three or four papers they have found on a topic area provide the whole picture. A common mistake made by these same students when they undertake their first research project is to assume that their work will make a much greater contribution to the knowledge base in the topic area than is actually the case!

When you read a description of a research study, you should set out to identify not just the research question that the authors sought to address, but also – and more fundamentally – the conceptual and theoretical basis of their study (to use the terminology I introduced in Chapter 2, which 'ology' does this study belong in – and is this the only or the most appropriate framing of the problem being addressed?). You should also have some wider questions in your mind such as 'What had previous research studies on the same topic shown (and what did any subsequent studies show)?' 'Why did the authors do *this* study rather than a different one?' and 'Overall, so what?' The examples in the chapters that follow should illustrate this important element of scholarship in the academic study of primary care.

The next four sections give a general outline of the different research designs relevant to primary care. They are not intended to be exhaustive or comprehensive but to serve as a preliminary map of the territory of what the primary care research literature contains.

3.2 Qualitative research

Qualitative research addresses questions that begin with 'How . . . ?' 'Why . . . ?' or 'In what way does . . . ?'. As with any research, good qualitative studies usually address clearly defined questions (e.g. 'What do children feel about having epilepsy?'[12] or 'What worries parents when their child is unwell in the night?'[3]), although the 'clearly focused question' printed in the published paper may have progressed substantially from the question that originally drove the research study.

Following are the characteristics of a good qualitative research study:
• It includes an unambiguous statement of whom the research relates to (in the two examples above, the research relates, respectively, to 'children with epilepsy' and 'the parents of pre-school children who have sought emergency out-of-hours treatment').
• It gives a clear statement of the setting and context of the research.
• It is not designed to confirm particular beliefs or prejudices of the researcher – that is, it is protected as much as possible from researcher bias.

Unlike quantitative research (see Section 3.3), for which there are a limited number of well-known study designs, qualitative research employs a wide range of designs. These are described in detail elsewhere,[13] but include:
• In-depth individual interviews, which are generally semi-structured – i.e. they include a list of open-ended questions but allow scope for the participant

to answer the question in their own words and include what is important to them. See Section 6.5 for an example of how interviews (in this case, narrative ones) were used to illuminate the key issues relating to interpreted consultations in primary care.

• Focus groups – meetings in which a trained facilitator uses the group interaction to test the extent to which views expressed by one individual are shared or contested by others. In Section 4.3, I briefly mention the use of focus groups as a method to identify the priorities of both patients and clinicians for diabetes research.

• Observation of events (e.g. sitting in on consultations or group meetings and making notes on what you see happening). In Section 10.3, I describe how observation of people using electronic health records informed the understanding of the work processes and routines that these records support.

• Participation in events (e.g. simulated patients who attend 'as if' they had a real illness and make note of their feelings and experiences). An example of this is described in Section 11.5.

• Shadowing (e.g. accompanying a district nurse on her rounds).

• Analysis of contemporaneous material (such as letters, e-mails, minutes of meetings, diagrams, flip chart paper and so on).

• Mixed-method studies employing more than one of the above – for example, Dopson and Fitzgerald used naturalistic methods (observation, shadowing, and other non-interventionist approaches) along with analysis of contemporaneous material in the study of the implementation of evidence-based practice described in Section 5.5.[14]

The strengths and limitations of qualitative research are shown in Box 3.3 (and, note, this is not an exhaustive list). Few researchers dismiss qualitative research entirely (though some do), but researchers are divided on the question of whether a qualitative study can ever stand alone or whether it should always serve as an adjunct to quantitative research. I am strongly of the opinion that qualitative research is valid and important in its own right, but I also see the value of mixed-method designs, in which qualitative studies supplement and enhance quantitative designs, most notably randomised controlled trials (see Section 3.3). In mixed-method studies, the qualitative elements can be divided into *exploratory* ('upstream' hypothesis-generating studies which identify key questions that quantitative studies may subsequently address), *explanatory* ('contemporaneous' qualitative studies undertaken alongside randomised trials to capture key process elements and help explain why the intervention did or did not prove efficacious) and *evaluative* ('downstream' qualitative studies undertaken after an intervention has been trialled and is being implemented in real-life practice; such studies can help explain the mismatch between the effect seen in the research trial and the actual impact observed in real-life). The role of qualitative studies in mixed-method research is illustrated in Figure 3.2.

But qualitative research can also influence clinical practice directly, simply by illuminating a problem and raising awareness of its existence. It can also

---

Box 3.3 Strengths and weaknesses of qualitative research in a healthcare setting.

Strengths

• Qualitative research allows the researcher to explore the meanings that respondents attach to particular experiences
• Qualitative research is open ended: respondents' own priorities are allowed to lead the data collection
• Small samples allow rich (i.e. detailed) data to be obtained
• Data are context-rich
• Multiple methods and data sources may be used, such as interviews, focus groups and observation
• Validity of data is established through confirmation with research participants

Weaknesses

• Data are context-specific and may not be generalisable to other contexts
• The researcher has an impact on the data collected
• Small samples mean that findings may be parochial and ephemeral

Implications for health professionals doing qualitative research

• Their identity and status will affect the nature of the data collected
• They may be driven, consciously or unconsciously, by their own professional beliefs and priorities
• The empirical orientation of most health services research may limit the analytical potential of the research

Adapted with permission from teaching materials produced by Jill Russell. See also Table 2.2.

---

follow logically from quantitative research rather than vice versa. For example, the question 'Why do patients delay seeking help when they have acute chest pain?' followed from quantitative studies that had demonstrated long delays in the time between patients developing chest pain and calling for help.[15] This question was addressed via an in-depth interview study of survivors of acute coronary events and provided considerable insight into reasons for delayed 'pain to needle time'.[4] The findings from this qualitative study prompted further quantitative research – for example, a survey that explored the association between age, gender and other variables and length of delay in heart attack patients[16] and another similar study of delayed presentation in stroke patients.[17] Taken together, these studies on delays in accessing health care had a profound influence on healthcare organisation and policy both nationally

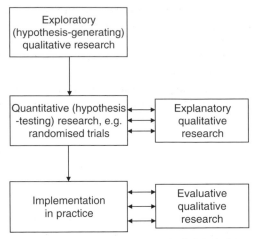

Figure 3.2 The place of qualitative research in mixed-method clinical trials.

and locally – including guideline development, organisational changes such as an extended out of hours telephone service, inclusion of brief advice on practice leaflets and education programmes for high-risk patients and their relatives. What the qualitative study on why patients delay seeking help when they have chest pain did not (and could not) answer was the quantitative question 'What is the chance that a person with chest pain will delay seeking help for more than four hours?' This, of course, requires a quantitative study (see Section 3.3).

In qualitative research, serious bias (i.e. distortion of findings or their interpretation) can occur when researchers do not critically examine their own perspective and the influence that they themselves might have had on the results. An example of this is the doctor or nurse researcher who asks a sample of patients what they think about conventional and alternative forms of hormone replacement therapy, but who does not sufficiently consider that their own position as an authority figure in conventional medicine might prejudice the interviewees' responses.

Qualitative research fits well within the interpretive approach to knowledge, in which the main goal is a search for meaning and understanding, but it is also used in research studies that take a more logico-scientific perspective, where the goal is establishing causality (see Table 2.2, page 47), as shown in the example of 'explanatory' research in Figure 3.2.

3.3   Quantitative research

Quantitative research in healthcare is almost always undertaken within a logico-scientific paradigm (see Section 2.7 and especially Table 2.2, page 47). All (or almost all) questions in quantitative research can be expressed in the general format 'What is the chance that ...' or 'What proportion of ...' – and hence can be answered by numerical measurements. Quantitative research is the cornerstone of epidemiology (see Section 8.1) – one of the key underpinning disciplines of primary care. As a rule of thumb, all epidemiological research addresses one of five types of question, and each of these questions has a preferred research design.

• *Prevalence questions* take the general format 'What proportion of the population suffers from disease X?' The prevalence of diabetes in the UK is about 2% – in other words, 2 in every 100 people are known to have the disease. The research method of choice for answering this sort of question is a simple counting exercise – or, to use its formal scientific name, a *cross-sectional survey*. Section 7.1 presents data on family structure that are based on the most ubiquitous cross-sectional surveys of all – the General Household Survey of England and Wales ('the Census'), which all citizens are asked to complete every 10 years. Section 9.1 describes how data from the same survey were used to generate the Index of Multiple Deprivation – an aggregate estimate of disadvantage. Note also that questionnaire studies, covered in Section 3.4, are also a form of cross-sectional survey – but instead of measuring what proportion of people have a disease, the questionnaire survey measures what proportion holds a particular attitude or opinion. The cross-sectional survey design is shown in Figure 3.3.

• *Incidence questions* take the general format 'What is the chance that a person will develop disease X in time period T?' Whereas prevalence expresses the total number of cases per unit of population, incidence measures the number of *new* cases over a given time period (usually per year). The incidence of multiple sclerosis in the UK is 4 per 100,000 – in other words, (on average) in a population

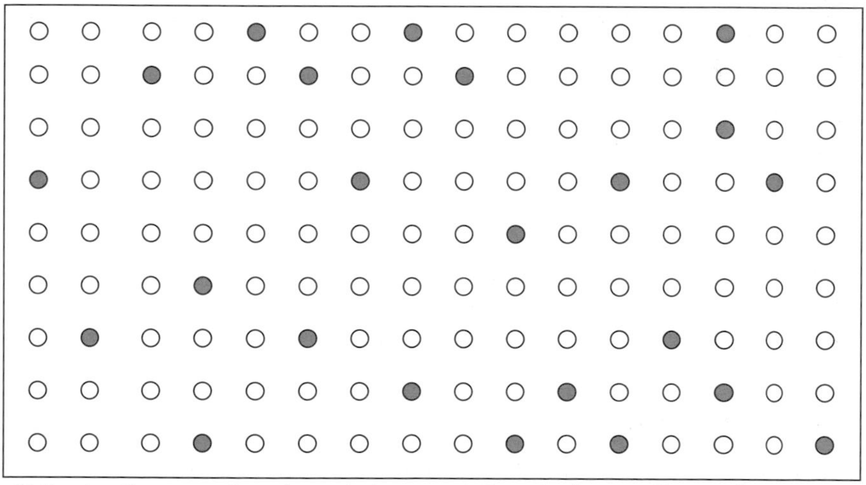

Estimates the proportion of people in a population who have a disease (prevalence study) or who hold a particular opinion (questionnaire survey)

Figure 3.3 Basic design for a cross-sectional survey.

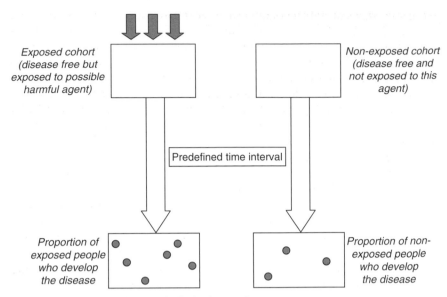

Figure 3.4 Basic design for a longitudinal cohort study.

of 100,000, 4 people will develop the condition over the next 12 months. The preferred research method for incidence questions is a careful follow-up of a population for a given period of time (i.e. a *longitudinal survey*), using validated diagnostic methods and criteria to pick up new cases. Section 8.3 describes a longitudinal survey that followed women up to find the outcome of different screening tests for Down syndrome. The longitudinal cohort design is shown in Figure 3.4.

• *Prognosis questions* take the general format 'What proportion of people with disease X will develop outcome Y over time period T?' For example, if a young woman develops breast cancer, her first question to the doctor (or perhaps the breast cancer support nurse) might be 'What is my chance of survival?'. The doctor or nurse cannot tell her her individual survival time (which is why patients have usually misunderstood their clinician when they say 'I've been given five years to live'). But epidemiology allows us to give patients' information on prognosis such as 'If 100 people with the same disease as you were left untreated, 50 would still be alive in five years'. Indeed, cancer prognosis is generally expressed in terms of 5-year survival (5YS), except in poor prognosis tumours when it is expressed in terms of 1-year survival (1YS). The research method of choice for prognosis questions is again a longitudinal survey – but this time our focus is not on the whole population (any of whom might develop a new disease) but on a group of individuals who already have a particular disease at a particular stage in its natural history – a group known as an *inception cohort*. Prognosis studies inform (indeed, are the basis of) the clinical prediction rules described in Section 5.2.

• *Harm questions* take the general format 'What proportion of people exposed to risk factor R will develop unwanted outcome O?' Risk factor R might be a drug, a vaccine, an environmental pollutant (including cigarettes), a be-haviour choice (e.g. riding a motorcycle), a surgical operation – indeed any-thing that might lead to an adverse outcome. The research method of choice for harm questions is often a longitudinal cohort study – of which post-marketing surveillance (i.e. keeping careful records of all patients prescribed a particular drug within 3 years of its release onto the market) is a good example. Thus, for example, patients in the USA taking the new parathyroid hormone ana-logue teriparatide, recently licensed for the treatment of severe osteoporosis, are routinely placed on a register and their doctors sent regular questionnaires to monitor any health problems. So far, not a single one of the 350,000 patients on this register has developed bone cancer (a theoretical risk from a drug that aggressively promotes bone growth).[18] Another useful method for exploring the link between exposure and harm is a case-control study, in which peo-ple who have developed an unwanted condition (e.g. autism) are carefully matched with people who have not, and these 'cases' and 'controls' carefully studied to compare their past exposure (or not) to the putative harmful agent. Parents contemplating the triple measles, mumps and rubella (MMR) vaccine for their child, for example, may ask 'What is the chance that my child will develop autism as a result of this jab?' – to which we can now say confidently 'No greater than their chance of developing autism if they do not have the jab' (see Section 8.2 for a full discussion of this example). The case-control design is shown in Figure 3.5.

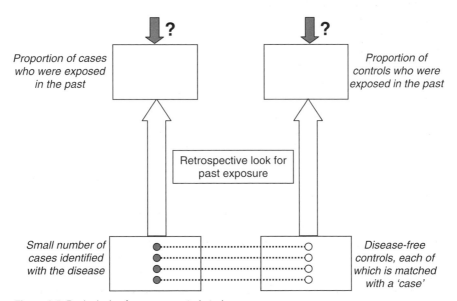

Figure 3.5 Basic design for a case-control study.

• *Therapy questions* take the general format 'what proportion of people with disease X and treated with treatment [e.g. drug or operation] Y will develop outcome O, compared with the proportion who get outcome O on no treatment [or on treatment Z]?' The comparison group is very important for therapy questions. Ninety-nine percent of children with mild sore throat who are given penicillin will be cured within 9 days, but a similar proportion will be cured on no treatment! The research method of choice for therapy questions is the randomised controlled trial, in which eligible participants are allocated randomly to either the intervention or the control group, so that (in theory at least) we start the trial with two groups who differ only in terms of the intervention being studied. Randomised controlled trials have traditionally been the province of secondary care (patients lying in their beds are more easily recruited and randomised than those in the community), but there is now a growing evidence base from high-quality randomised trials (and systematic reviews of such trials – see Section 3.8) that helps us address the bread-and-butter questions of primary health care such as whether (and in what circumstances) to give antibiotics for sore throats, what wound dressing to use for leg ulcers and so on. Rather than reference specific trials as examples, I strongly encourage you to check out the Cochrane Controlled Trials Register on http://www.nelh.nhs.uk/cochrane. The randomised controlled trial design is shown in Figure 3.6.

A particular form of prevalence study is the validation of a diagnostic or screening test, in which a new (perhaps cheaper, safer or more acceptable) test is compared with a recognised gold standard. Every participant in the

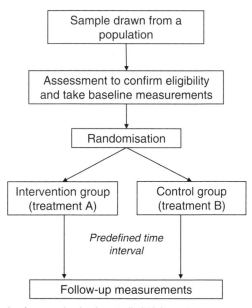

Figure 3.6 Basic design for a randomised controlled trial.

Table 3.2 Format for a 2 × 2 matrix for validation of a diagnostic or screening test.

		Result of gold standard test	
		Disease positive **a + c**	Disease negative **b + d**
Result of screening test	Test positive **a + b**	True positive a	False positive b
	c + d Test negative	c False negative	d True negative

Sensitivity = a/(a + c); specificity = d/(b + d); positive predictive value = a/(a + b); negative predictive value = d/(c + d) (see Section 3.3 for explanation of these terms).

study is offered both tests, and using a 2 × 2 matrix (Tables 3.2 and 3.3), the proportion of true and false positive results can be calculated. In the example shown in Table 3.3, the Helisal saliva test performs well but not outstandingly: it has a sensitivity of 88% (i.e. successfully picks up this proportion of people with *Helicobacter pylori*); a specificity of 70% (i.e. successfully excludes this proportion of people without the condition); a positive predictive value of 75% (i.e. if the test is positive the person has this chance of actually having the condition); and a negative predictive value of 85% (i.e. if the test is negative the person has this chance of not having the condition). In Section 8.3, I will discuss some more examples of how epidemiology can be used to screen pre-symptomatic people for disease.

It is important not to conflate quantitative research with the limited range of designs and techniques used in epidemiology. Whilst these are the main ones of relevance to clinicians, there are many other types of research that use quantitative data and many other ways of collecting and analysing such data. For example, social network analysis (see Section 9.2) is essentially a quantitative technique, as is the mathematical modelling that informs much economic analysis these days, and questionnaire research (see below) spans both qualitative and quantitative fields.

Table 3.3 Validation study for 'Helisal' saliva test for detecting *Helicobacter pylori* infection against established gold standard.[19]

		Result of gold standard test*	
		Disease positive	Disease negative
Result of screening test 'Helisal' saliva	Test positive	True positive 120	False positive 41
	Test negative	17 False negative	96 True negative

*Combination of three existing tests including urea breath test.

3.4   Questionnaire research

I learnt most of what I know about questionnaire research from my colleague Dr Petra Boynton, and I strongly recommend her series in the *British Medical Journal*.[20–22] Questionnaires are often thought of as an 'objective' means of collecting information about people's knowledge, beliefs, attitudes and behaviour (see Table 2.2, page 47). Are our patients satisfied with the care they receive? What is the quality of life of men with prostate cancer like? What proportion of the population would describe themselves as homosexual? Why don't doctors use guidelines? Of course, questionnaire research is only as useful and meaningful as the questions asked and the manner in which they are posed. Questionnaires may be used as the sole research instrument (e.g. in a survey) and are also increasingly used in mixed-method research – for example, to supplement data in randomised trials.

Inexperienced researchers may decide to use a questionnaire to answer a research question that is better suited to a different research design. Table 3.4 gives some real examples based on papers that have appeared in the published[26] and unpublished literature.

There are two essential ways to go about conducting a questionnaire survey:
• *Use an off-the-peg instrument*. The term 'instrument' in this context just means 'questionnaire', but it implies that the questionnaire has been formally developed and validated for its psychometric properties (e.g. what is the spread of responses in a particular population; are the responses normally or evenly distributed; do they represent the full range of possible answers; and so on). An off-the-peg instrument is greatly preferable both because it will save work and because the findings from any new study can be compared with the findings of previously published studies in similar or contrasting populations. Before selecting an off-the-peg instrument, you must identify what information you seek to gain from the study. For example, a clinician might be interested in studying the impact of an exercise programme on quality of life in cardiac rehabilitation patients – but a 'generic' quality of life measure such as the Medical Outcome Survey Short Form (universally referred to as the SF-36),[27] is likely to generate much less useful information than a quality of life measure specifically developed for people with cardiac disease.[28] See Section 11.1 for more on measuring quality of life in the healthcare context.
• *Develop a new instrument*. If no appropriate questionnaire is available in the literature, your first task (after identifying precisely what information you seek) is to explore the range of possible responses – e.g. by a qualitative study such as a series of semi-structured interviews, perhaps supplemented by an off-the-peg instrument that covers a closely related area of enquiry. From these exploratory data, you may develop a list of questionnaire items and pilot them on a representative sample of participants so you can calculate its psychometric properties.

Two important terms used when discussing questionnaire research are 'validity' and 'reliability'. A valid questionnaire measures what it claims to

Table 3.4 Examples of research questions for which a questionnaire may not be the most appropriate design.

Broad area of research	Example of research questions	Why is a questionnaire NOT the most appropriate method?	What method(s) should be used instead?
Burden of disease	What is the prevalence of asthma in schoolchildren?	A child may have asthma but the parent does not know it; a parent may think incorrectly that their child has asthma; or they may withhold information that is perceived as stigmatizing	Cross-sectional survey using standardised diagnostic criteria and/or systematic analysis of medical records
Professional behaviour	How do general practitioners manage low back pain?	What doctors say they do is not the same as what they actually do, especially when they think their practice is being judged by others[23]	Direct observation or video recording of consultations; use of simulated patients; systematic analysis of medical records
Health-related lifestyle	What proportion of people in smoking cessation studies quit successfully?	The proportion of true quitters is less than the proportion who say they have quit.[24] A similar pattern is seen in studies of dietary choices, exercise and other lifestyle factors[25]	'Gold standard' diagnostic test (in this example, urinary cotinine)
Needs assessment in 'special needs' groups	What are the unmet needs of refugees and asylum seekers for health and social care services?	A questionnaire is likely to reflect the preconceptions of researchers (e.g. it may take existing services and/or the needs of more 'visible' groups as its starting point), and fail to tap into important areas of need	Range of exploratory qualitative methods designed to build up a 'rich picture' of the problem – e.g. semi-structured interviews of users, health professionals and the voluntary sector; focus groups; and in-depth studies of critical events

Reproduced with permission from *Boynton and Greenhalgh*.[20]

measure. In reality, many fail to do this. For example, a self-completion questionnaire that seeks to measure people's food intake may be invalid, since in reality it measures what they say they have eaten, not what they have actually eaten.[29] Similarly, questionnaires asking GPs how they manage particular clinical conditions have been shown to differ significantly from actual clinical practice.[23] An instrument developed in a different time, country or cultural context may not be a valid measure in the group being studied.[22]

A reliable questionnaire yields consistent results from repeated samples and different researchers over time. Differences in the results obtained from a reliable questionnaire come from differences between participants, and not from inconsistencies in how the questions (known as 'items') are understood or how different observers interpret the responses. A standardised questionnaire is one that is written and administered in a strictly set manner, so all participants are asked precisely the same questions in an identical format and responses recorded in a uniform manner. Standardising a measure increases its reliability. Just because a questionnaire has been published in a peer-reviewed journal does not mean it is either valid (i.e. a good way to get the information the researchers were seeking) or reliable (i.e. that all participants answered consistently and all researchers interpreted responses in the same way). The detailed techniques for achieving validity, reliability and standardisation in questionnaire research are covered in specialist texts on the subject.[30,31]

Questionnaire research is often (wrongly) viewed as qualitative research. In fact, questionnaires may include closed items (e.g. 'tick on of the following five boxes to indicate how you feel') or open-ended ones (which invite free text responses). The former counts as quantitative research since it produces findings of the general format 'X percent of people strongly agree with the statement . . . ', whereas the latter counts as qualitative research since any meaningful analysis must involve the use of interpretive methods. See Section 4.3 for a topical discussion of a famous questionnaire – Prochaska and DiClemente's stages of change instrument which seeks to detect how much a person wants to give up smoking (or any other bad habit).

3.5 Participatory ('action') research

Action research has been defined by the British educationalists Carr and Kemmis as:

> 'A form of self reflexive enquiry undertaken by the participants in social situations in order to improve the rationality and justice of (a) their own social or educational practices; (b) their understanding of these practices; and (c) the situations in which these practices are carried out'.[32]

This definition of action research places it firmly in the territory of professional development and links with Schon's work on the reflective practitioner (see Section 11.4).[33] But an alternative definition, produced by researchers in the USA where action research had been closely linked to traditions of citizen and community action, is somewhat more politically loaded:

> 'the systematic collection of information that is designed to bring about social change'.[34]

Both these definitions place action research very firmly in the right hand column of Table 2.2 (page 47) – i.e. within an interpretive rather than a logicodeductive philosophical tradition.

Both the above definitions of action research embrace a tension between two competing commitments – to find some transferable (if not entirely

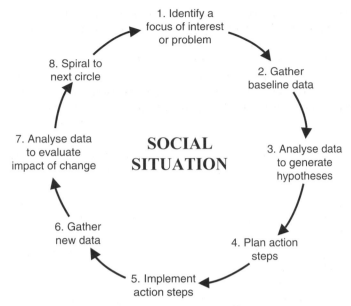

Figure 3.7 The action research cycle (adapted from Somekh[35]).

generalisable) truths through empirical research *and* to help individuals and communities find pragmatic solutions for local problems. The defining feature of action research, as shown in Figure 3.7, is a cycle (or more accurately, a spiral) in which the group systematically defines a problem, collects data to illuminate that problem, plans and undertakes an action and measures the impact of that action. The best way to develop an understanding of how action research is undertaken in practice is to read a worked example – see, for example, Ann Macaulay's diabetes prevention work with indigenous ethnic groups in Canada, described briefly in Section 9.5.

Because action research is *both* research *and* action, good action research must fulfil the criteria for good research outlined on page 50–60 and must also measure up on more pragmatic and local criteria (e.g. is it acceptable to the community, does it align with other key priorities and so on). The question of validity in action research is complex and beyond the scope of this introductory textbook but has been explored in detail by others.[36] The principles of action research are summarised in Box 3.4.

3.6 Research data – and analysing it

One of the key defining characteristics of research is the presence of a rigorous, consistent and – usually – reproducible approach to the collection and analysis of data. It is clearly important to identify which data to collect and how. As we

---

Box 3.4 Principles of action research.[36,37]

1 Action research has three key elements: partnership with the research participants; a developmental emphasis; and a commitment to both social science (theory) and social change (implementation in practice).
2 It has dual roots – in professional education and reflective practice, and in movements for social justice. It is particularly suited to exploring and meeting the needs of deprived, disempowered and marginalized groups.
3 The strength of action research is its ability to influence the particular situation being researched while simultaneously generating data that are applicable to a wider audience.
4 Action research should be judged not merely by the success of the local project but by the lessons learnt and their transferability to future research and wider service policy. There may be a tension between developing valid, generalisable knowledge and addressing local needs.

---

shall see in the examples in the chapters that follow, not all researchers manage to achieve this. In quantitative research, the research team must decide at the outset of the study what to count (or otherwise quantify) and what instruments to use to take the measurements. In qualitative research, the research team must decide whose experiences, opinions, attitudes or perspectives to tap into, and what form (tape-recorded accounts, written 'free text' responses to questions, pictures, real-world action) is most appropriate to capture those things.

Data analysis is an aspect of research where the novice often gets stuck – and it is also the aspect where the experienced researcher can add most value. To put it another way, one of the key differences between a novice and an expert researcher is in the quality of the analysis they can provide. So what is 'analysis' in this context?

The online dictionary Encarta offers a number of definitions of the verb 'analyse', including *'to study closely – i.e. to examine something in great detail in order to understand it better or discover more about it'* and *'to find out what something is made up of by identifying its constituent parts'*. I prefer the first of these definitions since the latter is somewhat reductionist – that is, it implies that we can understand something better by cutting it up into smaller parts, studying the parts, and then adding up our findings to understand the whole. That is sometimes true – but sometimes the understanding of the whole is greater than the sum of the parts and is best achieved by studying the whole!

The decision on what data to collect and how the analysis of data will be undertaken is part of the research design in any research project. In other words, the researchers' plan for how they will analyse their data should be set out in the *methods* section of the research proposal (and summarised in the methods section of the paper). This analysis section should, in general, address five questions:

1 What is the research question?
2 What data are needed, and at what level should they be collected (individual, group, population, etc.)?
3 What is the unit of analysis?
4 What is the method of analysis?
5 What degree of abstraction will the analysis aim for?

In order to explain these terms, let's consider a research project that aims to determine the impact of an educational programme intended to increase the number of GPs and practice nurses who follow evidence-based guidelines for diabetes care. Let us assume that the research team has developed an educational intervention to be delivered as a half-day course in the practice where the GPs and nurses work. Half the practices (the intervention group) will be randomised to receiving this package plus the diabetes guidelines, and half (the control group) will just get the guidelines.

The *research question* is, of course, what the researchers are trying to find out. It will provide insight into the focus of the study. For example, in the above scenario the research question might be (A) 'Do clinicians who receive education on evidence-based guidelines change their behaviour?' or it might be (B) 'Do the patients of such clinicians have better health outcomes?' or (C) 'Is a GP practice where staff have been trained in evidence-based guidelines more of a learning organisation [see Section 11.6]?' The focus of research in these three cases is different. In question (A), the focus is clinical behaviour (such as the recording and actioning of clinical data); in (B), it is patient outcomes (such as control of blood pressure or blood glucose levels); and in (C), it is practice culture.

The *data collected* in a research study might be at the level of gene (or genetic make-up), the cell, the organ, the individual, the group or team, the organisation (e.g. the GP practice) or the institution (e.g. the National Health Service). In the above examples, questions (A) and (B) require data collected at the level of the individual (the clinician and the patient, respectively). Question (C), which addresses the practice, considers, for example, whether it is the kind of practice where evidence-based decisions are promoted and supported, where staff are rewarded for making evidence-based decisions and where there is a training budget for developing staff in this area? Such questions will probably require many different types of data collected at individual, group, team and organisational level. Note that when the chosen level of analysis shifts from the individual to the organisation, the type of data (and how it is analysed) will also shift.

Note also that there is no universal 'best' type of data or level of analysis – the best data set for any piece of research is the one that is most appropriate to address the research question, given the focus chosen by the researchers. One of my biggest bugbears about the human genome project is the assumption that an analysis at the level of a person's genetic make-up will answer all the questions in health care! It will answer many important questions – but there are many other questions for which a different level of analysis is needed.

As we shall see in some of the examples in this book (see Section 9.3 for example), it is perfectly legitimate to collect and analyse data at more than one level – and indeed, complex phenomena are often best analysed in a multi-level framework. Incidentally, it is no accident that I have divided the remainder of this book primarily according to the main level of analysis of the research presented. I hope this will emphasise that different levels of analysis provide different (and complementary rather than contradictory) insights into primary care problems.

The *unit of analysis* is the key entity that you collect and analyse data *on*. If, when writing up research findings, the researcher writes 'we analysed a total of X things' – the unit of analysis is 'the thing'. In question (A) in the above example, a reasonable unit of analysis will be the individual clinician ('X% of clinicians who received the educational intervention subsequently followed the guideline'). In question (B), because patients generally attend more than one clinician for their diabetes care, the most appropriate unit of analysis is probably the practice ('X% of patients in practices who received the intervention had good diabetic control, compared to Y% of patients in control practices'). In question (C), the unit of analysis is also the practice. The choice of unit of analysis must be made at the time of designing the study since this will have important implications for the research design (in the above example, the unit of randomisation will be the practice, not the individual clinician, for example), and this in turn will have implications for sample size. Incidentally, another possible unit of analysis for this study could be the clinical decision (in X% of clinical encounters for diabetes, guidelines were followed).

Questions (B) and (C) above illustrate the principle that data generated at one level in a research study can inform an analysis at a different level. In question (B), for example, individual patient data on diabetes control can contribute to the analysis of the performance of the practice in controlling diabetes in its practice population. In question (C), individual semi-structured interviews with clinicians, field notes from observation of team meetings and aggregated data from patient satisfaction questionnaires can also contribute to a case study of practice culture.

A typical unit of analysis for a qualitative study might be the individual semi-structured interview. But other units of analysis might be appropriate – for example, if the qualitative study was collecting stories about clinical incidents, the unit of analysis might be the story. If one interviewee told three stories during the course of a single interview, each of these would be analysed as a separate unit. Other units of analysis in qualitative research include the interpersonal interaction, the social situation, the referral, the handover and so on.

The *method of analysis* is the technique used by the researchers to analyse their data. Poor quantitative research is often characterised by indiscriminate lists of figures without rigorous statistical analysis (as in '25% of patients got better'). It is almost always the case that quantitative data do not stand on their own, but need to be analysed using the appropriate statistical test (see Martin Bland's book for an excellent introduction to this[38]). At the very least, differences between two samples – before and after an intervention, or between an intervention group and a control group – must be shown to be both clinically significant (i.e. big enough to mean something to the patient) and statistically significant (i.e. big enough so that it is unlikely that the difference arose by chance). But 'statistically significant' findings *might* have arisen by chance, especially in small studies, and a study in which this has happened is more likely to have been written up and published, so 'significant' findings still need to be interpreted in context. Just as different statistical techniques are appropriate for different types of quantitative data, so there are different methods of qualitative analysis that are more or less appropriate for different qualitative data. The detail of how to analyse qualitative data is beyond the scope of this book, but I strongly recommend Cathy Pope and colleagues' introductory article on this topic.[39]

Figure 3.8 illustrates the final key dimension to be considered in data analysis, particularly qualitative analysis – the degree of abstraction involved. Qualitative data are virtually worthless if all the researcher has done is listed 'themes' (as in 'participants interviewed in this study talked about the following six things … ') or cherry-picked a few interesting quotes. One very useful approach to qualitative data analysis in healthcare research is thematic content analysis.[41] In this technique, the researcher reads the texts (interview transcripts, field notes and so on) and assigns preliminary *descriptive categories* (e.g. 'comments

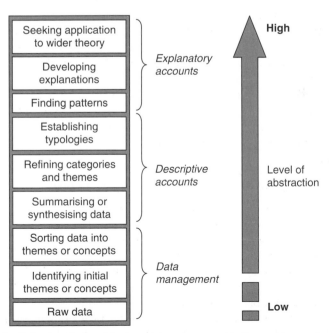

Figure 3.8 Analysis of qualitative data: from data management to theory-driven explanations. (Adapted from Ritchie and Lewis[40]).

on the physical surroundings of the clinic', 'comments on what the doctor said to them', 'comments on how they felt about the diagnosis'). After this first coding has been completed, researchers discuss amongst themselves and refer to relevant literature to develop some preliminary *theoretical categories* based on a pre-existing (or, more rarely, newly developed) explanatory model of what is happening. Typical theoretical categories might be, for example, 'patient centredness' (see Section 6.5) 'stage of change' (see Section 4.3), 'self-efficacy' (see Section 2.8), 'transference' (see Section 6.3) and so on. These preliminary theoretical categories are typically refined through discussion amongst the research team and/or by presenting the preliminary analysis to the people who provided the data (e.g. patients). For more on thematic analysis, see the excellent book on qualitative research by Green and Thorogood.[41]

Another common (and generally very respectable) method for analysing qualitative data is the 'framework' approach. This has considerable overlap with thematic analysis (some would say it can be thought of as an optional stage within thematic analysis, though not all researchers are agreed on this). Its particular characteristic is the use of a matrix (e.g. an Excel spreadsheet) to help sort out the data and compare themes across different units. Down the rows of the matrix are listed the units (e.g. 'Participant 1', 'Participant 2', etc., or 'Focus Group 1', 'Focus Group 2', etc.). Along the columns are listed the main emerging themes (e.g. 'comments on what the doctor said'). The framework approach, developed by Ritchie and Spencer, is often used by people who are new to qualitative research, who find it provides a helpful structure and starting point for 'taming' a vast and amorphous set of data.[42] But of course, a framework analysis is only as good as the themes and categories allocated to the columns and the researchers' ability to interpret the text appropriately within these themes and categories. In the end, there is always an element of interpretation in any qualitative analysis which takes the researcher from simply making an observation ('he stood up, leaned over and spoke loudly to her') to assigning a *meaning* to the observation ('he was trying to intimidate her') – and therein lies the challenge of qualitative data analysis. For more on this topic, and certainly if you plan to undertake a qualitative study yourself, I once again recommend Green and Thorogood's textbook.[41]

3.7 Critical appraisal of published research papers

As I have emphasised already, this is not a book on how to do critical appraisal (I have written a different book on that[2]). This section is intended to outline the very basics of how to approach any published paper describing research relevant to primary health care.

Critical appraisal means reading a research paper carefully, using a structured checklist to help address two key questions:
• Can I trust this paper?
• Is it relevant to the question I need to answer and the patient(s) I plan to treat?

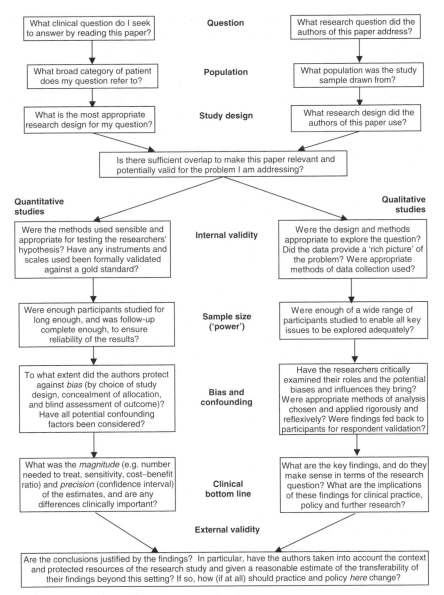

Figure 3.9 Flowchart for critical appraisal of a research paper.

Figure 3.9 presents a flowchart for evaluating the quality and relevance of published studies. This chart can be applied to both quantitative and qualitative papers, since the underlying question sequence is similar (though it is not so relevant to action research). For both types of research, the two main issues that determine whether a published paper is trustworthy are bias and internal validity.

Bias can be defined as '*any factor arising from the design and conduct of a study that skews the data in one particular direction, either away from or towards the "true" value that is being estimated*'. Examples of bias in quantitative research include selection bias (e.g. when sicker participants are allocated to active treatment and less sick ones to placebo); observer bias (when an assessor knows that a participant had the 'real' procedure or active drug and subconsciously assesses improvement as greater than it really is); withdrawal bias (when a high proportion of participants withdraw from study before it is completed, especially if they differ systematically from those who continue); measurement bias (caused by systematic errors in instruments used to assess outcomes); and publication bias (authors and editors keener to publish 'positive' results). One of the commonest forms of bias is confounding, or 'left out variable bias' in which the relationship between two measured variables (such as smoking and heart disease) is mediated via a third, unmeasured variable (such as social class).

In qualitative research, the term 'bias' is not generally used but it is widely recognised that the identity and background of the researcher, the selection of the sample, the context of the interview or other data collection and the selection of theoretical perspective to drive the analysis will all have a bearing on the findings. A different interviewer, seeking the same information but in a different context and from participants recruited in different circumstances, will find something different. There is no way of eliminating such influences since there is never a 'view from nowhere', but both researchers and the readers of published research must take account of these influences when they interpret the findings. Terms like 'researcher influence' or 'study context' often give a clue to how the findings may have been influenced.

Internal validity is the relevance of the actual measures used – either equipment (e.g. sphygmomanometers), questionnaire scales (e.g. the SF-36 as a measure of overall health status[43]), or the various techniques adopted by the qualitative researcher to develop a 'rich picture' of a problem – to the aspects of health or illness that the researchers claimed they wanted to measure. Poor internal validity arises when the measurements used do not accurately measure (or are irrelevant to) the outcomes and exposures of interest. One of the most widely cited examples of poor internal validity is the gap between what GPs *say* they do and what they *actually* do in clinical practice – which means that sending GPs a questionnaire asking how they treat condition X is not a *valid* way of establishing what goes on.[44]

External validity is another term for relevance. The findings of a study undertaken in another country, another region or even a general practice down the road may not be directly transferable to one's own practice. Figures for the prevalence of teenage pregnancy, or insights about why teenagers do not attend family planning clinics, in Epsom (an affluent middle class UK town with a stable, mainly white population) may not be transferable to Hackney (an inner London district with a highly mobile population and diverse ethnicity).

Much of the remainder of this book comprises worked examples of clinical and organisational issues in primary care in which I present my own critical appraisal of key research evidence. A more detailed discussion of bias, confounding and validity, as well as a full set of critical appraisal checklists can be found in specialised EBM textbooks.[2,45]

3.8 Systematic review

I have covered systematic review in detail elsewhere[2]; in this brief section I will do no more than introduce the principle. A systematic review is an overview and summary of primary studies (i.e. of papers reporting the kind of empirical research described in Sections 3.2–3.6) that has two key characteristics: (a) it contains a statement of objectives and methods; and (b) it has been conducted according to an explicit, transparent and reproducible method. In other words, a systematic review is an essay about a topic area in which the author has been systematic about what to include and how to assess the value and relevance of each study.

The most widely cited, and, for many research questions, the best quality systematic reviews have been undertaken according to the strict protocols of the International Cochrane Collaboration, a community of scholars committed to producing a database of summaries of biomedical research and focusing predominantly (though not exclusively) on meta-analyses (statistical summaries) of randomised controlled trials.[46] The mainstream Cochrane Collaboration takes an explicitly logico-deductive perspective on the nature of knowledge (see Section 2.7 and Table 2.2, page 47), defining quality in terms of objectivity and political neutrality of the researcher, the volume and robustness of quantitative data, the use of deductive methods to arrive at summary statistics and conclusions, the accuracy and precision of measures (such as the 'point estimate of effect' and the confidence interval surrounding it in a meta-analysis – see Figure 3.10) and the generalisability of the findings. There are fringe groupings within the Cochrane community who deviate from this general approach, but let's not muddy the waters too much. The Cochrane library (see http://www.cochrane.org/) is a superb resource of up-to-date summaries of quantitative research, including close on half a million clinical trials and around 5000 systematic reviews.

If you are interested in doing a Cochrane review yourself, you should first go on a course to learn the skills of focusing and refining your research question, searching electronic databases, critical appraisal of research papers (see Section 3.7) and the use of statistical software packages to produce the mathematical estimates illustrated in Figure 3.10. In the figure, studies A, B and C are all small or medium-sized randomised controlled trials which, although they favour the intervention, have produced estimates of impact that cross the line of no effect (i.e. they are compatible with the conclusion that there is no difference between intervention and control). The meta-analysis produces a

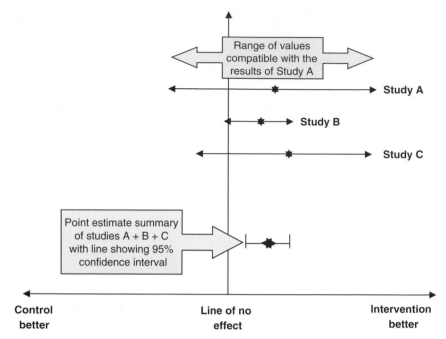

Figure 3.10 Diagrammatic representation of a meta-analysis.

statistical summary of the findings from all three trials with a narrower confidence interval that shows clear benefit from the intervention.

Cochrane reviews, and in particular meta-analyses of randomised controlled trials, have transformed knowledge management in healthcare.[47] The Cochrane library is almost always the best place to start, for example, if you are looking to summarise the evidence of effectiveness of treatment for a particular condition. But the Cochrane approach has its limitations if your goal is not to produce an objective and generalisable summary of quantitative evidence on a focused clinical question but to illuminate a complex topic area and summarise what are often disparate and heterogeneous qualitative studies, all of which have looked at the problem in a slightly different way.

Whilst the Cochrane Collaboration does have a qualitative methods group, there is also considerable work being done by other academic teams to develop methods for summarising and synthesising qualitative research that align with an interpretive perspective on knowledge (see Table 2.2, page 47) – i.e. which aim to achieve interpretation and understanding of an issue rather than accurate measurement of an effect of an intervention, and which are more concerned with informing specific local decisions than producing findings that are widely generalisable. Given that any text can generate multiple interpretations, it is inherent to interpretive synthesis that its outputs are not as precise and reproducible as the synthesis of quantitative data, and this may be no bad thing. If you would like to explore qualitative (and mixed qualitative and quantitative) systematic review further, see the paper by Nick Mays' team on combining evidence for management and policymaking[48]; my own team's work on meta-narrative review[49]; and Ray Pawson's realist review.[50] Mary Dixon-Woods has summarised a number of other methods in an excellent article.[51] All these approaches have more similarities than differences, in that they see systematic review as an interpretive (and fundamentally inductive) exercise rather than (purely) an exercise in measurement and deduction.

It is not always the case that a paper calling itself a systematic review is more reliable and rigorous than a paper describing a single empirical study. Flaws occur in systematic review just as they do in any research. In this book, I have drawn on systematic reviews in a number of places, including Section 4.3 on lifestyle choices, Section 4.4 on self-management of chronic illness, Section 5.2 when I discuss clinical decision tools and Section 5.5 when I consider intervention studies to encourage clinicians to follow guidelines.

3.9 Multi-level approaches to primary care problems

Having spent a substantial fraction of this book so far persuading you to be clear about the underpinning discipline and underlying theory which you are using to explain your observations or inform the design of an intervention, and about your research method and unit and level of analysis (see Section 3.7), I am now going to offer you examples of approaches that incorporate multiple theories and which also require multiple methods, multiple units of analysis and multiple levels of analysis. As a primary care practitioner, you are probably already well aware that a typical problem in your clinical practice might be addressed on a number of levels, and that the most effective intervention is likely to address more than one level. Multi-level theories are becoming very popular in epidemiological research following the failure of simple interventions in research studies. Here, I briefly introduce one multi-level theory to illustrate the power of the approach: Stokols' social ecology theory.

Social ecology theory, which has been widely used in studies of health promotion in primary care, was developed by (among others) David Stokols.[52] The term 'ecology' refers to '*the study of the relationship between organisms and their environments*'.[52] The theory includes an emphasis on biological processes, physical health, geographical space, psychological aspects of behaviour choices, individual identity and the wider social, institutional and cultural contexts of people–environment relations. It has close parallels with general systems theory and complexity theory, both of which use 'ecological' metaphors to describe the dynamic interrelationship of multiple variables at multiple levels (and the need for empirical and analytic methods that can embrace this complexity).

According to Stokols, social ecology theory is built on four principles:

• *Multiple facets:* multiple aspects of the individual (such as genetic predisposition and psychological traits), the physical environment (such as geography, architecture and technology) and the social environment (such as social networks) interact dynamically to produce an overall effect on individual behaviour. Examples of such multiple dimensions include physical health status, emotional well-being, social cohesion, development maturation. Human experience and behaviour in the real world cannot be meaningfully studied in terms of any one of these influences alone.

• *Multiple dimensions:* Environments may be characterised in terms of a number of dimensions such as: (a) physical and social features, (b) objective (actual) or subjective (perceived) qualities of these and (c) scale or immediacy to individuals and groups. Emotional well-being, for example, may be influenced not just by the physical aspects of people's environment but also by the perceived predictability, controllability, novelty and symbolic values of this environment.

• *Interdependence:* People influence their environment, which in turn influences the people who live there. The key to understanding transactions between people and their environments is grasping the recurrent (and often complex) cycles of mutual influence that occur.

• *Non-linearity*: Using a concept from general systems theory, the social ecological system contains multiple (positive and negative) feedback loops, which means that sometimes, small things can have big effects and vice versa. The effectiveness of an intervention directed at the health of a community can be increased substantially through the coordination of individuals and groups acting at different levels. Because of this, social ecological research generally requires diverse methods and multiple levels of analysis.

An important principle of social ecology theory, known as differential dynamic interplay, is that environmental factors may affect different people differently depending on such factors as personality, health practices, perceptions of the controllability of the environment and financial resources. Stokols proposed that the level of *congruence* (or compatibility) between people and their surroundings is an important predictor of well-being.

Because of its explicit inclusion of multiple perspectives (psychology, sociology, social geography, social epidemiology), social ecology theory is inherently interdisciplinary and requires the integration of multiple levels of intervention and analysis (e.g. 'macro' level preventive strategies at the level of fiscal policy and public health, as well as 'micro' level individual interventions in primary care). The approach is, as might be expected, methodologically diverse, including epidemiological surveys, environmental recordings, physical examinations, questionnaires and behavioural observations. In Section 8.4.3, I describe an adaptation of social ecology theory – Glass and McAtee's 'stream of causation' theory – in relation to a discussion on the social determinants of health. In Section 5.4, I discuss another important multi-level theory, Engel's biopsychosocial model of illness, which underpins the patient centred clinical method.

References

1 Bell J. *Doing Your Research Project*. Buckingham: Open University Press; 1999.

2 Greenhalgh T. *How to Read a Paper: The Basics of Evidence Based Medicine*. 3rd edn. Oxford: Blackwells; 2006.

3 Kai J. What worries parents when their preschool children are acutely ill, and why: a qualitative study. BMJ 1996;313:983–986.

4 Ruston A, Clayton J, Calnan M. Patients' action during their cardiac event: qualitative study exploring differences and modifiable factors. BMJ 1998;316:1060–1064.

5 Kavanagh AM, Broom DH. Women's understanding of abnormal cervical smear test results: a qualitative interview study. BMJ 1997;314:1388–1391.

6 Butler CC, Pill R, Stott NC. Qualitative study of patients' perceptions of doctors' advice to quit smoking: implications for opportunistic health promotion. BMJ 1998;316:1878–1881.

7 Shaw S, Boynton PM, Greenhalgh T. Research governance: where did it come from, what does it mean? J R Soc Med 2005;98:496–502.

8 Shaw S, Barrett G. Research governance: regulating risk and reducing harm? J R Soc Med 2006;99:14–19.

9 Slowther A, Boynton P, Shaw S. Research governance: ethical issues. J R Soc Med 2006;99:65–72.

10 Department of Health. *Research Governance Framework for Health and Social Care*. London: Her Majesty's Stationery Office; 2002.

11 Sackett DL, Haynes RB, Guyatt GH, Tugwell P. *Clinical Epidemiology: A Basic Science for Clinical Medicine*. Boston: Little Brown & Company; 1991.

12 Weinbren H, Gill P. Have I got epilepsy or has it got me? Narratives of children with epilepsy. In: Greenhalgh T, Hurwitz B, eds. *Narrative Based Medicine: Dialogue and Discourse in Clinical Practice*. London: BMJ Books; 1998.

13 Denzin M, Lincoln P. *Sage Handbook of Qualitative Research*. 3rd edn. London: Sage; 2005.

14 Dopson S, Fitzgerald L. *Knowledge to Action? Evidence-based Health Care in Context*. Oxford: Oxford University Press; 2005.

15 Heriot AG, Brecker SJ, Coltart DJ. Delay in presentation after myocardial infarction. J R Soc Med 1993;86:642–644.

16 Sheifer SE, Rathore SS, Gersh BJ, et al. Time to presentation with acute myocardial infarction in the elderly: associations with race, sex, and socioeconomic characteristics. Circulation 2000;102:1651–1656.

17 Williams JE, Rosamond WD, Morris DL. Stroke symptom attribution and time to emergency department arrival: the delay in accessing stroke healthcare study. Acad Emerg Med 2000;7:93–96.

18 Gold DT, Pantos BS, Masica DN, Misurski DA, Marcus R. Initial experience with teriparatide in the United States. Curr Med Res Opin 2006;22:703–708.

19 Reilly TG, Poxon V, Sanders DS, Elliott TS, Walt RP. Comparison of serum, salivary, and rapid whole blood diagnostic tests for *Helicobacter pylori* and their validation against endoscopy based tests. Gut 1997;40:454–458.

20 Boynton PM, Greenhalgh T. A hands-on guide to questionnaire research part one: selecting, designing, and developing your questionnaire. BMJ 2004;328:1312–1315.

21 Boynton PM. A hands-on guide to questionnaire research part two: administering, analysing, and reporting your questionnaire. BMJ 2004;328:1372–1375.

22 Boynton PM, Wood GW, Greenhalgh T. A hands-on guide to questionnaire research part three: reaching beyond the white middle classes. BMJ 2004;328:1433–1436.

23 Adams AS, Soumerai SB, Lomas J, Ross-Degnan D. Evidence of self-report bias in assessing adherence to guidelines. Int J Qual Health Care 1999;11(3):187–192.

24 Gariti P, Alterman AI, Ehrman R, Mulvaney FD, O'Brien CP. Detecting smoking following smoking cessation treatment. Drug Alcohol Depend 2002;65:191–196.

25 Little P, Margetts B. Dietary and exercise assessment in general practice. Fam Pract 1996;13:477–482.

26 Gillam B. *Developing a Questionnaire: Real World Research Series.* London and New York: Continuum; 2000.

27 McHorney CA, Ware JE, Jr, Raczek AE. The MOS 36-Item Short-Form Health Survey (SF-36): II: psychometric and clinical tests of validity in measuring physical and mental health constructs. Med Care 1993;31:247–263.

28 Hofer S, nelli-Monti M, Berger T, Hintringer F, Oldridge N, Benzer W. Psychometric properties of an established heart disease specific health-related quality of life questionnaire for pacemaker patients. Qual Life Res 2005;14:1937–1942.

29 Drenowski A. Diet image: a new perspective on the food-frequency questionnaire. Nutr Rev 2001;59:370–372.

30 Oppenheim AN. *Questionnaire Design, Interviewing and Attitude Measurement.* London and New York: Continuum; 1992.

31 Sapsford R. *Survey research.* London and New Delhi: Sage and Thosand Oaks; 1999.

32 Carr W, Kemmis S. *Becoming Critical: Education, Knowledge and Action Research.* Lewes: Falmer Press; 1986.

33 Schon D. *The Reflective Practitioner.* New York: Basic Books; 1983.

34 Bogden R, Biklen SK. *Qualitative Research For Education.* Boston: Allyn and Bacon; 1992.

35 Somekh B. Action research and collaborative school development. In: McBride R, ed. *The Inservice Training of Teachers: Some Issues and Perspectives.* Brighton: Falmer Press; 1989.

36 Waterman H, Tillen D, Dickson R, de koning K. Action research: a systematic review and guidance for assessment. Health Technol Assess 2001;5(23):3–157.

37 Meyer J. Using qualitative methods in health related action research. BMJ 2000;320: 178–181.

38 Bland JM. *An Introduction to Medical Statistics.* 3rd edn. Oxford: Oxford Medical Publications; 2000.

39 Pope C, Ziebland S, Mays N. Analysing qualitative data. BMJ 2000;320:114–116.

40 Ritchie J, Lewis J. *Qualitative Research Practice.* London: Sage; 2003.

41 Green J, Thorogood N. *Qualitative Methods for Health Research.* London: Sage; 2004.

42 Ritchie A, Spencer L. Qualitative data analysis for applied policy research. In: Bryman A, Burgess RG, eds. *Analyzing Qualitative Data.* London: Routledge; 2001.

43 Anderson RT, Aaronson NK, Bullinger M, McBee WL. A review of the progress towards developing health-related quality-of-life instruments for international clinical studies and outcomes research. Pharmacoeconomics 1996;10:336–355.

44 Eccles M, Ford GA, Duggan S, Steen N. Are postal questionnaire surveys of reported activity valid? An exploration using general practitioner management of hypertension in older people. Br J Gen Pract 1999;49:35–38.

45 Crombie I. *The Pocket Guide to Critical Appraisal.* London: BMJ Publications; 1996.

46 Alderson P, Green S, Higgins JPT. *Cochrane Reviewers' Handbook 4.2.6.* Chichester: John Wiley & Sons Ltd.; 2006.

47 Grimshaw J. So what has the Cochrane Collaboration ever done for us? A report card on the first 10 years. CMAJ 2004;171:747–749.

48 Mays N, Pope C, Popay J. Systematically reviewing qualitative and quantitative evidence to inform management and policy-making in the health field. J Health Serv Res Policy 2005;10(suppl 1):6–20.

49 Greenhalgh T, Robert G, Macfarlane F, Bate P, Kyriakidou O, Peacock R. Storylines of research in diffusion of innovation: a meta-narrative approach to systematic review. Soc Sci Med 2005;61:417–430.

50 Pawson R, Greenhalgh T, Harvey G, Walshe K. Realist review – a new method of systematic review designed for complex policy interventions. J Health Serv Res Policy 2005;10 (suppl 1):21–34.

51 Dixon-Woods M, Agarwal S, Young B, Jones D, Sutton A. *Integrative Approaches to Qualitative and Quantitative Evidence*. London: Health Development Agency; 2004.

52 Stokols D. Translating social ecological theory into guidelines for community health promotion. Am J Health Promot 1996;10:282–293.

CHAPTER 4

The person who is ill

Summary points

1 This chapter uses examples of five topics relating to individual illness and health-related behaviour to illustrate how an academic perspective can illuminate the problem and suggest possible ways of addressing it.

2 The sick role is a sociological concept about what an ill person is expected to do and what society is expected to do for them. Parsons' widely cited theory of the sick role, developed in the 1950s and based on a passive patient and paternalistic doctor, has been replaced by more contemporary theories that emphasise the need for the chronically sick to play an active part in society and for society to make efforts to accept them.

3 The illness narrative is a concept derived from literary theory in which an individual constructs a story with characters (heroes, villains, passive bystanders), trouble (the illness) and a particular plot (restitution, quest, chaos). The choice of literary devices (comedy, irony, metaphor and so on) can provide insights into the narrator's perception of what has caused the illness and what is needed to resolve, manage or cope with it.

4 People's health-related behaviour choices (diet, smoking, drug use, exercise and so on) may be considered using one of a number of psychological theories such as the stages of change theory or the theory of reasoned action. These theories, which assume rational and reasonably stable beliefs and attitudes, have been used extensively in the design and testing of interventions to help patients make healthy lifestyle choices. They have also been extensively criticised.

5 'Self-management' is a popular concept that is currently driving health policy in the UK and North America towards a more active role of patients in managing their own chronic illness. But the pragmatic term 'self-management' raises more academic questions about the meaning of the terms 'self' and 'management'. The extensive research literature is inconsistent in how these terms are defined and used, which has led to a large, heterogeneous and somewhat confusing array of clinical trials in this area. A theory-driven approach can help disentangle this literature and draw some conclusions for practice.

6 Low health literacy limits the ability of many individuals to participate actively in their own health care. Because of this, strategies based on information, empowerment and promotion of self-care are likely to have a differential impact on the articulate and well-educated middle classes than on disadvantaged

(Continued)

(*Summary points continued*)

> and socially excluded groups. Health literacy is generally researched as a biomedical notion of the ability to gain and use knowledge, but a more radical framing that includes 'critical consciousness' offers additional avenues for future research.

4.1 The sick role

This chapter is not intended to tell you everything you need to know about the person who is ill. In this chapter, as in all the remaining chapters in this book, I have selected a particular level of analysis (in this chapter, the individual) and offered various worked examples (such as 'self-management', 'understanding risk' and 'behaviour change') to illustrate how an academic perspective (see Section 1.2) and the judicious application of the concepts and theories represented in different disciplines (the 'ologies' – see Chapter 2) can enrich our understanding of primary care problems and suggest practical solutions. Because of the breadth of topics covered in this book, I have been unable to consider all possible themes that might have a bearing on the study of the person who is ill, for which you will have to consult the many other books and papers available on this topic. Note also that it is inherent to the nature of primary care problems that they are multifaceted and could legitimately be viewed through a number of different theoretical lenses. The perspectives on the individual set out below, and the perspectives on other levels of analysis set out in the chapters that follow, are not the only (or necessarily the most appropriate) ones for any particular problem. But they will, I hope, set you thinking.

Strictly speaking, the title of this chapter should be 'The person who is ill, believes themselves to be ill, or might become ill'. As any medical student knows, disease is defined as the formal, 'objective' diagnosis assigned by a doctor or other health professional, whereas illness is the subjective experience of being unwell and the associated change in social role. This section considers the individual who is (or is behaving) 'ill', and how the meaning of 'being ill' has changed as both society and the nature of disease have changed over time.

British sociologist Talcott Parsons developed his classic theory of the sick role (summarised in Table 4.1) in the 1950s.[1] In this theory, which has been widely cited and is still taught in British schools, doctors and patients were seen to exist in an 'exchange' relationship. The patients were excused from social duties (work, family obligations) and exempt from some self-care tasks; they were required to put their trust in professionals and relinquish an element of self-determination. The doctor, in turn, provided a professional level of care, assured confidentiality and was accorded high social status. A less well-known element of Parsons' work (published later and after criticism of his early work) was a revised concept of the sick role for chronic conditions,

Table 4.1 The sick role as originally proposed by Talcott Parsons.[1]

Patient		Doctor	
Social obligations	*Rights*	*Social obligations*	*Rights*
Want to get well Seek and follow medical advice Regarded as in need of professional care and unable to get well solely by his or her own decisions and will	Allowed to (and may be expected to) shed normal activities and responsibilities (employment, household tasks)	Be highly trained, technically competent and skilful Apply specialist knowledge and skill to the problems of illness (including legitimating a person's claim to the sick role) Act for welfare of patient and community rather than for self-interest, desire for money, advancement etc. Be objective and emotionally detached (e.g. should not judge patients' behaviour in terms of own value system or become emotionally involved with them) Be guided by rules of professional practice	May examine patients physically and enquire into intimate areas of physical and personal life Granted considerable autonomy in professional practice Occupies position of authority in relation to the patient

in which continuing to function socially and economically was an important aspect of the 'sick' person's identity and in which the person often developed considerable expertise in his or her condition.[2]

Subsequent sociologists have introduced a number of modifications to Parsons' original sick role to reflect new social roles and expectations (e.g. people often live very active lives with chronic illness, and a 'civilised' society is now expected to accommodate the sick or disabled individual). One notion, derived from symbolic interactionism (see Section 4.4), is the concept of 'self' developed by Erving Goffman.[3] Goffman reframed the notion of 'the self' from something internal to the individual to something that is actively presented and enacted to the external world, especially in our interactions with other people. The way we dress, our body language, our gestures and expressions, our leisure activities, the books we read and so on are all chosen partly to fit in with the sort of person we want others to believe we are – and, in presenting ourselves in a particular way, we become that person. Goffman used the term 'body idiom' to denote the sum total of artefacts and actions by which others may classify, label and judge us. The presentation of the self is a continuous and dynamic process that occurs in all our public (and private) interactions. It plays a crucial role in creating, maintaining and developing our identity.

Table 4.2 Trajectory model of chronic illness.

PHASE 1: Pre-trajectory	Before onset of symptoms: opportunity for prevention
PHASE 2: Onset (crisis)	Appearance of first symptoms and formal diagnosis of chronic illness poses a threat to social identity
PHASE 3: Acute	Onset may precipitate a period of illness that requires active intervention to control disease progression and prevent complications – often in an inpatient setting
PHASE 4: Stable	If interventions effective, a period of stability follows, requiring varying degrees of intervention to maintain individual health – usually in an outpatient setting
PHASE 5: Unstable	A series of challenges to recovery eventually ensues, which each requires reappraisal and adaptation of interventions to promote coping and stability
PHASE 6: Downward	Responses to challenges to recovery become increasingly unsuccessful
PHASE 7: Dying	Patient's condition becomes terminal

Adapted from Strauss[8] and Woog.[9]

Illness can be seen as interfering with this effort to 'present' the self, because physical or mental imperfections will (to a greater or lesser extent, depending on social norms and prejudices) classify the individual as 'spoiled'. Goffman's book *Stigma: Notes on the Management of Spoiled Identity*, published in 1963, is one of the all-time classic textbooks of medical sociology.[4] It exhibits the enduring characteristics of a good theory in that it can be applied to contemporary diseases such as AIDS[5] or chronic fatigue syndrome[6] as well as to those (such as epilepsy) for which Goffman originally developed it.[4,7]

Related to the notion of the 'spoiled self' is the idea of chronic illness as biography – that is an integral part of the life story. In the 1970s, Strauss developed a 'trajectory' theory of chronic illness (what we might today call 'the illness journey'), summarised in Table 4.2.* He emphasised the social as well as medical elements of chronic illness, including family stress, role disruption, economic loss and stigmatisation.[8] Along with Corbin, Strauss extended his theory in the 1980s to identify three lines of 'work' which the sick

---

*See also Figure 10.1, page 249, which is the model of chronic disease used in contemporary approaches to chronic disease management. Note the important difference in Strauss's original theory: the trajectory of *illness* (a sociological construct that emphasises the sick role and how the person is accepted and looked after by society) rather than the course of chronic *disease* (a biomedical construct that emphasises the progression of pathological processes and deterioration of the body), though of course each of these constructs embraces an element of the other.

person was faced with: 'illness work' (symptom control, crisis management, medication management), 'everyday life work' (employment, housework, childcare) and 'biographical work' (reconstruction of personal identity) – about which more in the next section.[10]

Michael Bury linked Parsons' concept of the sick role to that of the unfolding illness biography. He undertook studies of arthritis patients and identified three critical dimensions of what had previously been called the sick role: (a) *coping* with the effects of the illness and maintaining a sense of self-worth, (b) *strategy* (the actions taken to mitigate the effects of the illness) and (c) *style* (the way a person responds to the illness and treatment regimen – e.g. by social withdrawal).[11,12] All these dimensions are negotiated and shaped with reference to the family, friends, health professionals and others, but (as Bury and many others demonstrated, and as I explore in Chapter 7) the family is an especially important influence.

These classic theories of the sick role, stigma and illness biography underpin some important contemporary models of primary health care – notably the work on self-management of chronic disease, which is discussed in detail in Section 4.4.

4.2   The illness narrative

Arthur Frank, a professor of sociology who has written movingly about his own serious illnesses,[13] has suggested that literary theory (see Section 2.6) is a key lens through which to analyse patients' accounts of illness. Illness, he suggests, is an enacted story with characters, a plot and 'trouble'. He divides illness narratives into four broad genres:
• *Restitution* (the doctor-hero accurately diagnoses and treats the illness and/or the patient-hero successfully navigates a complex system of care to achieve the desired cure);
• *Tragedy* (the doctor-hero does his or her best but the patient nevertheless succumbs – or, perhaps, the patient-hero struggles unsuccessfully to survive and be heard in the face of medical incompetence or insensitivity);
• *Quest* (the patient-hero embarks on a journey to find meaning and purpose in his or her incurable illness);
• *Chaos* (the story is incoherent, unsatisfying and does not make sense).[13]

The transcript of the consultation in Box 4.1 (which is adapted from a real encounter with 'fictionalised' health problems to protect confidentiality)[14] includes a moving narrative by this elderly gentleman about the death of his son. I will not go into details about the clinical aspects of this consultation, but the wider life narrative is especially powerful. My patient's recounting of his painful story in the privacy of the consulting room, in a voice that was barely above a whisper, fits Aristotle's famous definition of tragedy: 'An action that is serious, complete, and of a certain magnitude; in language embellished with artistic ornament. [. . .] with incidents arousing pity and fear, wherewith to accomplish catharsis of the emotions'.[15]

Box 4.1 A GP–patient consultation.

TG   Hi, do come in Mr Brown.
[he enters slowly, and takes time to sit himself down]

JB   *[remains silent]*

TG   Chronic bronchitis check, isn't it? How've you been?

JB   Mmm

TG   *[there is silence for a while, while GP scrolls down the computer template for asthma check]*
Ah, Sandra's done most things and entered all the data. Looks like she's done all the checks and I just have to listen to your chest. Your peak flow rate's not too bad this time – that's a measure of your lung function. Need to keep a close eye on that. Symptoms – still coughing sputum most days. That's a pity. Blood tests last month fine. Those tablets aren't doing you any harm. Smoking. You're still smoking?

JB   I've told her and I'll tell you. I'm gonna live a short life and a happy one.

TG   Okay. I won't get onto you if that's how you feel. But you do know what it does to your lungs?

JB   You said my lungs were OK.

TG   I said they weren't too bad – but they could be a lot better. And smoking's also bad for your heart and your blood vessels. It makes you three times more likely to have a thrombosis. If you give up smoking your circulation will improve within 72 hours because once the poison is out of your body the blood will flow more freely.

JB   So you said last time.

TG   That's what I'm paid for. To nag you. The point is if your lungs get compromised much more, you may end up living a short unhappy life rather than a short happy one.

JB   *[does not react to this. GP notices that he is not engaging in their usual banter, and makes eye contact, raising her eyebrows as if asking if he's OK]*
Sorry, doc.

TG   I've got to examine your chest. You know you're on a monthly recall all through the winter for this.

JB   *[raising his shirt slowly and rather wearily]*
Go on then, doc.

TG   In and out, nice and deep.
[records on computer]
OK. It's not much worse than last time. Will you tell me if you change your mind about the smoking?

JB   Yeah

TG   How's the wife?

JB   Bad

TG   Her legs again?

JB   No

TG	What then? Just life?
JB	*[silence]*
TG	*[waits]*
	Go on.
JB	We lost a son.
TG	*[surprised]*
	Oh dear. I'm very sorry to hear that. What happened?
JB	*[pulling his chair close in to the doctor's desk, allowing him to talk in a low voice]*
	I did come in about it. But there was a locum. A locum in a hurry. You know.
TG	*[consulting paper record]*
	27th June. Dr McNair. He's normally very good. He looked in your ear.
JB	There was nothing wrong with my ear.
TG	So he said in the notes.
	[both laugh ironically]
JB	That was three days after it happened [...]
TG	Go on.
JB	The wife hasn't been out since.
TG	I'm not surprised. How old was he?
JB	43
TG	Same age as me.
JB	A good age.
TG	Mmm. What did he do?
JB	Graphic something or other. Had his own flat in Chelsea. Nice flat.
TG	Did he have a family?
JB	No, just the dog. But it was lucky he had the dog [...]
TG	Go on.
JB	He'd had this pain. Polyp or something, they told him. At least that was what the wife said it was.
TG	What symptoms did he have?
JB	Bellyache, awful bellyache. Spent a long time on the toilet. Came out black sometimes and he was too weak to get himself back to bed.
TG	Good grief. Why didn't he go to the doctor?
JB	*[wearily]*
	You tell me. Anyway, he wakes up one day and he's messed himself, and he's real weak and everything, and he can't get up to phone. And you know, that dog got out of the window in the kitchen, and he ran down the street to my son's friend's house, and he barked his head off until the friend came back with him, and the friend broke the door down, and by then my son was out for the count, but still breathing like, and the friend called the ambulance and they shipped him off, blue light and all, but when they got there he was already dead. They put him straight in the mortuary. [...]
	[looks at the doctor and they make eye contact for several seconds]

TG   *[remains silent, thinking there is probably more to come]*
JB   *[after a long pause]*
      He was just in like an old T-shirt. A ripped one. With some picture of a band on it, that he didn't even like any more. He'd had it years. And it was all blood and that on it.
TG   Mmm?
JB   And I'd got this suit like. Too small for me. The wife wanted to give it to Oxfam but I'd had this feeling for years I should keep it. Really good quality. Saville Row. Nice dark grey, with like a fleck in it. And a nice shirt and a tie to go with it. I'd kept them all on a hanger, with the tie rolled up in the pocket. All ironed and everything. And when I'd identified him, I came back straight away like, and I got this suit and the tie and all, and I took it back there and they put it on him. Now wasn't that lucky?
TG   Lucky you'd kept the suit?
JB   Yeah. It was a good suit. Probably the best I've ever had. No, definitely the best.
TG   Show your respects.
JB   Exactly. And lucky about the dog, being able to get out.
TG   Very lucky. So tell me about your wife.
JB   Nothing to say. She's at home.
      [He pushes his chair back, and makes to put on his jacket]
TG   Do you want me to visit?
JB   No.
TG   Or bring her in?
JB   Maybe.
TG   I need to check your chest again in about a month.
JB   Yeah, OK. I'll come in for that.
TG   Will you bring her?
JB   If she'll come.
TG   And I'll lay off nagging you about the smoking for a bit.
JB   Doesn't bother me doc. You got to do your job. Water off a duck's back.
TG   If you want to see me sooner you come in. OK?
JB   No, I'll be fine. See you after Christmas.

The patient, as far as I know, had had no training in literary theory, but he managed to engender a lot of emotion in his listener (me) – partly because the nature of what happened is inherently tragic, but also because of the way he told the story. The heroic efforts of the dog, for example, are used in this story as a literary trope to represent that someone cared and tried to help; something was done; the young man did not die abandoned. The presence of the dog is described, with heavy irony, as 'lucky' (a description that I am asked to affirm), presumably because the patient subconsciously seeks to achieve a level of moral order in the story. The efforts of the dog are symbolic of the efforts my patient would have made himself had he only known he was needed.

I have, somewhat unusually, chosen a narrative of an acute illness (death from a bleeding colonic polyp, told from the perspective of a grieving father) as an example of how a literary perspective may add value in studying how people cope with illness in themselves and their relatives. More usually, it is chronic illness that is studied using the tools of narrative analysis. Cancer, for example, is often presented as a personal tragedy that throws a family into a reluctant but unstoppable drama. When a patient or carer tells the story of cancer, the various relatives, friends, nurses, doctors and informal carers inevitably become characters in the drama – such as heroes, villains, clowns or bystanders. Acts or omissions of individuals (or the system, or the gods) may be presented (implicitly or explicitly, and justifiably or otherwise) as having 'caused' a particular turn in the story. The person cannot change the situation, but at least he or she can account for what has happened and key individuals can be depicted as virtuous (brave, selfless, devoted) and as following the expected social norms and conventions (e.g. the doctor demonstrated skill and judgement; the family pulled together).

I have written a separate monograph on how narrative analysis can inform and enrich the practice of medicine.[16] My own interest in narrative lies mainly with the medical management of physical illness and the ill person's use of narrative in coping with conditions such as cancer, diabetes, depression and other chronic conditions. Others, notably John Launer, have taken a more psychodynamic perspective on the application of narrative theory to illness – especially the use of narrative-based family therapy in the care of complex distress in primary care.[17]

4.3   Lifestyle choices and 'changing behaviour'

A few years ago, I was involved in a small project to identify the priorities of doctors, nurses and people with diabetes for diabetes research. We held a number of focus groups. In their groups, the doctors identified behaviour change as one of their top priorities. So did the people with diabetes. The difference was that in the view of doctors, it was patients' behaviour that needed to change (e.g. giving up smoking, taking more exercise, losing weight), whereas the people with diabetes felt that it was doctors' behaviour that should change (e.g. talking less, listening more, explaining better)! The nurses in the focus groups, incidentally, felt that the biggest research priority was improving communication all round. The other insight I gained from listening to the people with diabetes was just how offensive they found the expression 'behaviour change'! They felt patronised, stereotyped and misunderstood – especially in relation to complex lifestyle phenomena such as how to lose weight. Since that experience, I tend to avoid the term 'changing behaviour' because it has connotations of Pavolvian dogs being induced to jump through hoops and ignores the fact that 'behaviour' may be embedded in social and political structures that cannot be readily changed (see Section 8.5).

Here's an example: Wazim Maziak, writing in the British Medical Journal about the appallingly high prevalence of obesity (70%) and diabetes (24%) in the Arab world, says,

> 'Solutions for such health problems cannot necessarily be imported. For example, advocating diet and physical activity to combat the epidemic of obesity among women in Arab societies may be naïve. Overwhelmed by having to take care of large households, and deprived of basic knowledge and power to conceptualise life outside traditional frameworks, women may be unable to alter their lives'.[18]

I believe that the term 'supporting positive lifestyle choices' is generally preferable to 'changing behaviour', because it avoids victim blaming and also because it does not assume that the level of change has to be the individual (see Section 3.9). Providing women-only swimming sessions for Muslim (and other) women in local swimming pools, for example, is a different approach to supporting positive lifestyle choices. It does involve a change in the women's behaviour (more of them may now go swimming), but the problem was not the women's motivation or intention – it was the cultural appropriateness of the facilities available. Having voiced my reservations about targeting individual behaviour, let's briefly consider the academic basis of some commonly used behaviour change strategies aimed at patients. Incidentally, taking note of the patients' perspective set out in the first paragraph, I cover changing health professionals' behaviour in Section 5.4.

Prochaska and DiClemente's widely cited model of behaviour change[19] is more popularly known as the 'transtheoretical model'. I have placed the word 'transtheoretical' in quotation marks because it implies that the model transcends a number of different theoretical streams. In my own view, it can be explained largely in terms of mainstream cognitive theory (see Section 2.3). The core concepts are motivation, behaviour change (the former being seen as the key to the latter) and the sequential transition between 'stages' of motivation. According to the model, an individual faced with a behaviour change moves back and forth between five stages (Table 4.3): (a) pre-contemplative (in which they are not even considering the change), (b) contemplative (in which they are considering the change but not attempting to change), (c) preparation (in which they are getting ready to make the change), (d) action (in which they are actively making the change) and (e) maintenance (in which they are attempting to maintain the change). The model suggests different approaches to influence and support the patient depending on the stage of change, and the approaches are oriented to shift the individuals from their current stage to a higher one.

The stages of change model is used extensively by clinicians and clinical researchers to try to influence patients' success in changing their behaviour – most usually, in giving up unhealthy habits like smoking and excess drinking. The practical application of the model is that instead of giving the same health advice to everyone, this advice is tailored to the particular individual's stage of change. Thus, for example, a person who states that he or she

Table 4.3 The stages of change model and how to classify someone.

Stage	Descriptor	Defining question
Pre-contemplative	Not even thinking about changing	Have you thought about change at all in the last 6 months? [Answer: no]
Contemplative	Thinking about changing	Have you planned to change between 31 days ago and 6 months ago? [Answer: yes]
Preparation	Making plans to change	Have you planned to change in the past 30 days? [Answer: yes]
Action	Actively trying to change	Have you actually changed (even for a short time) in the past 6 months? [Answer: yes]
Maintenance	Having achieved the change, is trying to maintain it	Have you maintained the change for the past 6 months? [Answer: yes]

Summarised from Prochaska.[20]

has no intention of giving up smoking is simply informed of the dangers of smoking and told that more help is available if they change their mind; someone who admits to trying to give up is offered information on the different methods of achieving this and offered counselling, pharmacotherapy and so on.[20]

A systematic review of smoking cessation trials, which was helpfully summarised in the British Medical Journal,[21] showed that such tailored approaches work better than 'one size fits all' interventions. The stages of change model helps us understand *why* a tailored approach might be more successful, and it also guides the design of new interventions. But the model is not without controversy. Indeed, critics have described it as a fundamentally flawed model whose popularity far outweighs its credibility.[22] For one thing, claims West, the stages proposed are entirely arbitrary ('lines in the sand') which do not have a firm basis in cognitive psychology. For another, the theory behind the model assumes that individuals typically make coherent and stable plans – and thus, at any point in time a person can be confidently classified, for example, as being in the 'contemplative' stage as opposed to the 'action' stage. Empirical research, claims West, suggests the opposite – that most people's plans to quit smoking are unstable and may change on a daily basis. Finally, the stages of change model focuses on conscious, rational decision making whereas smoking (and other addictive behaviour) is often justified by recourse to non-rational explanations and hence may be relatively resistant to a rational treatment model.[23] Nevertheless, Prochaska and DiClemente's model is one of the most widely used in empirical research on patient behaviour change, so it's certainly worth knowing about.

The stages of change model was recently tested against conventional advice in a clinical trial.[24] We all know that eating several portions a day of fresh fruit and vegetables improves long-term health. But as clinicians we often feel that eating fresh food is a 'lifestyle' that some people (especially those from low-income families) choose not to follow. Clinicians are rightly cynical about dishing out lifestyle advice since it is increasingly evident that patients do not 'obey' the doctor, nurse or pharmacist – they make their own choices that may or may not be influenced by what the professionals say. This trial was a randomised design in which people from low-income groups were randomised to receive behavioural counselling based on the stages of change model or standard nutritional advice. Although both groups improved their intake of fruit and vegetables, the 'stages of change' group improved significantly more than the control group – a finding which suggests that the model has practical value, even though purists can find fault with its theoretical basis.

Another theory that primary care researchers increasingly draw upon in relation to behaviour change is the theory of reasoned action. Developed in the 1970s by Ajzen and Fishbein,[25] this theory has a number of core concepts: norms, attitudes, values and intention. The theory states that a particular behaviour is determined most immediately by the person's intention to behave in that way. Intention to behave is in turn determined by (a) subjective norms (beliefs about what behaviour is expected by significant others, and motivation to comply with these expectations); (b) attitudes towards the behaviour (based on beliefs about, and evaluation of, the likely consequences of that behaviour) and (c) the relative importance to the individual of norms versus attitudes. The theory of reasoned action was later extended to include non-voluntary behaviour (i.e. behaviour over which the individuals do not have complete control), and renamed the theory of planned behaviour.[26]

An example of how the theory of planned behaviour helps explain patients' health choices and inform primary care interventions is a study by Conner et al. on why women use dietary supplements.[27] Users of such supplements were significantly more likely to have positive attitudes about supplements, and to believe that the supplements would keep them healthy and stop them from getting ill. Takers of the supplements also believed that this behaviour was a norm (i.e. an expected and accepted behaviour) within their own social group. The implication of this theory in relation to reducing unnecessary (and potentially harmful) supplement use in certain groups includes the possibility of developing interventions to change attitudes towards as well as simply knowledge about such supplements, and of challenging prevailing norms in certain subgroups. Again, the theory is useful only to the extent that it explains the findings of research and helps us in developing new hypotheses to test. The theory of reasoned action has been used to develop targeted, theory-driven interventions aimed at reducing marijuana smoking[28] and increasing positive behaviours such as brushing teeth,[29] the use of condoms by high-risk drug addicts in sexual encounters[30] and patients' compliance with prescribed medication.[31]

Ogden has offered an incisive critique of the theory of reasoned action (and other theories in what is known as the 'social cognition' school).[32] First, such theories do not enable the generation of hypotheses because their constructs are not sufficiently specific to allow them to be tested. Second, their central tenet is often a near-circular argument (the fact that a person who intends to smoke is more likely to smoke than someone who doesn't intend to may be true – but it is true by definition, so it's not saying much!). Finally, questionnaires and other instruments designed to assess what people plan to do may influence those plans rather than being an unbiased measure of them. If you feel swayed by these arguments, you should also look up Ajzen and Fishbein's spirited response.[33] As with all theories, this one is useful for illuminating reality, but it is not a short cut to any simple truths. The quote from Maziak, earlier in this chapter, reminds us that there are other levels of intervention, and other theories about how interventions work, that may prove more fit for purpose in promoting behaviour change for positive health outcomes.

4.4 Self-management

Self-management is a popular concept in the UK and North America. Government policy in the UK seeks explicitly to promote self-management of chronic conditions from arthritis to depression by what are officially known as 'expert patients'.[34,35] The idea behind self-management (i.e. the notion that patients managing their own illness is a 'good thing') is worth studying, not merely as a contemporary policy theme in its own right, but also as an example of how a combination of different academic perspectives can help us build a rich picture of a complex and controversial subject area. This topic provides a good worked example of how systematic reviews (see Section 3.8) can provide useful summaries of a complex topic area but how such reviews often produce findings whose meaning is contested and lack an obvious 'evidence-based plan of action' for practice and policy.

Scholars from different academic disciplines have conceptualised and explained self-management differently, based largely on fundamentally different notions of the self (a 'cognitive self' capable of learning and executing a set of self-management tasks; a 'behaviourist self' whose performance in these tasks might be shaped by a system of rewards and punishments; or Goffman's 'sociological self', described in Section 4.1, who exists in a complex social context and unfolding life narrative) and of 'disease management' (e.g. obeying the doctor or building a meaningful life).

Given the diversity of academic perspectives underpinning research and practice in the field of self-management, it is not surprising that there is no universally agreed definition of the term. Some authors define it from a strictly biomedical perspective that emphasises the completion of disease-oriented tasks by the patient:

> *'active participation in self monitoring (of symptoms or disease processes), decision making (in relation to the disease or its impact), or both'.*[36]

Others take a more holistic view – for example,

> *'the individual's ability to manage the symptoms, treatment, physical and psychosocial consequences and life style changes inherent in living with a chronic condition. Efficacious self-management encompasses ability to monitor one's condition and to effect the cognitive, behavioural and emotional responses necessary to maintain a satisfactory quality of life. Thus, a dynamic and continuous process of self-regulation is established'.*[37]

The British government's perspective on self-management seems to fall midway between a narrowly biomedical view (health-enhancing 'behaviours') and a broader psychosocial one (actions to promote wellness and well-being):

> *'the actions individuals and carers take for themselves, their children, their families and others to stay fit and maintain good physical and mental health; meet social and psychological needs; prevent illness or accidents; care for minor ailments and long term conditions; and maintain health and wellbeing after an acute illness or discharge from hospital'.*[38]

In the field of epidemiology, numerous self-management programmes have been developed and tested, either in randomised controlled trials or using less robust study designs. Most such programmes are predicated to a greater or lesser extent on a biomedical model (Section 2.1) – that is, the individual receives training with a view to gaining the skills, motivation and confidence to undertake aspects of his or her medical care that were traditionally the province of health professionals, thereby gaining more control over the illness and its management, achieving greater well-being and (perhaps) freeing up public-sector health and social care services for other use. Four systematic reviews, described below, have each taken a slightly different approach to selection and analysis of empirical studies. A more recent review by the Picker Institute considers the implications for policy.[39]

Barlow and colleagues reviewed 145 trials of self-management interventions.[37] Of these, around half were randomised trials. The authors developed a provisional taxonomy based on the nature of the intervention, place (hospital, GP, home), group versus individual, disease, age of participants and so on. They commented that the interventions were highly heterogeneous in terms of the nature of the self-management intervention, with some programmes focusing on cognitive dimension (acquisition of knowledge) but others addressing skills (practical tasks) or motivational elements (confidence). Most trials had been conducted on adults with diabetes, asthma, hypertension or arthritis, delivered in groups by professionals and evaluated by physical (e.g. a blood test or examination finding) and/or psychometric (e.g. questionnaire) outcome measures. Most showed a statistically significant (but sometimes clinically marginal) impact of the self-management intervention. Overall, and contrary to prevailing policy fashion, programmes led by lay people did not appear more effective than professionally led ones. Whilst few studies had included formal measures of economic cost, group-based interventions appeared significantly cheaper.

Barlow et al.'s review identified several important methodological limitations of the primary studies (see Section 3.3): weak study design (uncontrolled before-and-after studies[†]), inadequate description of the intervention and its components, small sample size (typically 20–30 in each group), inappropriate choice of control intervention (e.g. waiting list), short follow-up (typically less than 6 months), unit of analysis errors (e.g. randomising by group but analysing data by individual) and lack of intention to treat analysis.

In another systematic review, Newman summarised 62 randomised controlled trials of self-management programmes for adults with type 2 diabetes, asthma and arthritis – published between 1997 and 2002.[40] Of these, 59 were professionally led. Again, these authors commented on the heterogeneity of the trials, the fact that many interventions were under-theorised (based, for example, on simple instructional models of change), and of variable methodological quality. Different studies had different objectives (e.g. to improve markers of progression of chronic illness, to avoid acute exacerbations, to improve daily functioning, to save money), and many failed to identify any explicit objective. They classified the different outcome measures used in the evaluation of self-management programmes:
• Clinical and laboratory assessments (e.g. blood pressure, HbA1c)
• Self-reported symptoms (e.g. pain scale)
• Self-reported functioning (e.g. activities of daily living)
• Psychological well-being (e.g. anxiety/depression scales and positive well-being scales)
• Quality of life (either generic or disease-specific: see Section 11.1)
• Behaviour (e.g. compliance with medication, exercise)
• Use of services (e.g. attendance at appointments)

The trials produced highly heterogeneous (and overall somewhat inconclusive) results. For example, of trials of self-management in diabetes in which HbA1c was measured, 61% showed 'some evidence of effectiveness at some point'. Of the arthritis trials, '40% of interventions showed some improvement in self reported symptoms'. Half the asthma studies that measured quality of life reported significant improvements with self-management training. And so on. The overwhelming majority of trials measured multiple outcomes, and there is a sense not just that publication bias has occurred but that previous editorials and commentaries (and perhaps certain policy decisions) have focused disproportionately on the 'positive' findings of primary studies.

[†]The problem with an uncontrolled before-and-after study is that all sorts of things may change between the 'before' data and the 'after' data, so any differences between the two sets of data may or may not be due to the self-management intervention.

Interestingly, Newman et al. noted numerous studies in which the putative mechanism of effect was not borne out (e.g. changes in clinical outcome measures in the absence of changes in knowledge or self-efficacy) and concluded that there is much we do not yet know about how self-management training achieves its impact. They recommended that in further research, particular approaches to self-management should be better matched with the type of disease, cultural background and learner profiles of a particular target group (e.g. adolescents or elderly).

Chodosh and colleagues published a meta-analysis of randomised controlled trials of self-management interventions in hypertension, diabetes and osteoarthritis.[36] They included 53 trials (which were heterogeneous in design) and showed a statistically significant overall impact of self-management training on the control of both diabetes and hypertension compared with 'usual care'. However, statistical tests for publication bias suggested that there may have been preferential publication of trials with positive results, so they advise interpreting the findings with caution. These authors used five specific predictions for hypothesis-driven statistical analysis:

• *Tailoring.* Patients who receive self-management interventions tailored to their specific needs and circumstances are more likely to derive benefit than those who receive generic interventions.
• *Group setting.* Group interventions (more than one patient with the same condition) are more effective than one-to-one interventions.
• *Feedback.* Patients are more likely to derive benefit if they receive a cycle of intervention followed by individual feedback on performance.
• *Psychological emphasis.* Interventions with some sort of psychological emphasis will be more efficacious than those without a psychological component.
• *Medical care.* Interventions delivered by physicians or primary care providers will be more efficacious than those delivered by other trainers.

Interestingly, whilst the above hypotheses are intuitively plausible as mechanisms for the success of self-management programmes, none was supported by the data – that is, there was no statistically significant difference between studies with and without the component. A post hoc analysis (i.e. one that was not planned at the outset) of a number of other components also failed to demonstrate conclusively that 'theory-driven' interventions work better than any other sort – but the authors comment that these interventions have a very complex mechanism of action and that many studies included insufficient detail for the theoretical mechanism to be unpacked by reviewers.

Bury and colleagues reviewed self-management programmes, focusing specifically on lay-led programmes.[41] Lay-led programmes have to some extent embraced the sociological self (rather than taking a purely behaviourist approach to teaching self-management 'tasks'). The theoretical benefits of lay-led programmes are that (a) the lived experience of illness is often far removed from the way the illness is framed (and managed) in the outpatient clinic or GP surgery; hence the lay person may be in a better position to identify and meet learning needs than the traditional medical expert and (b) social learning from peers is a particularly powerful mechanism for learning complex skills (see Section 2.8.2 which outlines Bandura's social learning theory). Bury et al. identified four key phases in lay-led self-management research:

• *Disease-specific lay-led self-management versus control group.* Many lay-led self-management programmes have been modelled on the seminal work of Kate Lorig and colleagues in the USA, whose 'landmark' randomised trial of self-management training in arthritis (Arthritis Self-Management Program or ASMP) back in 1986 had three arms: professional tutors, lay tutors and no training (control). Whereas professionally trained participants had the greatest increase in knowledge, lay-trained participants practised the self-management exercises (in this case, relaxation) more and reported greater reduction in disability. There were also significant cost savings in this group (presumably because the lay trainers were paid less than the professionals!).[42] Lorig et al. subsequently replicated this work on larger numbers of patients and used formal measures of self-efficacy and well-being, both of which increased in patients randomised to the lay-led training despite deterioration in the severity of their arthritis. The work was also replicated in a large UK study of 544 participants, in which the ASMP arm showed significantly better improvements in depression scores and quality of life (Euroqol) compared to waiting list controls.[43]

• *Disease-specific lay-led self-management versus 'personalised' package.* Lorig et al. recently published a randomised trial of their lay-led ASMP programme against a personalised package of advice (known as SMART – Self-Management Arthritis Relief Therapy) generated from the persons' medical record and mailed to them in the post.[44] The SMART intervention was tailored to the specific demographics, diagnosis, medication, self-efficacy and other personal characteristics of the participant. When compared with a control intervention, SMART led to greater self-efficacy, improved role function and lower disability scores at 1 year and 2 years, but not at 3 years. When compared with the lay-led ASMP, SMART led to improved disease severity at 1 year, but not at 2 or 3 years. These findings challenged the notion of some special 'essence' of lay-led training (e.g. the peer as a more credible or influential educator than the professional, or the crucial role of social modelling in learning self-management skills) and suggested that in arthritis at least, a personalised advice sheet might produce equivalent outcomes at lower cost. The fact that there seems little to choose between lay-led and personalised interventions may be because those who volunteer for such a trial may already be self-selecting for determination to self manage their condition effectively!

• *Generic lay-led self-management programmes.* Lorig and her colleagues worked with the US Health Maintenance Organisation Kaiser Permanente in the 1990s to develop a generic programme (Chronic Disease Self-Management Program or CDSMP).[45] The assumptions behind this programme were that (a) patients with different chronic diseases have similar self-management problems and disease-related tasks; (b) patients can (and, implicitly, should) learn to take responsibility for the day-to-day management of their disease(s) and (c) confident, knowledgeable patients practising self-management will use fewer healthcare resources. In the first trial, over 1000 patients (with heart disease, lung disease, stroke or arthritis) were randomised. Each CDSMP comprised 2.5 hours a week for 7 weeks and was delivered by two lay volunteer trainers (though in fact 23% of these described their job as 'health professional'). Overall, the CDSMP significantly improved 11 of 15 outcome variables compared to waiting list controls, though (curiously) psychological well-being did not improve. A 2-year follow-up of this programme suggested that many of the benefits were not sustained, though overall health status remained higher, and use of healthcare services lower, than the control group; and disability scores were actually higher in the intervention group at 1 year.[46]

• *'Hybrid' programmes (professionally supported, lay-delivered).* Many so-called lay-led self-management programmes are actually professionally supported and driven, but include lay people as peer educators. These are sometimes known as 'guided self-management'. The role of professionals in such programmes is ambiguous and variable, and no firm conclusions have been reached about their overall place in the range of self-management training options.[47]

Bury et al.'s review describes some 20 studies throughout the world of lay-led self-management programmes, many of which have broadly confirmed Lorig et al.'s findings – that such programmes are relatively low-cost, they improve self-efficacy and some intermediate clinical outcomes, but they do not dramatically alter the level of disability, they also describe additional studies which demonstrated no significant difference between lay-led and professionally led programmes except in terms of cost.[41] Bury et al.'s review also includes a large and well-designed study from the UK of generic chronic disease self-management programmes which had a much smaller impact on patients than the levels demonstrated in US studies by Lorig and colleagues, though some positive impact on clinical outcomes and self-efficacy was seen.[47]

In conclusion, there is currently a veritable industry of clinical trials of complex interventions to promote self-management. These were initially dominated by doctor – and nurse-led programmes predicated (implicitly if not explicitly) on a cognitive self which could be trained to complete biomedical tasks, thereby saving the professionals' time. More recently, lay-led programmes designed around a more sociological self living an active life in wider society and have delivered a broader programme of training oriented to this wider agenda – but these have not proved consistently better (or worse) than professionally led programmes. Clinical trials in this complex area have sometimes (though not always) been poorly designed, and insufficient detail is given in the papers to assess how the programme achieved (or failed to achieve) its intended outcomes. Psychological benefits (such as reduced anxiety or improved self-efficacy) are commonly seen in these programmes; physical benefits (such as reduced pain or improved mobility) are less consistently shown. Systematic reviews suggest that the selective publication of positive trials may explain part or all of the apparent benefit of self-management training on clinical outcomes.

4.5   Health literacy

Whilst (as discussed in the previous section) self-management is currently all the rage in policy circles, and published trials of 'empowering' interventions generally report positive findings, there is an alternative perspective to consider. Approaches that place so much responsibility on the patient are themselves inherently geared towards individuals who are educated, resourceful, capable and confident in whatever aspect of involvement is being promoted. I recently heard (verbally and 'off the record', so please interpret what I say in that context) that nurses in charge of implementing DESMOND,[48] a major diabetes self-management education programme in a deprived area of London, were asking clinics to 'send us the more intelligent people as we know it works better in those'.[‡]

There is no direct evidence of 'intelligence' being linked to the efficacy of the psychometrically robust and rigorously implemented DESMOND programme, but that is probably because no study has yet addressed that specific question. There is substantial evidence that both level of education and specific health literacy are highly correlated with getting diabetes in the first place and the control and outcome of diabetes once diagnosed.[51–55] There are certainly very plausible reasons why limited cognitive ability would attenuate the impact of a classroom-based education programme oriented towards the acquisition of facts and complex skills. In these days of patient-centred care and expert patients it is not very politically correct to suggest that many patients are not (and probably never will be) experts in anything, least of all in their own illness. This unsurprising fact is ignored by most policymakers and many academics, though a new literature is beginning to emerge – perhaps partly as a 'paradigm shift' research tradition following the disappointing impact of many self-management programmes outside the research setting. Let's take a look at this literature.

A US review found that 50% of all American adults have such limited literacy that they struggle to complete many daily tasks such as reading signs, filling out forms or following transport schedules.[56] An official report estimated that 20% of adults in the UK had 'severe problems' with basic literacy.[57] Formal tests of functional health literacy (see below) such as the TOFHLA (Test of Functional Health Literacy in Adults) and REALM (Rapid Estimate of Adult Literacy in Medicine) correlate closely with healthy lifestyle choices, compliance with medication, overall cost of health care, length of stay in hospital and outcome in a wide range of conditions from asthma to HIV.[56,58–61] The poor, the elderly and those with mental health problems are more likely to have limited health literacy.[56,58,62,63] Numerous epidemiological studies have identified low health literacy as the missing intervening variable linking education and health

---

[‡] What clinicians 'know' is, of course, very different from what has been demonstrated in clinical trials (see Section 5.3).[49,50]

outcome (and in some studies, socio-economic status and health outcome) in diabetes, cardiovascular disease, sexual health and HIV.[51–53,56,64,65] Many (and in some studies, all) ethnic differences in health outcome are explained by differences in health literacy.[52,55,59,66]

What exactly is health literacy? The World Health Organisation (www. who.org) defines it as

'the cognitive and social skills which determine the motivation and ability of individuals to gain access to, understand and use information in ways which promote and maintain good health'.

Caroline Spero has taken the concept apart and identified a number of key attributes including reading and numeracy in relation to health information, the capacity to use health information and the ability to 'perform in the patient role'.[61] These in turn rest on wider literacy and numeracy skills as well as health-related experience – the latter of which achieves two things: exposure to the medical vernacular and building the relevant cognitive schemas within which new health information makes sense. Ability to speak the language of the clinician is also, of course, important. My own team have found that different patients have different success in communicating through a professional interpreter, and one reason for this may be low health literacy in their native language (though our study was not designed to test this hypothesis).[67]

Nutbeam distinguishes three types of health literacy:

a Functional health literacy (basic skills in reading and writing to be able to function effectively in a health context);

b Interactive health literacy (more advanced cognitive, literacy and social skills to actively participate in health care);

c Critical health literacy (the ability to apply knowledge and skills in practical action to overcome barriers to accessing health care).[68]

Perhaps the most worrying aspect of the health literacy challenge is how poor clinicians are at spotting it and how little they generally do to 'meet patients halfway' with advice or information tailored specifically for low literacy. Empirical studies suggest that physicians only identify 20–50% of patients with limited health literacy and that a high proportion of patients find advice from clinicians and written educational materials incomprehensible.[56,58,69] A recent review by Angela Coulter and her team at the Picker Institute reviews the (currently sparse) evidence on interventions to address health literacy, mostly comprising randomised controlled trials of the impact of different types of low-literacy information resources on knowledge or clinical outcomes.[58] Broadly, the conclusion seems to be that research in this field is in its infancy and there are not as yet (and perhaps will never be) any clear or universal solutions.

My own view of this fascinating field is that it is currently unduly dominated by studies comparing 'plain English' information resources and decision aids (many of them technology-based, perhaps for no good reason) with more conventional information formats in a series of somewhat homogeneous and unimaginative randomised trials.[70] There appears to be remarkably little conceptual or in-depth qualitative work addressing *how* people might develop and make better use of their health literacy. Nutbeam's enticing notion of 'critical health literacy', which may offer the greatest potential for reducing health inequalities,[68] has not been widely taken up, and the WHO definition of health literacy seems to have been 'biomedicalised' by a focus on enhancing health knowledge at the expense of either motivation or social action. This narrow conceptual framing has shrunk the research agenda to the design and testing of literacy aids – a worthy project, but not by any means the whole story.

In his original paper, Nutbeam presented a deliberately ambiguous concept of critical health literacy. On the one hand, he used the word 'critical' as in 'critical appraisal', meaning an intellectual (but politically neutral) ability to evaluate information relevant to healthcare decisions. But in addition, he used the concept of critical consciousness, drawing explicitly on the work of Paulo Friere on the emancipatory, social and overtly political role of education in oppressed communities and groups.[71] With this latter framing, critical health literacy means much more than the ability to work one's way through a patient-focused decision support system that has been designed by a team of doctors, nurses and IT experts. It also means the ability to navigate through a potentially hostile health and social care system and demand one's fair share of society's resources!

Models of how people (and self-help groups and local communities) learn and change, especially the link between social learning and action (see Section 2.8), could enrich the theoretical basis of the emerging research tradition on health literacy. My own team is currently undertaking a trial of group-based oral storytelling in ethnic minorities with diabetes from socio-economically deprived backgrounds, many of whom are illiterate in any language. Preliminary data from that study suggest that learning in the group enables action because, as one participant commented, 'when we come to the group *we learn what to do*'.[72] Some of the actions that participants attribute to their membership of the story-sharing group, such as changing their diet or joining an exercise group, can be viewed via a traditional biomedical lens in which the purpose of educating patients is to change their behaviour towards health-positive lifestyle choices. But other actions, such as summoning the courage to challenge a GP who refuses to conduct an annual diabetes review, might be seen more through the lens of Friere's 'pedagogy of the oppressed'. This research is ongoing and we do not yet know the extent of the action (or positive change in health outcome) that occurs as a result of the story-sharing experience. Whatever the findings, a radical framing of Nutbeam's work (to what extent does health literacy develop, in what way is this health literacy critical and how is the oral exchange of stories instrumental or otherwise to this process?) may help explain them. If you are interested in this take on health literacy, watch the project website![§]

[§]See http://www.newhamuniversityhospital.co.uk/poseidon/.

References

1 Parsons T. *The Social System*. Glencoe, IL: The Free Press; 1951.

2 Parsons T. The sick role and the role of the physician reconsidered. In: Parsons T, ed. *Action Theory and the Human Condition*. New York: The Free Press; 1978.

3 Goffman E. *The Presentation of Self in Everyday Life*. New York: Penguin; 1969.

4 Goffman E. *Stigma: Notes on the Management of 'Spoiled' Identity*. New York: Prentice Hall; 1963.

5 Alonzo AA, Reynolds NR. Stigma, HIV and AIDS: an exploration and elaboration of a stigma trajectory. Soc Sci Med 1995;41:303–315.

6 Asbring P, Narvanen AL. Women's experiences of stigma in relation to chronic fatigue syndrome and fibromyalgia. Qual Health Res 2002;12:148–160.

7 Amoroso C, Zwi A, Somerville E, Grove N. Epilepsy and stigma. Lancet 2006;367:1143–1144.

8 Strauss AL. *Chronic Illness and the Quality of Life*. St Louis, MO: Mosby; 1975.

9 Woog P. *The Chronic Illness Trajectory Framework*. New York: Springer; 1992.

10 Corbin J, Strauss AL. Managing chronic illness at home: three lines of work. Qual Sociol 1985;8:224–247.

11 Bury M. Chronic illness as biographical disruption. Sociol Health Illn 1985;4:167–182.

12 Bury M. The sociology of chronic illness: a review of research and prospects. Sociol Health Illn 1991;13:451–468.

13 Frank A. *The Wounded Storyteller: Body, Illness, and Ethics*. Chicago, IL: University of Chicago Press; 1995.

14 Winter R. Fictional-critical writing: an approach to case study research by practitioners. Cambridge J Educ 1986;3:175–182.

15 Aristotle. *Poetics* (Translated by Malcolm Heath). London: Penguin; 1996.

16 Greenhalgh T. *'What Seems to Be the Trouble?': Stories in Illness and Health Care*. Oxford: Radcliffe; 2006.

17 Launer J. *Narrative Based Primary Care: A Practical Guide*. Oxford: Radcliffe; 2002.

18 Maziak W. Health in the Middle East. BMJ 2006;333:815–816.

19 Prochaska JO, DiClemente CC. *The Transtheoretical Approach: Crossing Traditional Boundaries of Therapy*. Malabar, FL: Kreiger Publishing; 1992.

20 Prochaska JO, Velicer WF. The transtheoretical model of health behavior change. Am J Health Promot 1997;12:38–48.

21 Lancaster T, Stead L, Silagy C, Sowden A. Effectiveness of interventions to help people stop smoking: findings from the Cochrane library. BMJ 2000;321:355–358.

22 West R. Time for a change: putting the transtheoretical (stages of change) model to rest. Addiction 2005;100:1036–1039.

23 Coxhead L, Rhodes T. Accounting for risk and responsibility associated with smoking among mothers of children with respiratory illness. Sociol Health Illn 2006;28:98–121.

24 Steptoe A, Perkins-Porras L, McKay C, Rink E, Hilton S, Cappuccio FP. Behavioural counselling to increase consumption of fruit and vegetables in low income adults: randomised trial. BMJ 2003;326:855.

25 Azjen I, Fishbein M. *Understanding Attitudes and Predicting Social Behaviour*. Engelwood Cliffs, NJ: Prentice-Hall; 1980.

26 Azjen I. The theory of planned behaviour. Organ Behav Hum Decis Process 1991;50:179–211.

27 Conner M, Kirk SF, Cade JE, Barrett JH. Why do women use dietary supplements? The use of the theory of planned behaviour to explore beliefs about their use. Soc Sci Med 2001;52:621–633.

28 Morrison DM, Golder S, Keller TE, Gillmore MR. The theory of reasoned action as a model of marijuana use: tests of implicit assumptions and applicability to high-risk young women. Psychol Addict Behav 2002;16:212–224.

29 Syrjala AM, Niskanen MC, Knuuttila ML. The theory of reasoned action in describing tooth brushing, dental caries and diabetes adherence among diabetic patients. J Clin Periodontol 2002;29:427–432.

30 Bowen AM, Williams M, McCoy HV, McCoy CB. Crack smokers' intention to use condoms with loved partners: intervention development using the theory of reasoned action, condom beliefs, and processes of change. AIDS Care 2001;13:579–594.

31 Ried LD, Christensen DB. A psychosocial perspective in the explanation of patients' drug-taking behavior. Soc Sci Med 1988;27:277–285.

32 Ogden J. Some problems with social cognition models: a pragmatic and conceptual analysis. Health Psychol 2003;22:424–428.

33 Ajzen I, Fishbein M. Questions raised by a reasoned action approach: comment on Ogden (2003). Health Psychol 2004;23:431–434.

34 Department of Health. *The Expert Patient: A New Approach to Chronic Disease Management for the Twenty-First Century*. London: Department of Health; 2001.

35 Donaldson L. Expert patients usher in a new era of opportunity for the NHS. BMJ 2003;326:1279–1280.

36 Chodosh J, Morton SC, Mojica W, et al. Meta-analysis: chronic disease self-management programs for older adults. Ann Intern Med 2005;143:427–438.

37 Barlow J, Wright C, Sheasby J, et al. Self-management approaches for people with chronic conditions: a review. Patient Educ Couns 2002;48:177–187.

38 Department of Health. *Self Care – A Real Choice*. London: Department of Health; 2005.

39 Coulter A, Ellins J. Improving self care. *Patient Focussed Interventions – A Review of the Evidence*. Oxford: Picker Institute; 2006.

40 Newman S, Steed L, Mulligan K. Self-management interventions for chronic illness. Lancet 2004;364:1523–1537.

41 Bury M, Newbould J, Taylor D. *A Rapid Review of the Current State of Knowledge Regarding Lay-Led Self-Management of Chronic Illness*. London: National Institute for Clinical Excellence; 2005.

42 Lorig K, Feigenbaum P, Regan C, Ung E, Chastain RL, Holman HR. A comparison of lay-taught and professional-taught arthritis self-management courses. J Rheumatol 1986;13:763–767.

43 Barlow JH, Turner AP, Wright CC. A randomized controlled trial of the arthritis self management program in the UK. Health Educ Res 2000;15:665–680.

44 Lorig KR, Ritter PL, Laurent DD, Fries JF. Long-term randomized controlled trials of tailored-print and small-group arthritis self-management interventions. Med Care 2004;42:346–354.

45 Lorig KR, Sobel DS, Stewart AL, et al. Evidence suggesting that a chronic disease self-management program can improve health status while reducing hospitalization: a randomized trial. Med Care 1999;37:5–14.

46 Lorig KR, Ritter P, Stewart AL, et al. Chronic disease self-management program: 2-year health status and health care utilization outcomes. Med Care 2001;39:1217–1223.

47 Wright N. Homelessness and primary care. Br J Gen Pract 2003;53:568–569.

48 Skinner TC, Carey ME, Cradock S, et al. Diabetes education and self-management for ongoing and newly diagnosed (DESMOND): process modelling of pilot study. Patient Educ Couns 2006;64:369–377.

49 Tannenbaum S. What physicians know. N Engl J Med 1993;329:1268–1271.

50 Benner P, Tanner C. Clinical judgment: how expert nurses use intuition. Am J Nurs 1987;87:23–31.

51 Schillinger D, Grumbach K, Piette J, et al. Association of health literacy with diabetes outcomes. JAMA 2002;288:475–482.

52 Schillinger D, Bindman A, Wang F, Stewart A, Piette J. Functional health literacy and the quality of physician–patient communication among diabetes patients. Patient Educ Couns 2004;52:315–323.

53 Schillinger D, Barton LR, Karter AJ, Wang F, Adler N. Does literacy mediate the relationship between education and health outcomes? A study of a low-income population with diabetes. Public Health Rep 2006;121:245–254.

54 Gucciardi E, Smith PL, Demelo M. Use of diabetes resources in adults attending a self-management education program. Patient Educ Couns 2006;64:322–330.

55 Borrell LN, Dallo FJ, White K. Education and diabetes in a racially and ethnically diverse population. Am J Public Health 2006;96:1637–1642.

56 Wilson JF. The crucial link between literacy and health. Ann Intern Med 2003;139:875–878.

57 Moser C. *Improving Literacy and Numeracy: A Fresh Start*. London: Department for Education and Skills; 1999.

58 Coulter A, Ellins J. Improving health literacy. *Patient Focussed Interventions – A Review of the Evidence*. Oxford: Picker Institute; 2006.

59 Sentell TL, Halpin HA. Importance of adult literacy in understanding health disparities. J Gen Intern Med 2006;21:862–866.

60 Andrus MR, Roth MT. Health literacy: a review. Pharmacotherapy 2002;22:282–302.

61 Speros C. Health literacy: concept analysis. J Adv Nurs 2005;50:633–640.

62 Wolf MS, Gazmararian JA, Baker DW. Health literacy and health risk behaviors among older adults. Am J Prev Med 2007;32:19–24.

63 Parker RM, Ratzan SC, Lurie N. Health literacy: a policy challenge for advancing high-quality health care. Health Aff (Millwood) 2003;22:147–153.

64 Kanjilal S, Gregg EW, Cheng YJ, et al. Socioeconomic status and trends in disparities in 4 major risk factors for cardiovascular disease among US adults, 1971–2002. Arch Intern Med 2006;166:2348–2355.

65 Rutherford J, Holman R, MacDonald J, Taylor A, Jarrett D, Bigrigg A. Low literacy: a hidden problem in family planning clinics. J Fam Plann Reprod Health Care 2006;32:235–240.

66 Sarkar U, Fisher L, Schillinger D. Is self-efficacy associated with diabetes self-management across race/ethnicity and health literacy? Diabetes Care 2006;29:823–829.

67 Greenhalgh T, Robb N, Scambler G. Communicative and strategic action in interpreted consultations in primary health care: a Habermasian perspective. Soc Sci Med 2006;63:1170–1187.

68 Nutbeam D. Health literacy as a public health goal: a challenge for contemporary health education and communication strategies into the 21st century. Health Promot Int 2000;15:259–267.

69 Rogers ES, Wallace LS, Weiss BD. Misperceptions of medical understanding in low-literacy patients: implications for cancer prevention. Cancer Control 2006;13:225–229.

70 McCray AT. Promoting health literacy. J Am Med Inform Assoc 2005;12:152–163.

71 Friere P. *Education for Critical Consciousness*. New York: Continuum; 1974.

72 Greenhalgh T, Collard A, Begum N. Sharing stories: complex intervention for diabetes education in minority ethnic groups who do not speak English. BMJ 2005;330:628–634.

CHAPTER 5

The primary care clinician

Summary points

1 The primary care clinician is a generalist. Generalist knowledge is characterised by a perspective on the whole rather than the parts; on relationships and processes rather than components and facts; and on judicious, context-specific decisions on how and at what level to consider a problem. Essential to performing effectively as a generalist are the contemporary academic skills of knowledge management, communication, teamwork and adaptability to change.

2 The rationalist approach to clinical method involves objectively assessing the patient's symptoms, physical signs and test results, and matching these with a textbook taxonomy of disease based on abstracted definitions. In recent years, epidemiological studies of the presenting features of disease have allowed us to develop clinical prediction rules based on Bayes' theorem, which reduce (but cannot eliminate) uncertainty in clinical diagnosis and prognosis.

3 Clinical method also depends on intuition – a rapid, unconscious process that integrates both objective and subjective reasoning. The intuitive imagination is essential to hypothesis generation in both clinical work (considering what may be wrong with the patient) and scientific research (considering what ideas to test through experiment and observation). In general, the novice (and the expert in unfamiliar situations) reason using logico-deductive methods whereas the expert in familiar situations reasons intuitively and heuristically by 'doing what normally works'. Moving judiciously between these two modes of reasoning is essential to clinical method, especially in primary care where the scope of work is broad and uncertainty high.

4 Increasingly, clinical decisions are (or should be) made according to evidence-based guidelines and protocols. An industry of research has emerged of how to influence clinicians to follow such guidelines, but until recently much of this work has been under-theorised and overly dominated by experimental studies. More recently, qualitative researchers have added to this literature by illuminating the process of influence and the phenomenon of resistance. Insights into how to influence clinicians to adopt new technologies and ways of working can be gained from beyond the health services research literature, especially from sociology (diffusion of innovations theory) and education (the Concerns Based Adoption Model).

(Continued)

(*Summary points continued*)

> **5** The 'good doctor' or 'good nurse' in primary care may be defined either in terms of virtues (intrinsic human qualities such as integrity and altruism) or in terms of performance (observable and measurable behaviours such as maintaining confidentiality). As society's trust in the professions has declined and the expectation of transparency, accountability and regulation have grown, so professionalism has come to be defined more in terms of measurable aspects of performance.

5.1   The role of the generalist

In his excellent book on family medicine, Professor Ian McWhinney described what he calls the 'lump fallacy' view of knowledge:

> '*Let us assume that the knowledge of one branch [of medicine] – pediatrics, for example – is at present of a quantity that can be covered by one physician. If [the quantity of] knowledge is exploding, then after n years, it will have to fragment into pediatric subspecialties, and after another interval each subspecialty will have to fragment again, and so on. . . . What we end up with, of course, is reductio ad absurdum*'.[1]

McWhinney listed six key fallacies about the nature of specialist and general knowledge (Table 5.1).

Contrary to popular belief, the knowledge of the generalist is not necessarily characterised by 'breadth rather than depth', since depth (quality of knowledge) is not the same as detail. Generalist knowledge is often highly strategic: the generalist must choose where to focus, through what conceptual lens, and at what level – hence the emphasis in this book on different theoretical perspectives and levels of analysis. The generalist seeks an understanding of the whole rather than the detailed workings of the parts – the patient rather than the organ, the team rather than the employee and so on. As befits the student of any organic system, he or she often focuses on linkages rather than components – that is on the relationships, interactions and patterns rather than the specifics of the things that are linked.[2]

The good generalist possesses the four contemporary academic skills, which I introduced in Section 1.2. First, he or she is skilled in the art of knowledge management – which can be defined as the ability to find, sort, index, store, evaluate, summarise, synthesise and share knowledge efficiently and effectively. The person who says 'I don't know the answer to your question – but I know where to look for it' has good knowledge management skills, as does one who can lay their hands on a key article copied from a journal several years ago. The student who cites long lists of facts but quotes them out of context and cannot link them to solve a multifaceted problem has poor knowledge management skills.

A seminal paper on knowledge management – and one that was pitched explicitly at the clinical generalist – was Alan Shaughnessy and David Slawson's

Table 5.1 Six fallacies about the nature of generalist and specialist medical knowledge.

Fallacy	Comment
A generalist has to cover the entire field of medical knowledge	The generalist's knowledge of any condition, like that of the specialist, is partial and selective. In meningococcal meningitis, for example, the generalist must identify possible cases at an early stage, so he or she must know the nature and predictive value of different combinations of non-specific symptoms in possibly ill patients.[104,105] The specialist needs different knowledge: how to assess severity and predict serious complications in a child who is definitely ill[106]
In any field, the specialist always knows more than the generalist	Actually, everyone becomes an expert in what he or she sees most of – which for the generalist is usually common variants of common conditions. The specialist may be less able than the generalist to manage a common condition that he or she rarely sees. For example, the family doctor or community nurse may have greater knowledge of how to treat the common forms of constipation in the elderly[107] than a specialist in neuromuscular disorders of the bowel[108]
By specializing, one can eliminate uncertainty	Arguably, the only way to eliminate uncertainty is to break down problems into simpler elements and isolate them from their surroundings. But in reality, all illness occurs in a complex system and impacts at multiple levels, so the challenge is not to eliminate uncertainty but embrace it appropriately in decision making
Only by specializing can one attain depth of knowledge	This fallacy confuses depth (high-quality knowledge, which both the specialist and the generalist may possess) with detail (the amount of information, which is mainly the province of the specialist). For example, the gastroenterologist who sees a schoolchild with abdominal pain and orders a dozen obscure blood tests and a colonoscopy may be showing less depth of knowledge than a school nurse who takes careful note of school pressures, family relationships, life events, associated symptoms and the patient's concerns and expectations[109]
As science advances, the information load increases	Actually, whilst scientific progress indeed involves the accumulation of more facts, good science also generates more sophisticated theories, which can make disparate and confusing findings fall into place – the scientific equivalent of Occam's razor (a single underlying diagnosis may explain multiple and apparently unrelated signs and symptoms)[110]
Error in medicine is usually caused by lack of information	Actually, very few errors are caused by lack of information. Most errors in primary care, as in secondary care, are caused by human failure and poor systems, and would not be prevented simply by making practitioners more knowledgeable or telling them more precisely what to do[111]

Adapted from McWhinney.[1]

'Feeling good about not knowing everything', published back in 1994.[3] In it, they argued that nobody (even a subspecialist) can keep abreast of the medical literature, and that we all need to develop skills in framing focused questions and searching for specific answers to these. Shaughnessy and Slawson also developed the notion of the POEM – patient-oriented information that matters – to help generalists target their search for tiny nuggets of useful information buried in vast medical databases.[4]

The second contemporary academic skill that marks out the generalist is the ability to communicate knowledge to the non-expert by contextualising, personalising and reframing it until it becomes meaningful to that individual. Thirdly, the generalist can work in a multi-disciplinary or multi-professional team, because he or she is aware, through an understanding of the big picture, of how their expertise links with that of other individuals with contrasting and complementary expertise. Finally, he or she is able to adapt appropriately to change rather than doggedly sticking to yesterday's approaches and models.

Whilst it is relatively easy to defend clinical generalism from a philosophical perspective, the argument begs the question of whether patients are better off if cared for by a generalist rather than a specialist. There is remarkably little evidence on this, but the little evidence that does exist tends to support the generalist role. Back in 1991, paediatrician David Morley and colleagues studied over a thousand sick and not-so-sick babies in both hospital and primary care. They checked various symptoms and signs and correlated these with four grades of illness severity. Most symptoms (slow feeding, sweating, crying, cough, rash and so on) were associated to some extent or other with all grades of illness. Only four symptoms were never reported in infants who turned out not to be sick: a fluid intake less than a third of normal, convulsions, frank blood in the stools and bile-stained vomiting.[5] From a Bayesian perspective (see Section 5.2), it is astonishing how much serious illness is detected promptly by GPs and how many not-ill infants are spared the traumas of hospital referral. Evidence also suggests that generalist care is more cost-effective than providing specialist investigations and treatment to the not-ill, not-yet-ill or not-very-ill.[6]

5.2   Clinical method I: rationalism and Bayes' theorem

Every textbook of medicine (invariably written by hospital doctors) contains a section on how to work out what is wrong with the patient and how to decide what to offer in the way of treatment. In general (but not universally), clinical method is presented in such textbooks as a rational process in which the doctor takes careful note of the patient's symptoms (what they feel), physical signs (what the doctor observes) and tests (what the instruments measure), adds these up and classifies the condition according to a formal taxonomy. Disease classification used to be a mystical and somewhat inconsistent art, passed down from one generation of doctors to another and largely withheld from non-doctors, but for over a century clinicians have worked to develop a classification of disease that is consistent across professions and internationally – the International Classification of Diseases (now in its 10th version, the ICD10).

Thus, if a patient has a productive cough on more than half the days in winter months, he or she can be said to be suffering from chronic bronchitis; if the cough isn't productive or it occurs on fewer than half the days, it (by definition) isn't chronic bronchitis. Similar clear definitions exist for everything from precocious puberty to schizophrenia, so in theory working out what's wrong with the patient should be pretty straightforward. You can download the ICD10 and read its fascinating history on the World Health Organisation website http://www.who.int/classifications/icd/en/. A comparable classification for primary care (the International Classification of Primary Care) has also been developed.[7] Whilst the formal classification and coding of disease against agreed standard definitions has important epistemological limitations (see below), it also has four important benefits[8]:
• It confers predictive power, allowing us to answer with greater accuracy the patient's question 'What is going to happen to me?'
• It points us to an effective treatment for the disease (should one exist);
• It gives us a common vocabulary and language with which to discuss our experiences with colleagues, both in the oral tradition ('grand rounds' and peer learning groups) and in the academic literature;
• Naming the condition may have important symbolic benefits for the patient, effectively 'taming' an incomprehensible and frightening set of symptoms.*

Having tried to sell the benefits of the rationalist approach, I must confess that it is also true that every textbook of general practice contains a section lamenting (or perhaps celebrating) the impossibility of such an approach to clinical method. Between 30 and 50% of all problems presenting in general practice are not classifiable using any known disease taxonomy.[1,9] The growing pressure on primary care clinicians to codify their diagnoses in the electronic patient record (using, e.g. the Read code, Snomed CT or ICPC systems)[7,10,11] frequently generates frustration because 'what is wrong with the patient' cannot be satisfactorily matched to the options on a pull-down menu.[†] Nurses have voiced similar protests about the impossibility of classifying 'what nurses do' and the judgments they make using an abstracted system of codes.[12,13] The initial response of technical designers (and 'techy' clinicians) was to introduce more options for coding diagnoses and clinical actions – encouraging general

---

*I cannot resist sharing the apocryphal example of the patient who went to his GP very anxious about a sore tongue. When he came home, his wife asked him if the doctor had been able to help. 'Yes,' he said, 'he told me I have glossitis'.
†My colleague Deborah Swinglehurst points out another problem. Different health professionals have different requirements for information, and therefore different priorities and taxonomies for coding. For example, it may be useful for a cardiologist to know that some one has an 'anterolateral myocardial infarction' but a general practitioner may be happy to code 'myocardial infarction' (MI) since at present our management of MI in the community is not substantially influenced by which part of the heart was affected by the MI. This has some interesting consequences for communication across professional boundaries and the vision of the universally accessible electronic patient record.

practitioners, for example, to move from three-digit Read codes such as G30 (acute myocardial infarction) to four-digit codes such as G300 (acute anterolateral myocardial infarction). But increasing the level of detail in clinical coding systems may not reduce the proportion of problems that are unclassifiable – if anything, they may increase it![14] Why is this?

To arrive at an answer, we must digress into philosophy. McWhinney describes two schools of thought from ancient Greece: the Cnidians and the Coans (he wisely omits a third school, the Aesculapians, who saw illness simply as a mystery and remedies as based purely on priestly authority). The Cnidians, who are seen as the forerunners of conventional biomedical reasoning and strongly influenced Galen, saw diseases as distinct from one another, and clinical method (though they didn't call it that) as essentially about separating out the different diseases from one another using abstract definitions that were independent of context (e.g. a myocardial infarction can be defined as such without reference to who is suffering from it). The Coans, on the other hand, who counted Hippocrates among their members, emphasised the essential unity of all disease and believed that disease presented differently depending on personal and environmental factors. The Coans saw clinical method as essentially about understanding the patient in his or her family and social context, and describing the particularities of how disease affected *this* person in *this* context, and at *this* time.

It is not quite true that Cnidian methods equate with objectivism and Coan with interpretivism (Table 2.2, page 47), nor that the Cnidian perspective underpins clinical method in secondary care while the Coan perspective underpins primary care, but that is not too far from the picture. Professor Marshall Marinker once described the task of hospital medicine, with deliberate irony, as '*distinguishing the clear message of the disease from the interfering noise of the patient as a person*'.[15] Of course, he was setting up a straw man, since few clinicians in either primary or secondary care are opposed to making diagnoses that are robust and reproducible (it is surely bad for business for a patient to be told by one doctor that he has chronic bronchitis and by another that he doesn't), and every competent clinician recognises that the 'same' disease will give different symptoms and induce a different illness response in different patients. All clinical work embraces the tension between diagnosis based on reason (Cnidian) and diagnosis based on experience and knowledge of the individual (Coan), and the skilful clinician moves judiciously between these two fundamentally different modes of reasoning.

I will return to the 'interfering noise of the patient as a person' in the Section 5.3 (on clinical intuition) and in Chapter 6 (on the clinician–patient relationship). For the remainder of this section, I want to focus on the rationalist approach to clinical reasoning and try to persuade you of its immense value – with the caveat that it should augment, not replace, what is coming later. Rationalist, disease-oriented decision making has recently become much more sophisticated by incorporating the tools of epidemiology and evidence-based medicine. How have these tools changed clinical method for the better? Mainly, as I explained in Section 2.2, by combining good old-fashioned clinical observation, the precision of modern tests and instruments, and the science of mathematics – in particular, Bayesian statistics (Box 5.1).

Box 5.1   Bayes, insurance premiums and clinical reasoning.

Thomas Bayes was an eighteenth-century clergyman with a side interest in mathematics and gambling. He made two statements about the 'science' of picking the winner in a horse race (called Bayes' First and Second Theorems)[112]:

1 Although no one can say for sure which horse will win any particular race, the chances of any horse winning are proportional to the presence of favourable features (such as size, strength, temperament, speed in training and so on) in the horse and jockey.

2 If a horse wins against the predictions based on such an assessment, the odds of that horse winning another race should be adjusted.

The first occupational group to use Bayes' theorem in reasoning was not the medical but the insurance profession. Historically, in order to charge large enough premiums to cover their losses (and hopefully make a profit), insurance companies used population-based ('actuarial') data to estimate the risk of future adverse events, from break-ins to hurricane damage. Using similar principles, though usually unconsciously rather than explicitly, gamblers have compared the odds of winning with those of losing in order to decide which way and how much to bet.

In the same way, evidence-based clinical reasoning involves estimating the likelihood of future events – both good and bad – in order to determine the best course of action.[113] Just as the informed gambler wants to know how often a horse has won races in the past before placing a bet, the evidence-based clinician (and, increasingly, the informed patient) wants to know the likelihood that the medicine she is about to prescribe is more effective, with fewer adverse effects, than alternative treatments (or no treatment). Taking such information into account before making a decision involves using 'conditional probability' because it requires predictions that are *conditional* upon a prior (i.e. pre-existing) feature in the situation you are assessing.

What does conditional probability look like in the clinic? Imagine you were about to call in your next patient, but had not yet looked at their notes or seen him or her in the waiting room. If you were to estimate that 'random' person's chance of dying from a stroke within 3 years, you might say something like 1 in 2000. But if, after reading the notes, you discover that your patient is 78 years old, a smoker, has had at least five small black outs over the past year, and has high blood pressure, you would probably adjust your estimate to something like one in five. Such Bayesian reasoning has been practised by clinicians for centuries – but as evidence-based medicine becomes an established science, this reasoning is increasingly formalized and quantified, as in Box 5.2.

Box 5.2 shows how epidemiology can refine the Bayesian approach to clinical reasoning, allowing the clinician to reduce (though importantly, never eliminate) uncertainty. Imagine a patient enters the consulting room complaining of red eye(s). From epidemiological studies, the clinician may be aware that the prior probability of any patient suffering from bacterial conjunctivitis in primary care is around 1 in 100. Even if the patient has red eyes, only around one in three has a bacterial cause (far more are due to allergy or physical irritants), which means that treating 'red eyes' with antibiotics is wasteful and may lead to unnecessary adverse effects. Remco Reitveld

---

Box 5.2 Using simple questions to inform Bayesian reasoning in primary care.[114]

In a patient complaining of a red eye, four questions can help substantially in discriminating between bacterial and non-bacterial conjunctivitis.

Question	Odds ratio	Score
Are both eyes glued together in the morning?	15	+5
Is one eye glued together in the morning?	3	+2
Do(es) the eye(s) itch?	0.5*	−1
Does the patient have a past history of conjunctivitis?	0.3*	−2

Total score	% that predicted a positive culture (regression analysis)	% correctly treated (sensitivity)[†]	% correctly untreated (specificity)[‡]
+5	77	9	100
+2	65	39	94
+3	51	39	92
+2	40	67	73
+1	27	84	38
0	18	89	22
−1	11	98	5
−2	7	98	4
−3	4	100	0

*i.e., in the presence of itch or a past history, the patient is *less* likely to have a bacterial cause than if these features are absent.

[†]i.e., if the score in this row was used as a cut-off for giving antibiotics, this percentage of all patients with bacterial conjunctivitis would correctly receive antibiotics.

[‡]i.e., if the score in this row was used as a cut-off for giving antibiotics, this percentage of patients without bacterial conjunctivitis would be correctly denied antibiotics.

and his colleagues undertook an elegant study in Dutch general practice, in which GPs carefully recorded the presence or absence of various factors – wearing contact lenses, bilateral symptoms, eyes glued in the morning, itch and so on. They then sent bacteriological swabs to confirm whether the patient actually had bacterial conjunctivitis. Computerised logistic regression analysis revealed the extent to which each of these factors contributed to the likelihood of bacterial conjunctivitis. After eliminating some questions which didn't predict one way or the other, they came up with three simple questions (Box 5.2) that usefully discriminated between bacterial and non-bacterial causes. Using a score derived from the contribution of each question in predicting the final diagnosis, the authors calculated that the optimum cut-off for offering an antibiotic is a clinical score of +2. This would mean that two-thirds of patients who could benefit from antibiotics would receive them and three-quarters of patients who would not benefit from antibiotics would not receive them.

If you found this example complex and are unimpressed that even with the benefit of a research study and statistical regression analysis, a substantial proportion of patients still get the wrong treatment, think how often you see a patient with a red eye and use little more than guesswork to decide whether or not to treat with an antibiotic. Remember also that in primary care, we see many patients with mild and often self-limiting illness, and many in the very early stages of more severe conditions. Distinguishing between people who should be actively treated and those who are best untreated is *inherently* impossible in many cases. We need more studies like that of Rietveld and colleagues to develop what are known as clinical prediction rules, even though such rules may only take clinical decisions in primary care from 'so-so' to 'pretty good' and never 'perfect'.

I strongly recommend that you look out research studies that have developed clinical prediction rules for some of the 'old chestnuts' in primary care: when to treat women with urinary tract infection[16]; when to give antibiotics for sore throat[17]; when to advise someone with back pain to return to work[18]; deciding whether a toddler's cough is serious[19]; and identifying the cause of chest pain in a newly presenting patient in primary care.[20] You should also note that clinical prediction rules such as the one shown in Box 5.2 only relate to the population and setting in which they were developed, and should not be used indiscriminately in a different set of patients or another country or region. In such circumstances your own intuition (see next section) may be more accurate than a rule developed elsewhere!

If you have read Section 2.7 on philosophy (particularly the part about epistemology and Table 2.2, page 47), you will recognise rational diagnosis as an example of the objectivist school, in which logico-deductive reasoning predominates. To the extent that diagnosis is ever objective, rational and deductive (and it often approximates to these descriptors), clinical prediction rules can be entered into computerised decision support systems and presented as algorithms to support diagnostic judgments in primary care.[21,22] The literature on computerised decision support systems is vast, but in a nutshell, such systems are generally expensive to develop and sometimes contain errors (e.g. the algorithms lack the latest evidence), but if clinically accurate and technically robust, they can greatly improve accuracy of diagnosis.[21–25] However, these systems may not fit well into the routines and work practices of clinicians, who may develop 'workarounds' to avoid using them. In some situations, and especially outside the research setting, paper-based decision support tools may be more acceptable and cost effective than their fancy electronic counterparts.[24,26] I return to the vexed issue of why clinicians resist using computers in Section 9.3 when I discuss socio-technical systems theory and its implications for the electronic patient record.

5.3   Clinical method II: humanism and intuition

Look back at the consultation shown in Box 4.1, page 95, which is based on a real encounter but fictionalised to protect the identity of the patient. If you are a clinician yourself, your professional response was probably charged with emotion. Most likely, you felt some degree of empathy with this poor elderly man, sadness at the personal tragedy he went through and increased motivation to be more alert in the future to subtle clues that a patient wishes to share an intimate secret. No amount of classifying and categorising of symptoms, no sophisticated diagnostic tests and no volumes of evidence-based medicine will ever capture this emotional dimension, because the nature of the knowledge you are using is humanistic rather than objective (Table 2.2, page 47).

The man who inspired evidence-based medicine's greatest achievement, the Cochrane Collaboration, was a British epidemiologist called Archie Cochrane. No doctor was ever more committed to the use of rational methods in clinical practice, but Archie Cochrane also knew their limitations. In this excerpt from his autobiography, he describes the last living moments of a patient to whom he briefly attended while the resident doctor in a prisoner of war camp:

> 'Another event at Elsterhorst had a marked effect on me. The Germans dumped a young Soviet prisoner in my ward late one night. The ward was full, so I put him in my room as he was moribund and screaming and I did not want to wake the ward. I examined him. He had obvious gross bilateral cavitation and a severe pleural rub. I thought the latter was the cause of the pain and the screaming. I had no morphia, just aspirin, which had no effect. I felt desperate. I knew very little Russian then and there was no one in the ward who did. I finally instinctively sat down on the bed and took him in my arms, and the screaming stopped almost at once. He died peacefully in my arms a few hours later. It was not the pleurisy that caused the screaming but loneliness. It was a wonderful education about the care of the dying. I was ashamed of my misdiagnosis and kept the story secret'.[27,p.82]

It is noteworthy that Cochrane only kept the story secret until he was released from the prisoner of war camp and had time for the honest reflection that is the hallmark of the professional clinician (see Sections 5.6, 11.3 and 11.4). From a philosophical perspective, humanistic clinical practice rests on the core concept of intersubjectivity – 'connecting with' the patient and being aware of this connecting. Different theoretical models have different perspectives on what exactly this 'connecting' entails, and how it might be analysed, and I introduce three examples of these in the next chapter (the sociolinguistic model of clinical interaction in Section 6.2, the psychodynamic model in Section 6.3 and the narrative model in Section 6.4).

It is also noteworthy that Cochrane's move from an 'evidence-based' approach (seeking opioid analgesia on the assumption that the patient's pain had not responded to aspirin) to an approach based on raw humanity (taking the dying man into his arms) was triggered by intuition. In the remainder of this section, I want to consider the phenomenon of intuition in more detail. As I argued in the previous section, clinical prediction rules, however evidence-based, are never going to eliminate uncertainty in primary care. General practitioners, nurses, pharmacists and others who work at the fuzzy coal face of primary care often advise their juniors to learn to 'fly by the seat of their pants' and trust their intuition. The nature of the judgments that allow GPs, most of the time, successfully to extract the 'seriously ill' needles from the haystacks of non-specific presentations are highly complex and require a judicious blend of both rationalistic *and* intuitive reasoning. Let's consider the latter here, based on a paper I published a few years ago in the *British Journal of General Practice*.[28] Note that whilst I have used the general practitioner as my example (because that's what I am), the theory behind this work was developed by a professor of nursing, Patricia Benner, who drew extensively on empirical work on how nurses make decisions.[29–31]

The story in Box 5.3 shows that intuitive insights are commonplace in general practice and they may or may not save lives. They are rarely as impressive as

---

Box 5.3 A story about clinical intuition.[28]

A few years ago, while doing a GP locum, I visited a 58-year-old man who had been complaining of abdominal pain for 3 days. He was on long-term steroids (which had probably been commenced decades ago for asthma). He was very overweight and lying the wrong side of a sagging double bed. His lifelong medical record consisted of a single page. Apparently, he had no previous medical history and had not consulted his GP for over 15 years. His wife was extremely anxious, because they were foster parents and due to take in a recently orphaned teenager. He had to be fit to drive the next day.

He admitted to being constipated, and his abdominal pain was probably no worse now than 2 days ago. Physical examination – inasmuch as I could complete one – was unremarkable. His abdomen was only mildly tender and the bowel sounds normal. He grunted a bit, but that was all. In view of the steroids, I sent him into hospital, and the registrar put him on 'fourly-hourly observations'.

That night, I went home and told my husband that I had seen a man who was going to die. He did indeed die, 4 days later, despite normal bloods and observation chart throughout. Post-mortem showed a strangulated volvulus.

the one I first heard quoted by Professor Nigel Stott (and which I subsequently analysed in detail[32]) from a GP in Cardiff: *'I got a call from a lady saying her three year old daughter had had diarrhoea and was behaving strangely. I knew the family well, and was sufficiently concerned to break off my morning surgery and visit immediately'*. This GP's hunch led him to diagnose correctly, and treat successfully, a case of meningococcal meningitis on the basis of two non-specific symptoms reported over the phone – an estimated 'hit rate' for that particular GP of 1 in 96,000 consultations. The intuitive judgments we make on a daily basis in clinical practice are generally less dramatic but no easier to explain on a rational level.

Few primary care clinicians dispute that intuition plays a part in their practice, but there has been relatively little formal research into how (and to what extent) intuition contributes to decision making in the clinical setting. Intuition has six key features:
• It is a rapid, unconscious process.
• It is context-sensitive.
• It comes with practice.
• It involves selective attention to small details.
• It cannot be reduced to cause-and-effect logic (B happened because of A).
• It addresses, integrates and makes sense of, multiple and complex pieces of data.

In one of the first of the *Sherlock Holmes* novels written by doctor-novelist Sir Arthur Conan Doyle, Holmes is asked to explain a particularly impressive and obscure feat of reasoning and responds as follows: *'From long habit the train of thoughts ran so swiftly through my mind that I arrived at the conclusion without being conscious of intermediate steps'* (my emphasis). Educationalists Hubert and Stuart Dreyfus, writing about intuition in industrial engineering, concluded that *'Experienced intuitive [practitioners] do not attempt to understand familiar problems and opportunities using calculative rationality.... When things are proceeding normally, experts don't solve problems and don't make decisions: they do what normally works'* (my emphasis).[33] Like Conan Doyle, Dreyfus and Dreyfus present intuition as a method of problem solving that marks the expert out from the novice, and they acknowledge the elusive nature of the intuitive method. Experts themselves can rarely provide an immediate, rational explanation for why they behaved in a particular way.

Table 5.2, which is based on real-life observations, shows excerpts from four clinical 'clerkings' taken a few years ago of a single patient with conjunctivitis (which, incidentally, are worth contrasting with the clinical prediction rule shown in Box 5.2). The different problem-solving approaches adopted by clinicians at varying stages of training illustrate stages in the classification that Dreyfus and Dreyfus derived from observations of professional engineers. According to them[33]:

The **novice** practitioner is characterised by:
• Rigid adherence to taught rules or plans
• Little situational perception
• No discretionary judgment

Table 5.2 Examples of clinical clerking styles of doctors at different stages of training and experience.

Third-year medical student	Fifth-year medical student
'Mr Brown is a 38 year old computer operator who attended the Accident and Emergency department with a bad feeling in his eye. The history of the presenting complaint was that it was there when he woke up at 7.15 am on Wednesday morning. When he was a little boy he had had an operation on his eyes for squint. He is up to date on his jabs. . . . '	'This 38 year old male attended with a feeling of grit in his right eye. The eye also had a yellow discharge. He could still read the paper with that eye. He had not had any previous episode like this. His visual acuity was 6/6 bilaterally. His pupils were equal, concentric responding to light and accommodation. . . . '

Casualty officer	GP
'38 year old male Gritty Rt eye 2/7; no h/o trauma Purulent discharge Vision 6/6, 6/6 No PMH of note Rx: G. chloramphenicol to Rt eye q.d.s. Review: See GP 1/52'	'Rt conjunctivitis Chloramphenicol drops See S.O.S.'

The **competent** practitioner:
- Is able to cope with 'crowdedness' and pressure
- Sees actions partly in terms of long-term goals or wider conceptual framework
- Follows standardised and routinised procedures

The **expert** practitioner:
- No longer relies explicitly on rules, guidelines and maxims
- Has an intuitive grasp of situations based on deep, tacit understanding
- Uses analytic (deductive) approaches only in novel situations or when problems occur

In general, we are at our most intuitive when doing our regular job and dealing with patients whom we know well. In unfamiliar situations, we resort to a more formal and rational approach based on explicit (and defensible) professional rules, as described in the previous section. The skill of the expert is to respond to the subtle cues that signal a need to shift between the two approaches. The GP who writes the single word 'conjunctivitis' in a medical record may live to regret it when the patient subsequently sues for a missed diagnosis of uveitis!

There are three widely held myths about clinical reasoning – first, that it is an entirely logical and deductive process; second, that experts think more logically than novices; and third, that more knowledge leads to better decisions. The research literature tells us otherwise. Firstly, the critical importance of experience, context and familiarity have been persuasively demonstrated by Kathryn Montgomery Hunter, a professor of literature who spent several years watching, and listening to, doctors going about their duties. As her detailed fieldwork showed, clinical decision making occurs by the *selective* application of general rules to particular individuals and contexts.[34] The uniqueness of the individual (comorbidity, values, context and the physiological idiosyncracies that give rise to murmurs in the normal heart and make one person's pain another's 'tingling' or 'pressure') preclude any purely rule-based method for assigning diagnoses or selecting treatments. Hunter concluded:

> *'Clinical education is preparation for practical, ethical action: what best to do, how to behave, how to discover enough to warrant taking action, which choice to make on behalf of the patient. [These] choices are governed not by hard and fast rules but by competing maxims.... As lawyers, literary critics, historians and other students of evidence know well, there is no text that is self-interpreting. As rules, these maxims are relentlessly contextual'.*[34]

Secondly, studies on the development of expertise in clinicians confirm the Dreyfus' taxonomy of problem solving: the more experienced a clinician gets, the less logical their decision-making processes are shown to be.[35] Thirdly, as the next section (on guidelines and changing clinical behaviour) shows, there is a striking absence of studies showing that knowledge per se improves decision making. As the example in Box 6.4 (page 161) shows, even in something as clinically clear-cut as a routine asthma check, the naïve application of 'evidence' without regard to the unique predicament and priorities of the individual patient soon makes the decision evidence-burdened rather than evidence-based.

A number of studies by cognitive psychologists and educationalists have begun to throw light on the process by which clinical expertise accumulates.[34,36–38] We start by learning detailed 'rules' about the cause, course and treatment of each condition. As we gain knowledge we convert these rules to stereotypical stories ('scripts'). We refine our knowledge by accumulating atypical and alternative stories via experience and the oral tradition (such as grand rounds, 'corridor consultations' and so on). Furthermore, there is growing evidence that clinical knowledge is stored in our memory *as stories* rather than as structured collections of abstracted facts. 'Doing what normally works' is an example of inductive reasoning (Table 2.2, page 47), based on the general principle that if the last 99 swans seen were white, the next swan will also be white.

I have separated rational deduction (Section 5.2) and intuition (this section) partly for the purposes of layout, since intuition is not necessarily irrational or humanistic! I sometimes despair of clinicians who believe that they must *either* be 'old-fashioned' practitioners whose decisions are based more or less on intuition or 'modern' ones who support the rational, explicit and systematic use of research evidence in the clinical encounter. Despite the fact that I have placed 'rational' and 'intuitive' clinical method in separate sections, there is actually no 'zero-sum' relationship (i.e. more of one implies less of the other) between the deductive steps of evidence-based decision making ('the science') and the contextual interpretation of the patient's illness story ('the art') in clinical encounters. On the contrary, as Medawar famously argued in relation to scientific induction, unique elements in the patient's personal story ignite the clinical imagination, producing entirely rational (but often intuitive) hypotheses about what might be wrong and possible options for management.[39]

Here's a worked example. Returning to the story in Box 5.3, my subconscious hypotheses about what *might* happen incorporated both generalisable, research-derived truths (such as the known masking impact of steroids and the low validity of physical signs elicited in less than ideal circumstances) and unique, contextual ones (including the lack of any previous consultations, the wife's profound concern and the patient's stoical 'grunt' on examination. When I predicted his impending death, I was not consciously aware of the intermediate steps that led me to my hypothesis, but when I learnt the outcome and sought a debriefing with his regular GP, the pieces of the jigsaw were revealed to both of us. The work of Patricia Benner[29] and Michael Eraut[37] (among others) suggests that the insight I gained from critical reflection and discussion with a professional colleague is to be expected. Reflecting retrospectively on the process of clinical intuition (asking, for example, 'Why did I make diagnosis X rather than diagnosis Y at that point?' or 'What prompted me to start/stop that drug?') is a powerful educational tool. In particular, critical reflection on past intuitive judgments highlights areas of ambiguity in complex decision making, sharpens perceptual awareness, exposes the role of emotions in driving 'hunches' (perhaps also demonstrating the fallibility of relying on feelings alone), encourages a holistic view of the patient's predicament, identifies specific educational needs and may serve to 'kick-start' a more analytical chain of thought on particular problems. I return to this theme in Section 11.4 when I consider learning and professional development.

Both this section and the previous one have taken the perspective that clinical method is something that occurs inside the clinician's head and without any significant interaction with the patient. Another view holds that clinical work is usually a dialogue, and the input of the patient has important influence on the diagnostic and treatment decisions made as well as on how these are communicated to the patient. Sections 6.2 (which takes a sociolinguistic approach to the clinical interaction), 6.3 (which covers Balint's psychodynamic approach) and 6.4 (which covers a 'literary' perspective on clinical interaction based on the notion of active listening) could all be classified as variants on clinical method as well as variants on the clinician–patient interaction.

5.4   Clinical method III: the patient-centred method

In this chapter, I have offered three 'takes' on clinical method – the rationalist approach (Section 5.2), the humanist and intuitive approach (Section 5.3) and the patient-centred method described in this section. I have already argued in the previous section that neither humanism nor intuition preclude or oppose the use of rational reasoning, and I now want to introduce one approach that attempts to unite them. It is important not to see the patient-centred method as something different from either a rationalist or a humanist approach. Patient-centred clinical method is the name given to an approach that *combines* both rational, objective reasoning *and* a humanist perspective towards the patient, *as well as* taking account of the wider social context that may have generated the illness and brought the patient into the consulting room in the first place. It is based on a multifaceted theory that incorporates both 'sides' of the epistemological divide in Table 2.2 (page 47), and which also takes a multi-level perspective on the nature of illness, considering both individual symptoms and behaviour and the wider context within which these occur (see Section 3.9).

The biopsychosocial model of illness is usually attributed to Professor Ian McWhinney and his team at the Department of Family Medicine at the University of Western Ontario; an excellent textbook summarises its origins, principles and applications.[8] These authors acknowledge the earlier work of George Engel, who was perhaps the first to apply systems theory (the notion that complex phenomena can be conceptualised as multiple interacting systems) to the diagnosis and management of illness (originally in psychiatry and subsequently in family medicine).[40,41] Engel recognised the multi-level nature of what doctors call illness, from the gene to the environment, and suggested that clinicians analyse problems on each of these multiple levels and then integrate insights from each. McWhinney's team also drew on Michael Balint's psychodynamic model of the doctor–patient interaction (see Section 6.3)[42] and Kleinman's study on patients' explanatory models of illness, undertaken from an anthropological perspective, which demonstrated that patients typically construct their illness very differently from health professionals.[43]

Figure 5.1 shows the biopsychosocial model in diagrammatic form. Let us work through one common problem in primary care – smoking-related illness – and see how this model may help illuminate the issues and inform the process of clinical reasoning. Why do people smoke? Perhaps, partly because smoking is an addiction that is to some extent inherited.[44] Pharmacological treatments for people seeking to quit smoking are designed at the level of the molecule and (in the future) may be specifically targeted (as in 'designer drugs') towards particular genetic variants of drug receptors.[45] At the level of the individual, interpersonal influence both from peers and within the family seems a critical factor prompting people to start smoking,[46,47] as does stress and traumatic life experience.[48] But poverty, too, is a strong influence on smoking behaviour, in that the lower a person's socioeconomic status the more likely they are to start smoking (and to resist advice to quit).[49–51] Some interventions aimed at reducing smoking have been designed at the level of economic policy and have had varying success.[52,53] Increasingly, research

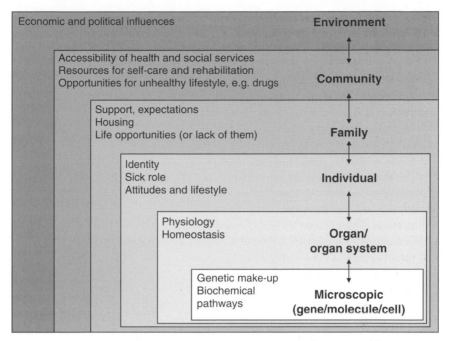

Figure 5.1 A biopsychosocial model of illness. (Adapted from Engel[41] and Stewart.[8])

into smoking behaviour and how to influence it uses multi-level theories that integrate the molecular, psychological, sociological and environmental influences on individual behaviour.[54,55]

In a recent review of the biopsychosocial model in the Annals of Family Medicine, Borrell-Carrio and colleagues remind us that this model, which has become especially popular in primary care in recent years, is not merely a practical clinical guide but also a philosophy of clinical care.[56] Epistemologically (see Section 2.7), the model contains what purists would see as incommensurabilities between mental and physical aspects of health (e.g. subjective experience depends on, but can never be reduced to, laws of physiology). But at a more practical level, it can usefully inform decision making within (and beyond) the clinical consultation.

The six interactive components of the patient-centred method are shown in Box 5.4. To some extent, the patient-centred method is not truly a multi-level approach since it begins and ends with the consultation – hence it can only bring in 'higher' levels (such as the social determinants of health) indirectly and partially. However, as the authors themselves emphasise, whatever the cause of an illness, the person who is ill tends to land up in the waiting room of the primary health care team, so it is probably not so unreasonable to take the clinical consultation as the focus of analysis.

Box 5.4 The six interacting components of the patient-centred clinical method.

1 Exploring and interpreting both the disease and the illness experience
   a Differential diagnosis (rationalist perspective)
   b Dimensions of illness, e.g. ideas, expectations, effects on function (humanist perspective)
2 Understanding the whole person
   a The 'person' (life history, personal and developmental issues)
   b The context (family, other support, physical environment)
3 Finding common ground with the patient about the problem and its management
   a Problems and priorities
   b Goals of treatment
   c Roles of clinician and patient (what will each be responsible for?)
4 Incorporating prevention and health promotion
   a Health enhancement
   b Risk reduction
   c Early detection of disease
   d Reducing the impact of disease
5 Enhancing the clinician–patient relationship
   a Aspects of the therapeutic relationship
   b Sharing power
   c Caring and healing relationship
   d Transference and countertransference (see Section 6.3)
6 Being realistic about time and resources
   a Time
   b Resources
   c Team building

Summarised from Stewart et al.[8]

In their '25 years on' review of the patient-centred method, Borrell-Carrio and colleagues suggest that whilst the humanistic and participatory approach to clinical method aligns with recent social and cultural changes in Western healthcare (see Box 1.2, page 7), such an approach may not be universally accepted. They propose a less culture-bound adaptation of this method whose pillars include: (1) self-awareness; (2) active cultivation of trust; (3) an emotional style characterized by empathic curiosity; (4) self-calibration as a way to reduce bias; (5) educating the emotions to assist with diagnosis and forming therapeutic relationships; (6) the use of 'informed intuition'; and (7) communicating clinical evidence to foster dialogue, not just the mechanical application of protocol.

One very important research tradition has stemmed directly from the Canadian work on patient-centred clinical method. It is built around the concept of 'shared decision making' – the active and equal involvement of the patient in decisions about his or her care, which requires effective communication about both the problem and the options for management, as well as mutual respect and trust and a recognition of the 'lifeworld' agenda (see Section 6.2) by the clinician.[57–64]

It is probably apparent from this brief section that there are many potential variations on the theme of the patient-centred method, and that all will include the judicious (rather than formulaic) application of rationalist approaches such as evidence-based medicine, the reflective use of subjectivity and intuition and a consideration of the social causes of illness and consulting behaviour.

5.5   Influencing clinicians' behaviour

As with efforts to change patients' lifestyle (see Section 4.3), interventions to change what clinicians do should be (but rarely are) based on robust theories about human behaviour, learning, influence and change. This section sets out some (but by no means all) theoretical perspectives relevant to influencing clinical practice. I have chosen to illustrate this very wide field of study using the example of how to get clinicians to follow evidence-based guidelines, partly because this is important territory in its own right, and partly because it illustrates very well how the 'ologies' introduced in Chapter 2 can inform and enrich our understanding of primary care.

There have been dozens of studies within evidence-based medicine (in a subtradition known as implementation research and led by, among others, Professor Jeremy Grimshaw) that have sought ways of improving clinicians' use of evidence-based guidelines. These have included mass media efforts to raise awareness of guidelines,[65] educational inputs of various kinds,[66–68] interventions led by designated 'clinical opinion leaders' (see below)[69] and incentives (typically, financial ones).[70] These studies were mostly randomised controlled trials of complex interventions, based on a design used by Sibley and Sackett back in 1982 ('intervention on' versus 'intervention off' and measuring a set of predefined outcomes, as illustrated in Figure 3.6, page 70).[71] Most such trials (including the early work done by Sackett's team), and with the possible exception of financial incentives, had surprisingly low success at inducing the hoped-for changes in clinical practice.

An overview by Richard Grol summarises the reasons why intervention trials to promote 'behaviour change' were so often only marginally effective (or ineffective).[72] Many evidence-based guidelines were ambiguous or confusing; they usually only covered part of the sequence of decisions and actions in a clinical consultation; they were often difficult to apply to individual patients' unique problems; they generally required changes in the wider health care system as well as doctors' behaviour; and their implementation was rarely cost-neutral (so may have required resources to be shifted from other activities that were equally 'evidence-based'). In other words, the underlying theory on which conventional intervention trials were built (epidemiological research → publication of evidence → implementation by clinicians[73]) was critically flawed and needed more than minor adjustment.

In the early days, writers had talked about objective and context-neutral evidence driving the evidence-into-practice cycle *'like water flowing through a pipe'*.[74] The problem of getting research evidence to influence routine clinical practice was couched initially as an 'evidence gap' (evidence on what works was lacking), then as a 'knowledge gap' (clinicians were ignorant of the evidence) and then a 'behaviour gap' (they failed to act on it and needed a stick or a carrot). One randomised trial after another sought to identify the efficacy of different packages designed to fill these gaps. But the entire paradigm was (in my view) flawed, since the 'gap' metaphor is *inherently* inappropriate, implying as it does an empty space that can be 'made good' with a cleanly defined, targeted intervention. A different theory (or theories) is required.

As far back as 1993, one of the editors of the *British Medical Journal*, Tony Delamothe, wrote a piece called 'Wanted: Guidelines that doctors will follow'.[75] His idea was that rather than simply bemoaning the stubbornness and conservatism of the medical profession, there might be some generic characteristics of clinical guidelines that could be improved in order to make them more appealing, more accessible, more understandable and more practicable. A more theoretical take on making guidelines 'easier to follow' is the idea that a guideline is a form of innovation, and spreading the use of guidelines is a specific example of a more general phenomenon – the diffusion of innovations. Classical diffusion of innovations theory, as set out by sociologist Everett Rogers, arose from empirical work undertaken in the 1940s which demonstrated a consistent pattern of adoption of new ideas and practices over time by people in a social system.[76] The theory's central tenet is that the adoption of new ideas in a population follows a predictable pattern. There is a slow initial (lag) phase, followed by an acceleration in the number of people adopting in each time period, followed by a corresponding deceleration and finally a tail as the last few individuals who are going to adopt finally do so (Figure 5.2).

Rogers, whose distinguished academic career spanned five decades, was a rural sociologist – that is he mainly studied farmers and farming practices. He undertook his PhD in the early 1950s looking at the adoption of 'modern' agricultural methods (such as powerful chemical fertilisers) in the somewhat conservative state of Iowa. These modern methods had been developed in universities and government-funded centres of excellence. The farmers' reluctance to take up new agricultural technologies has many parallels to the resistance of modern-day clinicians to the adoption of evidence-based guidelines. Based on some 300 observational studies of the adoption (and non-adoption) of different innovations, Rogers distilled out some general principles about the *attributes* of innovations – that is, the characteristics which (in the eyes of potential adopters)

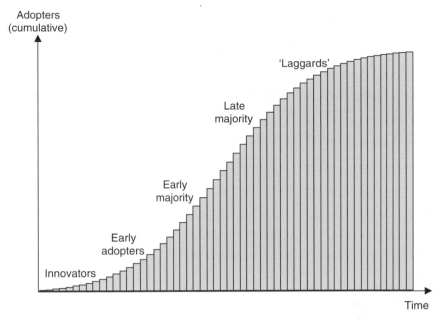

Figure 5.2 The S-curve in diffusion of innovations.

made them more or less likely to be taken up and sustained. Six attributes have been consistently shown to be linked to the rate and completeness of adoption (i.e., the gradient and final height of the curve in Figure 5.2):

• *Relative advantage* – if the innovation is seen to have a clear advantage over current practice;

• *Compatibility* – if the innovation is compatible with the values and norms of potential adopters;

• *Low complexity* – if the innovation is simple (or can be broken down into simple components);

• *Observability* – if the impact of the innovation is readily observable;

• *Trialability* – if the innovation can be tried out on a small scale before the adoption decision is made;

• *Potential for reinvention* – if the innovation can be customised to make it fit for purpose in a particular situation.

Roberto Grilli and Jonathan Lomas evaluated 23 separate studies of the extent to which doctors followed clinical guidelines and found a total of 143 recommendations. They assessed each one for three attributes: complexity, trialability and observability ('relative advantage' was assumed in that the guidelines were evidence-based so by definition better than standard practice; 'compatibility' could only be assessed by asking the doctors, which was not possible in this study design; and 'potential for reinvention' had not yet been identified as important). They found that observability was hard to assess, but that low complexity and trialability together accounted for up to 47%

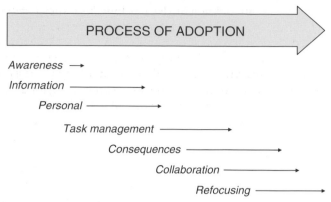

Figure 5.3 Hall and Hord's Concerns Based Adoption Model.

of doctors' non-compliance with guidelines. A clear message then: guideline developers should make their recommendations simple and trialable!

Another theory in innovation research, also highly relevant to the adoption of clinical guidelines, is the Concerns Based Adoption Model of Hall and Hord. Based on empirical study of teachers' efforts to adopt new educational technologies, they proposed that when individuals adopt an innovation, three sets of concerns must be addressed (Figure 5.3)[77]:

• *Concerns in the pre-adoption stage.* Important prerequisites for adoption are that the intended adopter is *aware* of the innovation; has sufficient *information* about what it does and how to use it; and is clear how the innovation would affect them *personally*, e.g. in terms of costs.

• *Concerns during early use.* Successful adoption is more likely if the intended adopter has continuing access to *information* about what the innovation does, and to sufficient training and support on *task issues*, i.e. about fitting the innovation in with daily work.

• *Concerns in established users.* Successful adoption is more likely if adequate feedback is provided to the intended adopter on the consequences of adoption, and if the intended adopter has sufficient opportunity, autonomy and support to adapt and refine the innovation to improve its fitness for purpose.

Note that whereas a simplistic 'behaviour change' theoretical lens glosses over the clinician's concerns and assumes that he or she can be rewarded, punished or otherwise incentivised to behave to order, the Concerns Based Adoption Model acknowledges 'resistance to change' as potentially well grounded in legitimate concerns of various types. As Figure 5.3 shows, this model also offers a time dimension – adopters' concerns change as the process of adoption unfolds, and the design of packages to promote guideline use should reflect this.

Another relevant component of diffusion of innovation theory is social influence. We copy some people more readily than we copy others. The US sociologists of the 1950s demonstrated some key characteristics of a person who is likely to be copied (an 'opinion leader') include high social status, greater knowledge (more years of education), 'cosmopolitanism' (makes visits to the local market town more often) and wide social networks (is known and named as a friend by more people).[76,78] The original research studies on opinion leadership were largely interview-based and involved asking professionals who influenced them (e.g. when deciding to prescribe a new drug for the first time). More recently, a fascinating series of ethnographic studies, in which qualitative researchers shadowed and observed clinicians and managers going about their work, has explored opinion leader influence in a real-world setting. I recommend the excellent summary of this literature by Louise Locock[79] and the book by Sue Dopson and Louise Fitzgerald about evidence-based medicine in context.[80] In brief, the naturalistic work on opinion leadership suggested that the social influence of certain individuals is often very profound – either positively if they support an innovation or negatively if they oppose it or are lukewarm. But such influences are subtle and tied to particular innovations and contexts. A person (e.g. an older experienced GP) may be a highly influential opinion leader for one aspect of clinical practice (such as how to handle difficult patients or manage staff) but not influential at all in others (such as how to treat hypertension). Furthermore, the qualitative studies have shown that opinion leadership is not static – the question of who influences us and by how much changes with time and perhaps even with what mood we are in. In other words, social influence is a complex phenomenon and it is perhaps small wonder that clinical trials of 'opinion leader on' versus 'opinion leader off' did not have a dramatic impact on practice.[69]

In summary, the numerous trials of interventions to make clinical practice more evidence-based through the use of guidelines are somewhat under-theorised. There are neither 'magic bullets' (complex interventions that are guaranteed to work in every setting) nor 'magic targets' (individuals, behaviours or situations where efforts should be concentrated).[81,82] The research agenda on implementing guidelines has begun (not before time) to be reframed from a rather Pavolvian goal of 'changing clinicians' behaviour' to 'improving the attributes of guidelines', 'identifying and addressing clinicians' concerns' and 'exploring the complexity of social influence in the real world of clinical work'.

5.6   The 'good' clinician

No chapter entitled 'the clinician' in the twenty-first century would be complete without a section on professionalism, the standards we expect of ourselves and how to promote and enforce these. Box 5.5 gives two examples of 'bad' clinicians and reminds us that we now live in an era when public trust in health professionals, which was once something that came with the job, has to be earned and retained. Trust, which was the subject of an excellent series of Reith Lectures by Onora O'Neill a few years ago (which were published as a book[83]), is closely linked to professionalism. Indeed, a working party of

Box 5.5 Bad clinicians.

Dr Harold Shipman, a general practitioner in Greater Manchester, was viewed by his patients as a kind, sympathetic, competent and thorough family doctor. In reality, he was Britain's worst ever serial killer. Following his trial for the murder of one of his patients in 2000, forensic enquiries indicated that he was probably responsible for an estimated 235 more. Yet many of his patients refused to accept that someone who had been such a 'good doctor' could possibly have committed murder. Patients were typically killed in the afternoon on surgery premises. A taxi driver dropped a fit-looking 56-year-old lady off for her routine appointment returned to pick her up an hour later, and was told that the woman had died while being treated by Dr Shipman. He became suspicious and began to make a list of other regular customers who had died recently – all of whom were patients of Dr Shipman. But he was reluctant to come forward. Who would believe the word of a taxi-driver over that of a doctor? An undertaker became alarmed at her colleagues' references to the phrase 'another one of Shipman's'. His patients were all found dressed, relatively healthy and the death was sudden and unexpected. When the undertaker voiced her concerns to her peers they were ignored and she was warned not to go public for fear of liability. It was 2 years – and around 80 more murders – later before Shipman was finally arrested.

   Beverley Allitt, or the 'Angel of Death' as she became known, is one of Britain's most notorious female serial killers. She murdered four of her child patients and attempted to murder nine others. At the same time, she befriended the parents of her victims with her caring and solicitous manner and the identity she projected as an experienced and highly trained nurse (in fact, she was neither). Allitt was an unhappy teenager given to self-harm, who became overweight as an adolescent and developed attention-seeking behaviour and aggression towards others. She went on to train as a nurse and was suspected of odd behaviour, such as smearing faeces on walls in a nursing home where she trained. Despite her history of poor attendance and repeated failure of her nursing examinations, she was taken on a temporary 6-month contract at the chronically understaffed Grantham and Kesteven Hospital in Lincolnshire in 1991, where she began work in the Children's Ward. There were only two trained nurses on the dayshift and one for nights. Her first victim, 7-month-old LT, was admitted with a chest infection. Allitt went out of her way to reassure his parents that he was in capable hands and persuaded them to go home to get some rest. When they returned, Allitt advised that LT had had a respiratory arrest but had recovered. She volunteered for extra night duty so she could watch over the boy, who had a further 'respiratory arrest' in the night and spent several days on a ventilator with severe brain damage before his parents made the agonising decision for it to be switched off. Several more victims followed, in similar circumstances.

the Royal College of Physicians recently defined medical professionalism as *'a set of values, behaviours, and relationships that underpin the trust the public has in doctors'*.[84] In this section, I will unpack and challenge this definition of professionalism, drawing on a number of recent reviews and commentaries.[84–86]

Sociologists define professions in terms of social roles and relationships. Creuss et al., for example, propose three defining features of any profession:
- Mastery of a complex body of knowledge and skills;
- Use of this knowledge in the service of others;
- A 'closed shop' whose members are governed by codes of ethics and make a commitment to competence, integrity, altruism and the promotion of the public good.

These commitments, they suggest, form the basis of a social contract between the profession and society, which in return grants the profession three things:
- A monopoly over the use of its knowledge;
- The right to autonomy in practice;
- The privilege of self-regulation.

I find this definition somewhat old-fashioned. To put it another way, I wonder whether medicine truly fulfils the definition of a profession in the twenty-first century. Most medical knowledge these days, for example, is available to anyone who bothers to look for it on the Internet. Whilst medical professionals may use this knowledge in the service of others, so increasingly do others – most notably the voluntary sector and self-help groups. Following an ethical code and maintaining competence is now not so much a professional commitment as a statutory duty enforced by the machinery of public accountability. Even 'self-regulation', the checks and balances initiated from within the profession (e.g. the General Medical Council[87,88]), has shifted subtly from the voluntary promotion of norms and values to the development and implementation of legally binding codes, procedures and compulsory checks.[89]

This change in the level of autonomy and independence accorded to doctors, and in how they are regulated – and a similar change in the nursing profession, both of which are paralleled in almost every western country – is (arguably) the result of a fundamental change in the nature of society. The current historical period in western society, known to sociologists as 'late modernity', is characterised by diminution of state regulation, growing consumerism, rapid technological change and increasing influence of globalisation, all of which have impacted on public trust in the state and its capacity for governance, as well as in science and technology. Life is more fluid; we can access knowledge ourselves; we trust the state – and the professions – less.[90,91] As a result, we increasingly expect them to be transparent, accountable and externally regulated.

The shift from an 'internal' view of professionalism (based on the person's commitment to professional values and codes) to an 'external' one (based on accountability to the state and the public, and the implementation of formally agreed, approved and measurable standards, as in – but not restricted to – clinical governance[92–94]) also reflects a very different theoretical model of 'the good clinician' (and, incidentally, a philosophical shift from humanism to objectivism as illustrated in Table 2.2, page 47). To caricature somewhat, in the good old days a 'good doctor' was one who had taken the Hippocratic Oath and believed it from the bottom of his heart; nowadays he or she is someone who has passed an OSCE (objective structured clinical assessment) in 'professional behaviour' (with marks for making eye contact, breaking bad news sensitively and not accepting excessive gifts from drug reps), completed the annual paperwork mountain for revalidation and blows the whistle on an underperforming colleague through the official channels. The underlying philosophical difference here in the nature of 'goodness' (see Section 2.7) is between professionalism as *virtue* (embracing, e.g. integrity, commitment and altruism, which like all virtues, can only be measured indirectly[95,96]), and professionalism as *performance* (e.g. 'maintains confidentiality', 'prescribes controlled drugs responsibly' and so on, which can be measured directly[87]). The tension between a humanistic (virtue-based) definition of professionalism and a objectivist or behaviourist (performance-based) one lies at the heart of the stormy debates currently raging about how to teach (and assess) professionalism in both medicine[86,97–100] and nursing.[101–103]

Leaving aside whether professionalism is mainly about the sort of person we are (humanist) or the way we perform (behaviourist), there is also the question of what domains 'professionalism' should cover. In the old days, and especially general practice and traditional nursing practice in the UK, professionalism focused mainly if not exclusively on the clinician–patient relationship and addressed issues such as respecting autonomy, not judging the patient's lifestyle or values, caring selflessly and maintaining confidentiality. But this is only one level at which professionalism needs to operate. Based on a qualitative research study of real examples of professional practice, Apker has argued that professionalism in contemporary nursing practice (characterised relentlessly by teamwork and interfaces) is as much to do with communication with other health professionals as it is to do with the nurse–patient relationship.[103]

The Royal College of Physicians working party on professionalism (see above) echoed this wider perspective, stating that professionalism implies multiple commitments – to the patient, to fellow professionals and to the institution or system within which healthcare is provided, to the extent that the system supports patients collectively.[84] Rather than a characteristic of the individual practitioner, professionalism is becoming a 'corporate' goal for healthcare organisations. This, of course, is the basis of clinical governance – a theme I return to in Section 10.4 where I also reflect further on the changing nature of trust.

The question of how we acquire and maintain professionalism is part of continuing professional development, which I address in Chapter 11 (especially Section 11.4).

References

1 McWhinney IR. *A Textbook of Family Medicine*. 2nd ed. Oxford: Oxford University Press; 1997.

2 Plsek PE, Greenhalgh T. Complexity science: the challenge of complexity in health care. BMJ 2001;323:625–628.

3 Slawson DC, Shaughnessy AF, Bennett JH. Becoming a medical information master: feeling good about not knowing everything. J Fam Pract 1994;38:505–513.

4 Slawson DC, Shaughnessy AF, Ebell MH, Barry HC. Mastering medical information and the role of POEMs – patient-oriented evidence that matters. J Fam Pract 1997;45:195–196.

5 Morley CJ, Thornton AJ, Cole TJ, Fowler MA, Hewson PH. Symptoms and signs in infants younger than 6 months of age correlated with the severity of their illness. Pediatrics 1991;88:1119–1124.

6 Baicker K, Chandra A. Medicare spending, the physician workforce, and beneficiaries' quality of care. Health Aff 7 April 2004:W4–W196.

7 World Organization of National Colleges of Physicians. *ICPC-2-R: International Classification of Primary Care*. Oxford: Oxford Medical Publications; 2005.

8 Stewart M, Brown JB, Weston WW, McWhinney IR, McWilliam CL, Freemna TR. *Patient Centred Medicine: Transforming the Clinical Method*. London: Sage; 1995.

9 Fry J, Sandler G. *Common Diseases: Their Nature, Prevalence and Care*. London: Petroc Press; 1993.

10 Peden AH. An overview of coding and its relationship to standardized clinical terminology. Top Health Inf Manage 2000;21:1–9.

11 Hofmans-Okkes IM, Lamberts H. The International Classification of Primary Care (ICPC): new applications in research and computer-based patient records in family practice. J Fam Pract 1996;13:294–302.

12 Henry SB, Mead CN. Nursing classification systems: necessary but not sufficient for representing 'what nurses do' for inclusion in computer-based patient record systems. J Am Med Inform Assoc 1997;4:222–232.

13 Moen A, Henry SB, Warren JJ. Representing nursing judgements in the electronic health record. J Adv Nurs 1999;30:990–997.

14 Slee VN, Slee D, Schmidt HJ. The tyranny of the diagnosis code. N C Med J 2005;66:331–337.

15 Marinker M. The chameleon, the judas goat, and the cuckoo. J R Coll Gen Pract 1978;28:199–206.

16 Fahey T, Webb E, Montgomery AA, Heyderman RS. Clinical management of urinary tract infection in women: a prospective cohort study. J Fam Pract 2003;20:1–6.

17 McIsaac WJ, Goel V, To T, Low DE. The validity of a sore throat score in family practice. CMAJ 2000;163:811–815.

18 Dionne CE, Bourbonnais R, Fremont P, Rossignol M, Stock SR, Larocque I. A clinical return-to-work rule for patients with back pain. CMAJ 2005;172:1559–1567.

19 Hay AD, Fahey T, Peters TJ, Wilson A. Predicting complications from acute cough in pre-school children in primary care: a prospective cohort study. Br J Gen Pract 2004;54:9–14.

20 Cayley WE, Jr. Diagnosing the cause of chest pain. Am Fam Physician 2005;72:2012–2021.

21 Wyatt JC. Decision support systems. J R Soc Med 2000;93:629–633.

22 Brokel JM, Shaw MG, Nicholson C. Expert clinical rules automate steps in delivering evidence-based care in the electronic health record. Comput Inform Nurs 2006;24:196–205.

23 Liu JL, Wyatt JC, Deeks JJ, et al. Systematic reviews of clinical decision tools for acute abdominal pain. Health Technol Assess 2006;10:1–186.

24 Coiera E, Westbrook J, Wyatt J. The safety and quality of decision support systems. Methods Inf Med 2006;45(suppl 1):20–25.

25 Sanders DL, Aronsky D. Biomedical informatics applications for asthma care: a systematic review. J Am Med Inform Assoc 2006;13:418–427.

26 Liu J, Wyatt JC, Altman DG. Decision tools in health care: focus on the problem, not the solution. BMC Med Inform Decis Mak 2006;6:4.

27 Cochrane A, Blythe M. *One Man's Memoirs.* London: BMJ Publications; 1989.

28 Greenhalgh T. Intuition and evidence – uneasy bedfellows? Br J Gen Pract 2002;52:395–400.

29 Benner P. *From Novice to Expert: Excellence and Power in Clinical Nursing Practice.* Menlo Park, California: Addison-Wessley; 1984.

30 Thompson C. A conceptual treadmill: the need for 'middle ground' in clinical decision making theory in nursing. J Adv Nurs 1999;30:1222–1229.

31 Paley J. Intuition and expertise: comments on the Benner debate. J Adv Nurs 1996;23:665–671.

32 Greenhalgh T. Narrative based medicine in an evidence based world. BMJ 1999;318:323–325.

33 Dreyfus HL, Dreyfus SE. *Mind Over Machine: The Power of Human Intuition and Expertise in the Era of the Computer.* Oxford: Blackwells; 1986.

34 Hunter K. 'Don't think zebras': uncertainty, interpretation, and the place of paradox in clinical education. Theor Med Bioeth 1996;17:225–241.

35 Boreham NC. Models of diagnosis and their implications for adult professional education. Stud Educ Adults 1988;20:95–108.

36 Cox K. Stories as case knowledge; case knowledge as stories. Med Educ 2001;816–818.

37 Eraut M. Non-formal learning, implicit learning and tacit knowledge. In: Coldfield F, ed. *Informal Learning.* Bristol: The Policy Press; 1999.

38 Macnaughton J. Anecdote in clinical practice. In: Greenhalgh T, Hurwitz B, eds. *Narrative Based Medicine: Dialogue and Discourse in Clinical Practice.* London: BMJ Publications; 1998.

39 Medawar P. *Induction and Intuition in Scientific Thought.* London: Methuen; 1969.

40 Engel GL. The biopsychosocial model and family medicine. J Fam Pract 1983;16:409,412–413.

41 Engel GL. The need for a new medical model: a challenge for biomedicine. Science 1977;196:129–136.

42 Balint M. *The Doctor, his Patient and the Illness.* London: Routledge; 1956.

43 Kleinman A, Eisenberg L, Good B. Culture, illness, and care: clinical lessons from anthropologic and cross-cultural research. Ann Intern Med 1978;88:251–258.

44 Al KN, Tyndale RF. Genetic influences on smoking: a brief review. Ther Drug Monit 2005;27:704–709.

45 David S, Lancaster T, Stead LF, Evins AE. Opioid antagonists for smoking cessation. Cochrane Database Syst Rev 2006;(4):CD003086.

46 de VH, Engels R, Kremers S, Wetzels J, Mudde A. Parents' and friends' smoking status as predictors of smoking onset: findings from six European countries. Health Educ Res 2003;18:627–636.

47 Madarasova GA, Stewart R, van Dijk JP, Orosova O, Groothoff JW, Post D. Influence of socio-economic status, parents and peers on smoking behaviour of adolescents. Eur Addict Res 2005;11:204–209.

48 Hapke U, Schumann A, Rumpf HJ, John U, Konerding U, Meyer C. Association of smoking and nicotine dependence with trauma and posttraumatic stress disorder in a general population sample. J Nerv Ment Dis 2005;193:843–846.

49 Haustein KO. Smoking and poverty. Eur J Cardiovasc Prev Rehabil 2006;13:312–318.

50 Jefferis B, Graham H, Manor O, Power C. Cigarette consumption and socio-economic circumstances in adolescence as predictors of adult smoking. Addiction 2003;98:1765–1772.

51 Warren CW, Jones NR, Eriksen MP, Asma S. Patterns of global tobacco use in young people and implications for future chronic disease burden in adults. Lancet 2006;367:749–753.

52 Buck D, Godfrey C, Sutton M. Economic and other views of addiction: implications for the choice of alcohol, tobacco and drug policies. Drug Alcohol Rev 1996;15:357–368.

53 Wild TC. Social control and coercion in addiction treatment: towards evidence-based policy and practice. Addiction 2006;101:40–49.

54 Greenbaum L, Kanyas K, Karni O, et al. Why do young women smoke? I: Direct and interactive effects of environment, psychological characteristics and nicotinic cholinergic receptor genes. Mol Psychiatry 2005;11:312–322.

55 Lerer E, Kanyas K, Karni O, Ebstein RP, Lerer B. Why do young women smoke? II: Role of traumatic life experience, psychological characteristics and serotonergic genes. Mol Psychiatry 2006;11:771–781.

56 Borrell-Carrio F, Suchman AL, Epstein RM. The biopsychosocial model 25 years later: principles, practice, and scientific inquiry. Ann Fam Med 2004;2:576–582.

57 Charles C, Gafni A, Whelan T. Shared decision-making in the medical encounter: what does it mean? (or it takes at least two to tango). Soc Sci Med 1997;44:681–692.

58 Elwyn G, Edwards A, Wensing M, Hood K, Atwell C, Grol R. Shared decision making: developing the OPTION scale for measuring patient involvement. Qual Saf Health Care 2003;12:93–99.

59 Makoul G, Clayman ML. An integrative model of shared decision making in medical encounters. Patient Educ Couns 2006;60:301–312.

60 Royal Pharmaceutical Society of Great Britain. From Compliance to Concordance. *Achieving Shared Goals in Medicine Taking.* London: RPSGB; 1997.

61 Stevenson FA, Barry CA, Britten N, Barber N, Bradley CP. Doctor-patient communication about drugs: the evidence for shared decision making. Soc Sci Med 2000;50:829–840.

62 Suurmond J, Seeleman C. Shared decision-making in an intercultural context. Barriers in the interaction between physicians and immigrant patients. Patient Educ Couns 2006;60:253–259.

63 Edwards A, Elwyn G. *Evidence Based Patient Choice.* Oxford: Oxford University Press; 2001.

64 Murray E, Charles C, Gafni A. Shared decision-making in primary care: tailoring the Charles et al. model to fit the context of general practice. Patient Educ Couns 2006;62:205–211.

65 Grilli R, Freemantle N, Minozzi S, Domenighetti G, Finer D. Mass media interventions: effects on health services utilisation. Cochrane Database Syst Rev 2000;(2):CD000389.

66 Davis D, O'Brien MA, Freemantle N, Wolf FM, Mazmanian P, Taylor-Vaisey A. Impact of formal continuing medical education: do conferences, workshops, rounds, and other traditional continuing education activities change physician behavior or health care outcomes? JAMA 1999;282:867–874.

67 Freemantle N, Harvey EL, Wolf F, Grimshaw JM, Grilli R, Bero LA. Printed educational materials: effects on professional practice and health care outcomes. Cochrane Database Syst Rev 2003;(2):CD000172.

68 Zwarenstein M, Reeves S, Barr H, Hammick M, Koppel I, Atkins J. Interprofessional education: effects on professional practice and health care outcomes. Cochrane Database Syst Rev 2001;(1):CD002213.

69 Thomson O'Brien MA, Oxman AD, Davis DA, Haynes RB, Freemantle N. Local opinion leaders. Cochrane Database Syst Rev 2000;(2):CD000125.

70 Grimshaw JM, Thomas RE, MacLennan G, et al. Effectiveness and efficiency of guideline dissemination and implementation strategies. Health Technol Assess 2004;8(6):iii–iv, 1–72.

71 Sibley JC, Sackett DL, Neufeld V, Gerrard B, Rudnick KV, Fraser W. A randomized trial of continuing medical education. N Engl J Med 1982;306:511–515.

72 Grol R. Improving the quality of medical care: building bridges among professional pride, payer profit, and patient satisfaction. JAMA 2001;286:2578–2585.

73 Haines A, Jones R. Implementing findings of research. BMJ 1994;308:1488–1492.

74 Dawson S. Never mind solutions: what are the issues? Lessons of industrial technology transfer for quality in health care. Qual Health Care 1995;4:197–203.

75 Delamothe T. Wanted: guidelines that doctors will follow. BMJ 1993;307:218.

76 Rogers EM. *Diffusion of Innovations*. 5th ed. New York: Free Press; 2003.

77 Hall GE, Hord SM. *Change in Schools*. Albany, New York: Stata University of New York Press; 1987.

78 Coleman JS, Katz E, Menzel H. *Medical Innovations: A Diffusion Study*. New York: Bobbs-Merrill; 1966.

79 Locock L, Dopson S, Chambers D, Gabbay J. Understanding the role of opinion leaders in improving clinical effectiveness. Soc Sci Med 2001;53:745–757.

80 Dopson S, Fitzgerald L. *Knowledge to Action? Evidence-based Health Care in Context*. Oxford: Oxford University Press; 2005.

81 Oxman AD, Thomson MA, Davis DA, Haynes RB. No magic bullets: a systematic review of 102 trials of interventions to improve professional practice. CMAJ 1995;153:1423–1431.

82 Dopson S, Fitzgerald L, Ferlie E, Gabbay J, Locock L. No magic targets. Changing clinical practice to become more evidence based. Health Care Manage Rev 2002;37:35–47.

83 O'Neill O. *A Question of Trust: The 2002 Reith Lectures*. Cambridge: Cambridge University Press; 2002.

84 Doctors in society. Medical professionalism in a changing world. Clin Med 2005;5(suppl 6):S5–40.

85 Hafferty FW. Definitions of professionalism: a search for meaning and identity. Clin Orthop Relat Res 2006;449:193–204.

86 Cruess SR, Johnston S, Cruess RL. 'Profession': a working definition for medical educators. Teach Learn Med 2004;16:74–76.

87 General Medical Council. *Good Medical Practice*. London: GMC; 2006.

88 General Medical Council. *A Licence to Practise and Revalidation*. London: GMC; 2003.

89 Pringle M. Regulation and revalidation of doctors. BMJ 2006;333:161–162.

90 Giddens A. *The Consequences of Modernity*. Cambridge: Polity Press; 1990.

91 Beck U. *Risk Society: Towards a New Modernity*. London: Sage; 1992.

92 Donaldson LJ. Clinical governance: a mission to improve. Clin Perform Qual Health Care 2000;8:6–8.

93 Rosen R. Clinical governance in primary care. Improving quality in the changing world of primary care. BMJ 2000;321:551–554.

94 Huntington J, Gillam S, Rosen R. Clinical governance in primary care: organisational development for clinical governance. BMJ 2000;321:679–682.

95 Vernon G. Virtue ethics. Br J Gen Pract 2003;53:60–61.

96 Armstrong AE. Towards a strong virtue ethics for nursing practice. Nurs Philos 2006;7:110–124.

97 van de CK, Vernooij-Dassen M, Grol R, Bottema B. Professionalism in general practice: development of an instrument to assess professional behaviour in general practitioner trainees. Med Educ 2006;40:43–50.

98 Winter RO, Birnberg BA. Teaching professionalism artfully. Fam Med 2006;38:169–171.

99 Stark P, Roberts C, Newble D, Bax N. Discovering professionalism through guided reflection. Med Teach 2006;28:e25–31.

100 Faunce T. Developing and teaching the virtue-ethics foundations of healthcare whistle blowing. Monash Bioeth Rev 2004;23:41–55.

101 Furlong E, Smith R. Advanced nursing practice: policy, education and role development. J Clin Nurs 2005;14:1059–1066.

102 Kidder MM, Cornelius PB. Licensure is not synonymous with professionalism: it's time to stop the hypocrisy. J Nurs Educ 2006;31:15–19.

103 Apker J, Propp KM, Zabava Ford WS, Hofmeister N. Collaboration, credibility, compassion, and coordination: professional nurse communication skill sets in health care team interactions. J Prof Nurs 2006;22:180–189.

104 Granier S, Owen P, Pill R, Jacobson L. Recognising meningococcal disease in primary care: qualitative study of how general practitioners process clinical and contextual information. BMJ 1998;316:276–279.

105 Wells LC, Smith JC, Weston VC, Collier J, Rutter N. The child with a non-blanching rash: how likely is meningococcal disease? Arch Dis Child 2001;85:218–222.

106 Casado-Flores J, Blanco-Quiros A, Nieto M, Asensio J, Fernandez C. Prognostic utility of the semi-quantitative procalcitonin test, neutrophil count and C-reactive protein in meningococcal infection in children. Eur J Pediatr 2006;165:26–29.

107 Hsieh C. Treatment of constipation in older adults. Am Fam Physician 2005;72:2277–2284.

108 Remes-Troche JM, Rao SS. Defecation disorders: neuromuscular aspects and treatment. Curr Gastroenterol Rep 2006;8:291–299.

109 Zimmermann PG. Assessment of abdominal pain in school-age children. J Sch Nurs 2003;19:4–10.

110 Drachman DA. Occam's razor, geriatric syndromes, and the dizzy patient. Ann Intern Med 2000;132:403–404.

111 Sandars J, Esmail A. The frequency and nature of medical error in primary care: understanding the diversity across studies. J Fam Pract 2003;20:231–236.

112 Anonymous. The science of making mistakes. Lancet 1996;345:871–872.

113 Ashby D, Smith AF. Evidence-based medicine as Bayesian decision-making. Stat Med 2000;19:3291–3305.

114 Rietveld RP, ter RG, Bindels PJ, Sloos JH, van Weert HC. Predicting bacterial cause in infectious conjunctivitis: cohort study on informativeness of combinations of signs and symptoms. BMJ 2004;329:206–210.

CHAPTER 6

The clinical interaction

Summary points

1 This chapter presents four contrasting perspectives from which to conceptualise and analyse the clinician–patient relationship: interaction analysis, sociolinguistic analysis, psychodynamic analysis and narrative analysis. A final section illustrates how a topic (in this case, the interpreted consultation) can be richly illuminated by drawing on all these perspectives (and others).

2 Interaction analysis (Section 6.1), which has roots in cognitive psychology, owes much to the work of Debra Roter whose coding system is extensively used in the analysis of clinician–patient consultations. Using transcripts or videotapes of interviews, sections of text (and, potentially, non-verbal communications too) are coded first into 'socio-emotional' and 'task-oriented' and then into more refined categories such as 'shows concern' or 'gives information'. In this way, the consultation can be classified according to the proportion of time spent on each type of interaction. Research using interaction analysis systems can correlate such findings with process variables such as consultation length and outcome measures such as patient satisfaction.

3 Conversation analysis (Section 6.2), whose theoretical roots are in discourse analysis and sociolinguistics, arguably takes a more critical view of talk, which is seen as not always what it appears to be. Based on the work of critical philosophers (notably Habermas) and sociologists (notably Scambler and Britten), conversation analysis seeks to interpret talk within its wider context, especially the power relations of the clinical relationship and the social system, through close analysis of words chosen, pauses, interruptions and so on.

4 Psychodynamic analysis of the clinical consultation (Section 6.3) is based on the work of Michael Balint, who believed that trivial and 'inexplicable' complaints are the main vehicle through which emotional problems are presented to the doctor. The key to healing in this type of illness is the persona of the doctor and the quality of the therapeutic relationship: the so-called 'doctor as the drug' effect.

5 A narrative perspective on the clinical interaction must go beyond the idea that the patient has a story to tell. The illness narrative is a dialogue, not a monologue, and therein lies its transformative potential. The patient constructs a more coherent, illuminative, hopeful and courageous narrative – and may even create a different self – through his or her awareness of, and trust in, the perspective of the clinician who is privileged to hear his or her story.

(Continued)

(Summary points continued)

6 An increasing proportion of consultations in primary care occur across a language (and cultural) barrier. Such consultations can be analysed through a number of different theoretical lenses, including biomedical, psychological, sociological and economic. I argue that a sociological analysis of the interpreted consultation is particularly illuminating because of the complex power relations and role ambiguities involved.

6.1   The clinical interaction I: a psychological perspective

Both the doctor–patient relationship, traditionally defined in terms of curing, and the nurse–patient relationship, traditionally defined in terms of caring, are easily romanticised. McWhinney talks of the family doctor's 'healing involvement', defined in terms of 'attention' and 'presence' and of the 'spirituality' (i.e. 'a sense of awe and deep meaning'), that characterises in the bond between clinician and patient.[1] Nursing academics have talked variously about 'caring presence',[2] 'nurturance'[3] and 'therapeutic touch'.[4] Psychotherapists such as Carl Rogers seek 'client-centredness' – a combination of empathy, respect, genuineness, unconditional acceptance and warmth.[5] Medical sociologist Arthur Frank celebrates 'just listening'[6] and physician WL Miller describes the 'clinical hand', including the symbolic opening of the hand to allow power-sharing, the 'palm of hope' and the 'fingers of direction'.[7] Is there more to all this than a warm feeling inside? What are the appropriate theoretical lenses through which to study the clinician–patient interaction? How should we conceptualise this interaction – and how might we research it?

One of the most widely used research designs for studying clinical interaction is interaction analysis. The underlying conceptual model here, which has its roots in cognitive psychology, is that any contribution to an interpersonal communication (a statement, a question, a particular body language) can be classified in terms of the purpose it serves. Very broadly, interaction in the clinical consultation can be divided into (a) 'care' talk – affective or socio-emotional interaction, for example, building the therapeutic relationship and (b) 'cure' talk – instrumental or task-focused interaction oriented to preventing, diagnosing or treating disease. Different interaction analysis tools use different modifications of this basic classification. The most popular instrument in healthcare research, the RIAS or Roter interaction analysis system (see www.rais.org), developed by US psychologist Debra Roter, is shown in Box 6.1. Most research based on RIAS analyses verbal interaction using either audiotaped or videotaped consultations, but if videotape is used, non-verbal communication (e.g. smiling, eye contact) can be coded using the same system.

The RIAS has been used in over 100 research studies on doctor–patient (and occasionally, nurse–patient) communication. If you plan to use this approach in your own research, you should study the online manual carefully before embarking on any fieldwork. You should also look up examples of previous research studies that have used RIAS, for example,

---

Box 6.1 Examples of coding categories in the Roter interaction analysis system.

Socio-Emotional Exchange

Personal remarks, social conversation
Laughs, tells jokes
Shows concern or worry
Reassures, encourages or shows optimism
Shows approval
Shows disapproval
Shows agreement or understanding
Asks for reassurance

Task-Focused Exchange

Structural
– Gives orientation or instructions
– Paraphrases or checks for understanding
– Medical condition
– Gives information
– Asks open question
– Asks closed question
Therapeutic regimen (subcategories as above)
Lifestyle (subcategories as above)
Counsels or directs behaviour (subcategories as above)
Asks for medication

This list, given for illustration, is not exhaustive and should not be used to code research data. Interested readers should consult the RIAS website www.rias.org.

• A study of 'hand on the doorknob...' behaviour – that is interaction in the closing moments of a consultation when the doctor thinks the encounter is finishing but the patient still has business to raise[8];
• A study from the USA of how the balance of different types of interaction in the consultation is linked to malpractice claims (in a nutshell, clinicians who had never been sued tended to use more humour, gave more orientation so that the patients knew what to expect, encouraged patients to talk more and checked understanding more)[9];
• An example of how the RIAS can be used in professional assessment – in this case, using simulated cancer patients to assess nurses' communication skills[10];
• A large study based on over 2000 videotaped consultations across six countries, comparing communication styles of doctors and relating these to diagnostic category of the main complaint[11];
• Studies of triadic consultations such as clinician–patient-relative[12,13] or clinician–patient-interpreter[14] (see Section 6.5 for further discussion of the latter);

• Studies of how clinician–patient interaction changes with the use of technology[15,16];
• Studies of patient-centredness based on Stewart and McWhinney's patient-centred clinical method.[17,18]

To some extent, different interaction analysis tools are distinguishable mainly by the extent to which they emphasise the instrumental or 'cure' aspects of the exchange over the affective or 'care' aspects. Instruments developed within mainstream cognitive psychology, with some exceptions, have tended to see the clinical encounter as largely task-oriented and emphasise 'cure' exchanges; those developed by clinicians (especially by nurses and general practitioners) tend to be more care-oriented. Table 6.1 shows some examples of different interaction analysis systems; for a more detailed taxonomy of such instruments, see two excellent reviews.[25,26]

In my view, all the tools listed in Table 6.1, and the many more covered in the above reviews, have more similarities than differences. Whilst research has shown very clearly that they are measuring different things (i.e. scores on any of these instruments correlate poorly with one another), they are all psychometric tools of one sort or another and they all involve a researcher coding clinical talk or non-verbal behaviour into a set of finite categories based on a cognitive-psychological classification system. 'Quality' in this sort of research is defined using psychometric terms such as

• Construct validity: Does the instrument measure what it sets out to measure – for example is 'patient-centredness' as measured by the Henbest and Stewart instrument really a measure of how far the patient is central in an interaction in the study?
• Content validity: Does what the instrument measures map to what is needed in the real world – for example, does patient-centredness as measured with this instrument in a research study correlate with what real patients see as 'putting them in the centre' in real consultations?
• Reliability: Does the instrument give the same score when used by different researchers (inter-rater reliability) or by the same researcher on different days (intra-rater reliability)?
• Parsimony: Is the instrument as short and user-friendly as it can be?

Interaction analysis tools are often used in combination with other psychometric instruments – notably patient satisfaction questionnaires[27–29] – which can also be 'quality-assured' in relation to the psychometric dimensions of validity and reliability and which can serve as an outcome measure in intervention studies to improve the quality of the clinician–patient interaction. Two alternative research designs within this tradition, for example, might be (a) an observational study in which audiotaped consultations are scored for patient-centredness and patients also asked to complete a satisfaction questionnaire; correlation analysis would test the hypothesis that patients who had more patient-centred interaction would be more satisfied or (b) a trial in which clinicians were randomised to receive training in patient-centred consulting, with patient satisfaction as an outcome measure.

Table 6.1 Examples of interaction analysis tools for analysing the clinician–patient consultation.

Name of tool	Key characteristics	Comment
Roter interaction analysis system[19]	Designed by a US psychologist for general medical and primary care consultations; distinguishes social/affective vs. task-oriented interactions. See Box 6.2 for examples of coding categories	The most widely used tool for analysing doctor–patient interaction. See text for examples
Verona psychiatric interview classification system[20]	Designed by Italian psychiatrists for mental health consultations	Used in training GPs in care of mental health patients
Patient-centredness instrument[17,18]	Based on Stewart et al.'s 'holistic' framework for patient-centred medicine (see Section 5.4); classifies consulting style into 'doctor-centred' and 'patient-centred'	Used extensively in primary care research
Communication scale for observational measurement (RCS-O)[21]	As above, but focusing on non-verbal communication. Developed by educators for use in objective structured clinical examination (OSCE) examinations, hence uses observer evaluations rather than analysis of recorded text	New instrument; used in teaching and assessment of medical students
Four habits coding scheme[22]	Another OSCE-oriented tool. Considers four 'habits': (a) Invest in the beginning (i.e. establish a good relationship), (b) elicit the patient's perspective, (c) demonstrate empathy, (d) invest in the end (i.e. achieve satisfactory closure)	Used extensively by Kaiser Permanente in USA to develop doctors' communication skills
OPTION scale of patient involvement[23]	Based on the model of shared decision making developed by Edwards and Elwyn,[24] evaluates level of patient involvement in clinical decisions in four dimensions: (a) defining and agreeing on the problem, (b) explaining that legitimate choices exist, (c) portraying options and communicating risk, (d) making or deferring the decision	Recently developed scale with promising psychometric properties

See Ong et al. for a more comprehensive taxonomy.[25]

Critiques of interaction analysis tools that are published from within the discipline of cognitive psychology (or a secondary discipline derived from its theories) tend to question the psychometric properties of a particular instrument or suggest how it might be adapted or refined.[30] More fundamental critiques of these tools, which generally come from disciplines outside psychology, question the worth of any psychometric instrument in assessing the complexity of clinician–patient interaction or meaningfully influencing it. Scambler and Britten, for example, have criticised psychologically driven research on doctor–patient consultations for being both under-theorised (studies are driven by a somewhat naïve and positivist search for a list of 'factors' that predict particular 'outcomes') and de-contextualised (the consultation is taken as a fixed unit of analysis without regard to the social or institutional context within which it is embedded).[31] Ong et al.'s review, for example, undertaken from a cognitive perspective, discusses such psychometric constructs as 'privacy behaviour', 'controlling behaviour', 'use of medical vocabulary', 'patient recall of information' and 'patient satisfaction'.[25] But such constructs do not allow for 'upstream' questions such as 'what is the nature of the social context that engenders the use of controlling behaviour?', 'what is not being said here and why?' and even 'who has not consulted the clinician at all, and why?'.

In other words, if the research question concerns the interaction within the clinical consultation *and nothing more*, the approaches described in this section are ideal for addressing it – but they have less utility in other contexts. In the next three sections, I will consider some alternative approaches to analysing clinical interaction – using sociolinguistic, psychodynamic and literary perspectives – which offer the opportunity to move the level of analysis of the consultation from the clinical dyad itself to the context in which that dyad is nested.

6.2   The clinical interaction II: a sociolinguistic perspective

A related, but I believe conceptually and theoretically distinct, approach to the study of clinical interaction is sociolinguistic analysis, which draws on the interface between sociology (the study of social roles, identity and interaction) and linguistics (the study of language). As with interaction analysis (see previous section), the focus of research is typically the consultation, and the usual research method is analysis of audiotaped or (preferably) videotaped encounters. The key theoretical difference between sociolinguistic analysis and psychological interaction analysis is that in the former, talk is seen as fundamentally *social*, and the researcher consciously and explicitly asks *why* particular utterances were made in a particular way at a particular time. Such questions require that the analysis move beyond what is said within the consultation itself to consider the social context and power relationships within which 'what is said' gains a particular, contextual meaning.

One theoretical perspective relevant to the study of meaning in human interaction is symbolic interactionism, most commonly associated with the name of George Herbert Mead. It was Herbert Blumer who took Mead's embryonic theory and developed it into one that had depth and coherence. In Blumer's words:

> 'The term 'symbolic interaction' refers, of course, to the peculiar and distinctive character of interaction as it takes place between human beings. The peculiarity consists in the fact that human beings interpret or 'define' each other's actions instead of merely reacting to each other's actions. Their 'response' is not made directly to the actions of one another but instead is based on the meaning which they attach to such actions. Thus, human interaction is mediated by the use of symbols, by interpretation, or by ascertaining the meaning of one another's actions. This mediation is equivalent to inserting a process of interpretation between stimulus and response in the case of human behavior'.[32,p.180]

The theory of symbolic interactionism rests on three core concepts. The first is that of meaning. Humans act towards people and things based upon the meanings that they have given to those people or things. Meaning is thus central to human behaviour. This may not seem so surprising, but when Mead originally introduced this idea, psychology (including social psychology) was still focusing mainly on stimulus–response theories. The concept of meaning required the 'stimulus' to be interpreted before the response was initiated. The second core concept is language. Language gives humans a means by which to negotiate meaning through symbols. This meaning is assigned through naming and engaging in 'speech acts' – that is a socially meaningful act that a speaker performs when making an utterance (such as conferring a knighthood with the command 'rise, Sir Lancelot', or terminating a consultation with the words 'here's your prescription Mrs Brown'). It is by engaging in speech acts with others (symbolic interaction) that humans come to identify meaning and develop discourse. The third core concept in symbolic interactionism is that of thought. Thought modifies each person's interpretation of symbols. Thought, which is of course based on language, is a mental conversation or dialogue that requires role taking or imagining different points of view. Whilst remarkably few research studies in primary care draw explicitly on the theory of symbolic interactionism, the notion that clinical talk is imbued with symbolic meaning (and must be studied closely, and in context, to draw out that meaning) is fundamental to the sociolinguistic study of the consultation.

   Another theory that can be applied to the sociolinguistic study of the consultation, for example, by sociologists Nicky Britten and Graham Scambler,[31,33] is the theory of communicative action developed by the German philosopher and social theorist Jurgen Habermas. Like the symbolic interactionists, Habermas believed that talk must be interpreted within its wider social context and was especially interested in the power relations of the interpersonal relationship and in the wider social system that generated and legitimated these power relationships. He is not the easiest of modern philosophers to comprehend (indeed, he has been described as one of the most impenetrable) but I believe that his theory of communicative action is crucial to understanding the primary care consultation, so I will spend some time explaining it here.

In the theory of communicative action, Habermas makes three important distinctions:
• Between communicative and strategic action;
• Between lifeworld and system;
• Between 'micro' (interpersonal) and 'macro' (socio-political) levels of analysis.

Communicative action is talk that is sincere and which has mutual understanding and consensus as its goal. Strategic action, on the other hand, has a more devious purpose. It occurs when at least one party instrumentalises speech for what might be called an ulterior motive. There are two types of strategic action: (a) open, in which a speaker openly pursues an aim of influencing the hearer(s), and there is an associated claim to power (as in giving an order to a subordinate) and (b) concealed, in which there is confusion between actions oriented to understanding and actions oriented to success, resulting in what Habermas calls communication pathologies. It usually involves either conscious or unconscious deception.

Let's assume for the moment that an instance of communicative action is occurring. The parties will make various claims whose validity is criticisable – that is, it will be possible to claim for each communication that it is true or not true, appropriate or inappropriate, justifiable or unjustifiable (all of which can be argued out through counter-claims), and also that it is sincere or not sincere (which may require practical demonstration or some other external evidence). In other words, if (and only to the extent that) talk is characterised by genuine communicative action on both sides, in a context in which each trusts the sincerity of the other, the questions and statements exchanged are likely to increase mutual understanding and bring the parties towards consensus (even if that consensus is agreeing to differ).

Let me give you some hypothetical examples. When I telephone my mother, who is a churchgoing 80-year-old, and ask what she has been doing today, I'm pretty sure I can count on her to tell the truth, and also to select aspects of her day that I would be interested in. That's because I know from years of phoning up my mother that she has never yet misled me about her activities, nor do I know of any reason why she might do so. Most of the time, our conversation can be described as communicative action – with an exception being perhaps when my mother has been out to buy me a birthday present but does not want to spoil the surprise, so she pretends to have been at home all day. On these rare occasions, she would be engaging in strategic action (not by lying, but by steering the conversation away from things she doesn't want me to ask about).

When I ask my son what happened to him at school today, I am less confident that I will hear an account that he views as the whole truth and nothing but the truth. He might, for example, wish to cover up the fact that he has flunked a test. He would then engage in concealed strategic action ('concealed' because I am not aware of his motives or strategies – but he is) by telling me all sorts of irrelevant news and deliberately withholding the fact that he has taken a test. If I later discover (perhaps from checking his books) that my son has indeed flunked a test, I might order him to his bedroom, thereby using my power as a parent to engage in open strategic action ('open' because both he and I are well aware that I am instrumentalising speech for the purpose of inflicting a punishment).

There is one more type of strategic action, which is especially important to the study of communication between doctors and patients, which is when there is deception going on but the deceiver is not consciously aware of it. Let's say my mother has been having some chest pains, but as someone who lived through the Second World War, she holds the view that one should not bother the doctor unnecessarily and, more generally, that one should not make a fuss about trivial matters. When my mother attends the doctor for a blood pressure check, she might be asked very explicitly if she has been having any chest pain, and might say something like 'Oh no dear, nothing serious', believing this statement to be entirely genuine. This is an example of *unconscious* deception, also termed 'systematically distorted communication' by Habermas. It occurs when at least one party is deceiving themselves that they are acting with an attitude oriented to the success of the conversation – and, as you might imagine, it is more common when there are large power differentials and when people's perceptions have been influenced by wider social forces.

Now, let us consider Habermas' distinction between 'lifeworld' and 'system', which has had considerable influence in primary care research. 'The lifeworld' represents family and household and is generally characterised by communicative action. 'The system' is the world of economy and state, characterised by strategic action oriented around money and power, respectively. When economy and state intrude in inappropriate and unaccountable ways into the lifeworld, they can be said to 'colonise' it.

The final contribution of Habermas' theory of communicative action is its ability to bring together the 'micro' of interpersonal relationships with the 'macro' of society and state. In other words, a Habermasian analysis of the consultation looks at both the clinician–patient interaction *and* the wider socio-political context within which that interaction is nested. I discuss this in more depth in Section 6.5 in relation to interpreted consultations. For a more in-depth analysis of the work of Habermas in relation to primary care, see Graham Scambler's excellent book.[33]

If we accept that conversation is not always what it appears to be and that there are situations where the researcher should 'zoom out' from the text of the consultation and ask what might be called political questions, how might he or she go about this? One technique that is becoming popular in primary care research is conversation analysis (which is one application of a wider technique called discourse analysis). Conversation analysis was first applied to clinical consultations by sociologist Elliot Mishler, whose elegant demonstration that the patient's lifeworld is partially colonised by the 'voice of medicine' (an example of encroachment by the state into the personal world) is one of the all-time great studies in medical sociology.[34] A subsequent paper by Barry et al. both confirmed and refined Mishler's original model.[35]

Box 6.2 An example of conversation analysis.

001	M1	D	Hm Hm... now what do you mean by a sour stomach?
002		P	......what's a sour stomach? A heartburn, like a heartburn or something
003	M2	D	[Does it burn over here?
005		P	Yea:h. It li- I think I think it like- if you take a needle and stick
006			ya right ... there's a pain right here
007		D	[Hm hm Hm hm [Hm hm
009		P	and and then it goes from here on this side to this side
010	M3	D	Hm hm. Does it go into the back?

....

016	M	D	How- how soon after you eat it?
017	M	P	.... Wel:l
018			......probably an hour .... maybe less
			[
019	M	D	About an hour?
020		P	Maybe less
021	L		................I've cheated and I've been drinking which I
022	L		shouldn't have done
			[
023	M	D	......Does drinking make it worse

See Box 6.3 for a glossary of notation.
From Mishler[34] (page 84), reproduced from original citation in Barry et al.[37]

Box 6.3 Symbols used in conversation analysis.

- Brackets containing a stop (.) indicate a pause of less than two seconds
- Numerals in round brackets indicate the length in seconds of other pauses
- Square brackets [ ] contain relevant contextual information or unclear phrases
- Italicized square brackets *[.]* describe a non-verbal utterance
- The symbol [in between lines of dialogue, indicates overlapping speech
- Underlining signifies emphasis
- An equal sign = means that the phrase is contiguous with the preceding phrase without pause
- A colon : indicates elongation of the preceding sound
- D is the doctor
- P is the patient

Mishler uses the notation 'L' for the voice of the lifeworld and 'M' for the voice of medicine.

Reproduced with original authors' permission.[38]

A characteristic of conversation analysis that distinguishes it from the inter-action analysis systems described in Section 6.1 is the level of detail required for coding and analysing each utterance, which Mishler saw as essential to the quality of the research.[36] Box 6.2, for example, shows a consultation frag-ment originally published in Mishler's early work on conversation analysis and subsequently quoted by Barry et al., who comment as follows:

> '. . . the [apparently] unremarkable interview, while appearing coherent and fluent on the surface, fragments meaning by means of frequent interruption, lack of acknowl-edgement of responses and shifts of topic with no reason given. The doctor is in control as both first and last speaker in each exchange. Only the doctor is involved in devel-oping the topic of talk, by asking a series of seemingly (to the patient) disconnected questions. This inhibits the patient from playing a role in maintaining conversational flow. Through these structures the doctor maintains a strong control over the devel-opment of the interview. However, the cost is a loss of context in terms of how the problem developed (the history and course) and the effects on the patient's life'.[37]

This commentary illustrates how a sociolinguistic analysis of the consulta-tion can reveal a political (i.e. relating to power) dimension to the consulta-tion. Such a dimension is largely, though not entirely, inaccessible using the more conventional interaction analysis described in Section 6.1. I discuss the power dimension again in Section 6.5 when I talk about interpreted consul-tations. The technical detail of how to undertake a sociolinguistic analysis of a transcript of an interaction – and even how to transcribe the interaction in the first place – is beyond the scope of this book, but if you are interested in pursuing this approach, I recommend Elwyn and Edwards' introductory chapter,[38] Mishler's methodological textbook[36] and the paper by Barry et al. which offers a perspective that builds on Mishler's original approach.[37] If you are confused by the idea of a political analysis of the consultation and are look-ing for a very basic introduction to sociolinguistic conversation analysis, try the recent paper by Maynard, which was written for an audience of medical educators.[39]

6.3   The clinical interaction III: a psychodynamic perspective

The model of clinical interaction most closely associated with British gen-eral practice is a psychodynamic one, developed by Hungarian psycholo-gist Michael Balint and based (very broadly) on psychoanalytic concepts and theories.[40] Because most people have firm (and perhaps stereotypical) views on what a psychoanalytic perspective is, it may be helpful to start by being clear about what it isn't. The conventional psychological perspective that underpins the approach described in Section 6.1 is essentially cognitive in nature – that is, it implies a rational self that weighs up pros and cons of potential actions, makes a decision how to act and then takes action. Cognitive theories in general are based on the assumption that such things as beliefs, attitudes, values and desires can be readily articulated and measured (e.g. by asking people what they believe, value or desire). Psychoanalytic theory is very different. Although the term often conjures up images of middle-class Victorian women reclining on couches recounting bizarre sexual fantasies in an old-fashioned, paternalistic and somewhat obscure clinical context, sex per se is not a fundamental tenet of psychoanalytic theory. Let me try to explain what the fundamentals really are.

Psychoanalysis was a practice before it was a theory. Freud's clinical experiences in managing hysterical paralysis and other clinical problems led him to develop a theoretical framework for analysing the behaviour of individuals,[41] groups[42] and society[43] which included the following key concepts:

• *The unconscious* – forces which lie beneath the conscious, knowing self has a powerful influence on both feelings and behaviour;

• *The role of emotion* – in linking unconscious forces and enacted behaviour – we act (or fail to act) because we feel anxious, angry or desperate for love;

• *The powerful influence of the past* – particularly that experiences in infancy and early childhood produce unfulfilled desires that drive behaviour;

• *Free association* – the unconscious can be accessed via a technique in which the patient relaxes and reports whatever ideas come up spontaneously;

• *Symbolism in dreams* – the symbolic, manifest content of a dream provides clues to its latent content of uncomfortable or frightening unconscious impulses;

• *Repression* – painful impulses are forced aside before we become aware of their existence;

• *Neurosis* – repressed impulses are expressed as maladaptive behaviour which the individual is unable to control or explain;

• *Transference* – in all emotionally charged situations we treat people in ways that are coloured by early emotional experience.

Freud proposed that human motivation can be explained in terms of the unconscious conflict between the pleasure principle of immediate gratification (the libido drive) and the reality principle which demands adjustment to an external world (the ego drive). We do things either to gain pleasure or to survive. Whether the darker side of the unconscious is chiefly concerned with the gratification of genital sex (as Freud believed), the oral gratification of the breast (Klein), social success and influence (Adler), life energy in general (Jung) or language and symbolic power (Lacan), psychoanalysis holds that something beyond reason and rationality determines much of human behaviour.

Psychoanalytic theory – in an adapted form – underpins the famous work of Michael Balint on the doctor–patient relationship. Balint was a Hungarian refugee who fled to Britain during the Second World War and rose to become President of the British Psychoanalytic Society. With his wife Enid Balint, he ran the famous Discussion Group Seminars on Psychological Problems in General Practice (universally referred to as 'Balint groups') for general practitioners (GPs), in which they were encouraged to reflect on cases they had seen in order to reveal the hidden meaning of the emotions they had felt and the behaviour that had been exhibited by both doctor and patient. Balint's contribution to the academic basis of general practice was immense, since he was (arguably) the only leader around when British general practice was emerging as a discipline in its own right and defining itself as separate from hospital medicine. As Osborne has observed, Balint's input was so influential that it can be thought of as 'highlighting ... the psychotherapeutic aspects of general practice so that they became actually definitive of general practice itself'.[44]

There were three key elements to Balint's application of psychoanalytic theory to general practice:

a Unlike hospital medicine, general practice is flooded with what a psychoanalyst would call 'neurotic illness' – that is, with symptoms that can be traced back to repression of one sort or another;

b Trivial and 'inexplicable' complaints are the main vehicle through which this type of illness is presented to the doctor; and

c The key to healing in this type of illness is the persona of the doctor and the quality of the therapeutic relationship – that is, such patients need, more than anything else, a dose of Balint's famous remedy 'the doctor as the drug'.[40] In his words (cited in Osborne[44]):

> '*I wish to state that the tool in psychotherapy – the counterpart to the surgeon's knife or the radiologists's X-ray apparatus – is the doctor himself ... he must learn to use himself as skilfully as the surgeon uses his knife, the physician his stethoscope and the radiologist his lamp*'.[40]

Balint, who was based at London's famous Tavistock Centre for most of his professional life, was well aware that in the clinical relationship, objectivity is not merely an over-rated virtue but inherently impossible to achieve; it is the doctor's *subjectivity* that is the key to both making the diagnosis and defining an appropriate treatment. When the doctor feels angry during a consultation, or when he or she observes anger in a patient, that emotional response should (if you will forgive me for borrowing some terminology from epidemiology) be treated as 'data'. Statements such as 'I experience your story as painful' or 'You seem to be disappointed' will begin to expose the emotions that may, in turn, lead to the underlying neurosis being revealed. The key to effective clinical interaction in general practice, Balint believed, is a complex dialogue held over time and in an atmosphere of trust, which will reveal to both doctor and patient insights into the nature of the illness and offer scope for its cure.

Balint believed passionately that all GPs must take part in research. But what he meant by 'research' was a continuous and searching reflection on their own personality as it influences their clinical relationships – in other words, the GP must go through a limited course in psychoanalysis in order to discover what sort of doctor he or she really is. Osborne cites this perspective on professional development as an example of what Max Weber called 'charismatic education' – instead of seeking to acquire specific knowledge or technical skills, GPs should focus on the controlled cultivation of personal qualities.

The detailed theory of psychoanalysis and how it can be applied in primary care is beyond the scope of this book. For the interested reader, I recommend Osborne's article[44] as well as Michael Balint's original textbook,[40] Enid Balint's research study of doctor–patient interaction in general practice,[45] John Launer's *Narrative Based Primary Care* which takes a psychotherapeutic view of narrative[46] and a recently published textbook on emotional problems in primary care.[47] There is also a large literature on counselling, with which I am not familiar, which I suspect will contain much of relevance to this perspective.

Whether or not you are naturally drawn to the psychoanalytic perspective on the consultation, you will probably see the value of such a perspective in two very practical areas of primary care. The first is the challenge of 'connecting' with the patient. In your clinical work, you will almost certainly have found that you 'click' better with some patients than with others, and that in a few cases (usually people you are seeing for the first time) you fail to connect at all. Why does the interpersonal bond that we sometimes refer to as 'reciprocity' sometimes prove so elusive? Psychoanalytic theory would say that before all else, we must demonstrate our humanness. McWhinney describes a surgeon colleague whose own son sadly died of a sarcoma in his own hospital. Years later, he was facing an elderly lady, inconsolable over the death of her daughter and lacking the will to go on living. Having made several attempts to connect with her, the surgeon suddenly disclosed, 'Do you know, my son died in this room'. The next day, the woman got dressed, put on her make-up and walked out of the hospital to get on with her life. Michael and Enid Balint would call this turning point a 'flash' – a connectional experience of profound closeness and intimacy. We have probably all experienced such moments, which are difficult to articulate, and perhaps a psychoanalytic perspective comes closest to offering a plausible explanation for why they are so powerful.

The other area where a psychoanalytic perspective may prove especially useful is in the study of 'difficult patients', who might be defined as those we find it impossible to connect with and where 'flash' moments are especially sparse. In an article that would now be classified (rightly!) as politically incorrect, Groves originally labelled such individuals as 'hateful patients' and produced a taxonomy of four categories: dependent clingers (excessively dependent on the doctor and tend to use flattery to get what they want), entitled demanders (articulate, demanding, view the doctor as the barrier to them receiving 'rightful' specialist referrals or prescriptions), manipulative help-rejectors (persist in seeking help but if a treatment if offered, find a way of blocking it) and self-destructive deniers (refuse to change an unhealthy lifestyle).[48] This early classification, though often cited, has a weak intellectual basis and is (arguably) little more than the ossified prejudices of a paternalistic physician. But Groves did have the insight to comment that *'The physician's negative reactions constitute important clinical data that should facilitate better understanding and more appropriate psychological management for each'*.

Subsequent work on 'heartsink' patients included systematic studies of precisely what sort of patients doctors found 'difficult' (to which the answer was

often those with chronic unhappiness, complex psychosocial issues, medically unexplained symptoms or all of the above)[49–51] and what measures
might be taken to support doctors in looking after such patients.[52,53] More
recently, efforts have been made to theorise the symptoms of heartsink patients (often described as 'somatising'), the clinical interaction with such patients, and 'diagnostic' reasoning using concepts derived from (or aligned to)
psychoanalysis.[54–56] In short, the kind of reflexive self-awareness prompted
by Balint and his successors may make the clinician better able to manage the
encounter with a patient with medically unexplained symptoms – and perhaps
move the clinical relationship towards productive dialogue.

6.4   The clinical interaction IV: a literary perspective

It is no coincidence that 'the case' as recounted in story form was the focus of
discussion in Balint groups,[40] nor that Arthur Frank views illness in terms of
story, and story not as a disembodied text but in terms of a narrator–listener
relationship.[6] In this section, I offer a different theoretical perspective on the
clinician–patient interaction, which draws centrally on literary theory. As other
sections in this chapter show, this is not the only (nor indeed the most commonly used) approach to the study of clinical interaction, but it is one that I
find particularly revealing in both clinical practice and research.

  Box 6.4 shows a fictionalised (and much shortened) version of a real consultation between a patient (Mrs Dunn) and her GP (Dr Patel), which I first used
in a monograph on narrative in illness and healthcare.[57] It illustrates the point
that what is increasingly referred to as 'the patient's narrative' is a dialogue,
not a monologue. At the beginning of the consultation, Mrs Dunn appears lost
for words. Dr Patel invites her to tell her story but she has, it seems, no clear
story to recount. Her non-specific symptom (tiredness) is linked with a general sense of confusion about associated events ('this and that'). The GP offers
a nudge ('Mmmh?') and then a prompt ('How's the family?'), to which she
responds in a poignantly non-committal way. The GP then attempts to lead
the narrative along the lines of a routine biomedical check-up (in this case, for
asthma), but Mrs Dunn inserts a cue ('I didn't keep the appointment [because]
I wasn't feeling well'), which indicates that she does not intend this to be a
straightforward 'check-up' narrative. Indeed, Mrs Dunn's implication that not
feeling well required her to miss the asthma check-up suggests quite explicitly
that the illness to be attended to was not asthma. The doctor picks up on the
cue ('Uh-huh?') and using various follow-up prompts ('Oh yes' and 'Tell me
more') supports the patient in constructing the beginnings of a very different
narrative – that of domestic violence.

  In this example, Dr Patel is neither conventionally 'directive' (asking a series of questions which the patient is expected to answer) nor conventionally
'non-directive' (allowing the patient to make every move in the conversation).
Towards the end of the excerpt, for example, he asks very directly, 'Did anyone hit you?', a question which Mrs Dunn appears not to resent (indeed, according to qualitative research studies on the topic, she probably welcomes

---

Box 6.4 A consultation fragment.

Dr Patel	Hello Mrs Dunn, what can I do for you?
Mrs Dunn	*[pause]*
	To be honest I'm not sure. Tired all the time, this and that.
Dr Patel	Mmm?
Mrs Dunn	*[silent]*
Dr Patel	How's the family?
Mrs Dunn	Oh, so-so.
	[another pause]
Dr Patel	Is this a routine asthma check?
Mrs Dunn	*[shakes head]* I know I'm due for that but...
Dr Patel	...Yes, you are. We changed your inhalers last time, didn't we? And I asked you to see the nurse.
Mrs Dunn	*[looking down]* I didn't keep that appointment. I wasn't feeling well....
Dr Patel	Uh huh?
Mrs Dunn	...No. I'd hurt my eye.
Dr Patel	Oh yes?
Mrs Dunn	Just a bit of bruising, nothing too serious. It's better now.
Dr Patel	*[putting his pen down and looking at her]* Tell me more.
Mrs Dunn	*[cries]*
Dr Patel	Did anyone hit you?
Mrs Dunn	*[pause]* Only the once...

---

being asked).[58] Until we reach the disclosure that Mrs Dunn has been hit, the doctor has contributed little to the conversation except 'Uh-huh'! Yet his role has been far from passive. This is not non-directive consulting but interactional narrative, of which a crucial feature is perhaps simple curiosity – wanting to know (and caring about) the next part of the story.[46]

The Russian philosopher and linguist Mikhail Bakhtin made a key contribution to narrative theory with his claim that all text is dialogical. What he meant by this was that every utterance – even 'uh-huh' – is made in response to (or anticipation of) some other utterance. The audience, claimed Bakhtin, is centrally involved in creating the meaning of the texts they read or hear. Without an audience, the text has no meaning. In Bakhtin's words:

> *'Human thought becomes genuine thought, that is, an idea, only under conditions of living contact with another and alien thought, a thought embodied in someone else's voice'.*[59]

In Bakhtin's view, the role of the listener is not merely to absorb a story passively, but to provide a separate perspective – something which Frank describes as *critical distance*.[6] Drawing on Bakhtin, Frank takes issue with conventional biomedical perspectives on patients' stories (see, e.g., *The Illness Narratives*[60]) in which doctors are encouraged to use listening as a diagnostic tool for extracting information that can contribute to a problem-solving sequence. In such an approach, he claims, 'the [patient] remains the object of the professional's privileged subjectivity: there is no relationship in the sense of reciprocated feeling for one another'.[6] But in a Bakhtinian framing of clinical interaction, the role of the clinician is to provide the subjective 'otherness' for an interactional narrative in which the patient will construct, and make sense of, his or her illness narrative.

In the exchange shown in Box 6.4, Dr Patel does not 'take a history' of domestic violence using conventional diagnostic questions. Indeed, in the remainder of this consultation (not shown) he is careful not to ask any more direct questions about the domestic incident. The doctor's input is both less and more than that of a conventional diagnostician: He provides the curiosity and critical distance that allow the patient to construct the first fragment of her painful and shocking story. Over the next few months, and within the protected confines of the consulting room, Mrs Dunn's domestic violence story will unfold gradually, alongside her asthma narrative and her wife-and-mother narrative. All three will be subtly woven into a wider tapestry of seemingly inconsequential story fragments – her young daughter's hay fever, her son's eczema – that make up the bread-and-butter of general practice consultations – and which, as Balint (see previous section) demonstrated, are often the presenting complaint that gets the patient through the door with his or her 'hidden agenda'.[40]

In Section 2.6, I introduced Jerome Bruner's notion of the narrative truth derived from a good story as distinct from the logico-deductive truth derived from scientific method. As I argued in Section 5.2, rigorous and conscientious application of logico-deductive reasoning (as in evidence-based medicine) is a critical dimension of good clinical care. Equally critical, however, is the recognition of narrative truth – the empathetic bearing of witness to the patient's story, and especially to his or her account of personal trouble and heroic efforts to face and resolve it. This witness-bearing is a complex exercise in intersubjectivity and equates to what Arthur Frank (with deliberate irony) has called just listening.[6]

Just listening encompasses not only the various forms of talking therapy offered to those with distress or mental illness, but also the intermittent dialogue of long-term continuing care for patients with chronic illness, and the especially intimate story shared with a patient who is, or might soon be, dying. The accumulation of (often brief and disjointed) clinician–patient encounters over time constitutes above all else just listening to an unfolding restitution, tragedy or quest narrative (see Section 4.2). If the chronic illness story unfolds in what Frank would call a chaos narrative, just listening provides the opportunity for both parties to co-construct a new narrative that holds some meaning for the patient and can begin to unfold for better or worse, but as a story should. The GP who invites the patient to 'come and see me again in a couple of weeks to tell me how you're getting on' and the cancer nurse who offers to 'pop in when I'm next passing' have recognized that the central purpose of the encounter is not for a diagnosis, a procedure, or a prescription – but simply, and crucially, for another instalment in the story.

Dr Patel's interjections in the example in Box 6.4 illustrate that just listening to a chaos narrative is a complex skill that goes beyond being present at its pouring-out. The American physician and narratologist Rita Charon has developed both a theory and a practical training for just listening. In her words, *'The effective practice of medicine requires narrative competence, that is the ability to acknowledge, absorb, interpret and act on the stories and plights of others'.*[61]

Charon's notion of narrative competence is more than the skills required in models of medical consulting that are based on psychological models of interaction (such as 'concordance'[62] or 'shared decision making'[63]). She argues at a higher level of abstraction that the practice of medicine is comparable to reading (i.e. immersion in and interpretation of) a text. The link is not merely logical (sickness calls forth stories, so the clinician must be able to hear and understand them), but also allegorical (sickness *is* a text that must be read).

In a different version of the consultation between Mrs Dunn and her doctor – one that was not merely evidence-based but naïvely evidence-driven – Dr Patel would have followed the pop-up prompt on his computer screen that told him that this patient's peak flow rate was overdue for checking. In doing so, he would have obtained a clinically important item of data at the expense of the trust we see being built through the subtle exchange of 'uh-huhs' and 'this and thats' in the consultation fragment in Box 6.4. He would also have failed to incur the ethical obligation that we see emerging when, at the end of this stop–start exchange, Mrs Dunn's shameful secret is disclosed. Such trade-offs will never be quantifiable, but Scandinavian GP Karl-Edward Rudebeck, (cited in Iona Heath's excellent monograph *The Mystery of General Practice*[64]) has argued passionately that general practice must not be pushed into *'defining itself at its own margins, leaving its very centre, its specific priorities, unfathomed by both critics and spokesmen'.* In other words, whilst evidence-based medicine (Section 2.2) and the rational clinical method (Section 6.2) are critical components of good primary care, they should supplement, not replace, just listening.

In Section 5.2, I referred to Marshall Marinker's satirical critique of specialist medicine, which sought to *'distinguish the clear message of the disease from the interfering noise of the patient as a person'.*[65] In Section 6.3, I referred to patients with medically unexplained symptoms, whose illness fails to fit a conventional diagnostic category. These patients include those who are 'inexplicably sick' as well as those whose illness is compounded by loneliness, social exclusion, stigma or lack of support. In such contexts (where the core business of contemporary primary health care surely lies), the patient's story – fragmented, incomplete and inconsistent though it is – may be a more helpful unit of analysis than the textbook disease category or evidence-based management protocol.[46] That is not to say that evidence-based medicine has nothing to offer the consultation in Box 6.4 – see, for example, the entry in Clinical Evidence on interventions that improve outcomes in domestic violence.[66] But note that in this example, just listening was what set the stage for the all-important disclosure. In his time-less treatise *Rhetoric*, Aristotle wrote that one of the key skills of argumentation (which he, like many ancient Greeks, viewed as a highly scholarly activity) is the imaginative and intuitive decision of *where to begin*.[67] Had Dr Patel begun his evidence-based decision making at the obvious place (with asthma or hypertension), he would have short-changed his patient. Because he placed high priority on the quality of the interactional narrative, and was sensitive to the new story that was tentatively emerging, he discovered the starting point at which his patient – probably unconsciously – sought to begin their dialogue. This is an example of the use of clinical intuition which I discuss in more detail in Section 5.3.

As illness in general becomes more complex, more multifaceted and more long-term (see Section 10.1), a 'literary' approach to clinical interaction (Charon's 'narrative competence') is likely to become increasingly important in clinical practice. A working definition of such an approach might be that:

• Narrative competence views the illness, and the patient's efforts to deal with it, as an unfolding story within his or her wider lifeworld.

• It acknowledges the patient as the narrator of the story and the subject (rather than the object) of the tale, and hence gives central importance to the patient's own role in defining, managing and making sense of the illness.

• It recognises that a single problem or experience will generate multiple interpretations and that the key version to be addressed is the one framed and developed by the patient.

• It embraces both trust (the patient makes herself vulnerable and stakes confidence in the clinician in the act of telling her story) and obligation (the clinician incurs ethical duties in the act of hearing it).

• It views the spoken (and enacted) dialogue between health professional and patient as an integral part of the clinical management.

But as I hope I have shown in this section, narrative competence does not absolve the clinician of the duty to base his or her recommendations on the best available scientific evidence. Indeed, I believe passionately that the narrative-competent clinician will be better able to draw appropriately and judiciously on the tools and techniques of evidence-based medicine, to apply sensitivity and common sense to the application of evidence to this particular case and to communicate the 'evidence' to the patient in a way that is personally relevant and culturally congruent.

6.5   The interpreted consultation

This section considers an increasingly common situation in contemporary primary heath care: the tripartite consultation in which communication is facilitated by the presence of an interpreter or advocate. Like all primary care challenges, the interpreted consultation can be viewed through multiple conceptual and theoretical lenses. Furthermore, because of the complexity and multifacetedness of the interpreted consultation, it cannot be fully understood unless more than one such lens (and perhaps multiple lenses) are used. Table 6.2 shows a number of different approaches that have been taken to the academic study of the healthcare interpreting. You will see that some have taken a level of analysis above that of the individual consultation (e.g. the organisation, the professional group or the healthcare system) and are beyond the scope of this chapter on clinical interaction. I will consider below those traditions that have addressed healthcare interpreting at the level of the interpersonal interaction.

The most obvious (and, some would argue, the least well-theorised) approach to studying interpreted consultations is to assume that the problem is purely one of translation. The interpreter is seen (in the words of one interpreter interviewed in my own research – see below) as a 'bilingual parrot'. What is said individually by doctor and patient is assumed to be what each of them wanted to say, and the big research question is whether the interpreter has correctly bridged the communication gap between them. Such research, which assumes a narrowly biomedical framework (the patient generally enters the consulting room with a 'disease' that needs to be diagnosed and treated, and must be given instructions about how to take the medication, etc. – see Section 2.1), is best undertaken by collecting audiotaped (or videotaped) consultations and getting an independent translator to 'mark' the quality of translation in each direction. Such studies have generally demonstrated that translation errors are common in some professionally interpreted consultations[73] and even more common when the interpreter is untrained (e.g. family member interpreting or using bilingual staff).[70-72] Most such studies conclude that the solution to this problem is to ensure that professional interpreters are more highly trained, that lay interpreting is discouraged (or even outlawed) and that standards for translation quality are developed and implemented.

As ever with the biomedical model, this approach to the interpreted consultation is very worthy, within the constraints of its world view. But research from the interaction analysis tradition (see Section 6.1) throws additional light on the interpreted consultation. Not only are such consultations often characterised by inaccurate translation, but they are also different in other ways from language-concordant consultations. In particular, as Ludwein Meeuwesen and her colleagues have shown, consultations across a language barrier with immigrant patients are more likely to be shorter and to contain fewer words of welcome, less empathy and less orientation (e.g. telling the patient what to expect); and immigrant patients show less assertiveness (and less emotion in general) than indigenous ones.[74,75] These findings add another dimension of quality in interpreted consultations to the metaphor of the bilingual parrot! Note that these findings do not *contradict* research on accuracy of translation – the latter is indeed a critical issue – but they are based on a different conceptualisation of the problem and hence start to add richness to the overall picture.

Another conceptualisation of the interpreted consultation sees it primarily as a complex social situation and is centrally interested in the presentation of self and the power relationships (and linked trust relationships) between clinician,

Table 6.2 Different research traditions that have studied healthcare interpreting.

Disciplinary roots	Main focus of research	Goal	Main level of analysis	Main research methods	Quality in this research tradition defined mainly in terms of	Examples of studies in this tradition
Epidemiology	Mapping the language need of a population	To inform planning and provision of interpreting services	Population	Epidemiological surveys	Needs assessment (language need is mapped accurately, including relevant dialects, and changes with time are captured promptly)	Baker & Eversley (London),[68] McPake (Scotland)[69]
Biomedicine	Assessing accuracy and completeness of translation in a clinician–patient exchange	To improve accuracy of diagnosis and efficacy of treatment	Interpersonal interaction	Cross-checking translation of audiotaped consultations	Accuracy of translation (phrases used by interpreter match those chosen by an independent translator; there are no omissions or embellishments)	Cambridge (UK),[70] Pöchhacker (Austria),[71] Elderkin-Thompson (USA),[72] Angellelli (USA)[73]
Psychology	Measuring type of communication that occurs in interpreted consultations and comparing this with non-interpreted ones	To inform training and practice of clinicians	Interpersonal interaction	Interaction analysis (see Section 6.1)	Proportion of the consultation that is spent on, e.g., welcoming the patient, orienting the patient, checking understanding, giving information, etc.	Meeuwesen (Netherlands)[74,75]

Medical sociology/ sociolinguistics	Exploring clinician– patient-interpreter interaction in its social context, with emphasis on identity, social roles and power relationships	To illuminate the social complexity of the interpreted consultation	Interpersonal interaction in its wider social context	In-depth qualitative analysis of transcripts or narratives	Open communicative action (both clinician and patient seek mutual understanding and work towards this). Voice of the lifeworld is heard and attended to (see text). Interpreter moves judiciously and appropriately between translator and advocacy roles	Roberts (UK),[76] Robb (UK),[77,78] Green (UK),[80] Leanza (France)[79]
Economics	Estimating costs and benefits of different service models of providing interpreters	To improve cost-effectiveness of services	Healthcare system	Economic modelling and evaluation	Accuracy, sensitivity and transferability of economic model	Jacobs (USA)[81]

(Continued)

Table 6.2 (Continued)

Disciplinary roots	Main focus of research	Goal	Main level of analysis	Main research methods	Quality in this research tradition defined mainly in terms of	Examples of studies in this tradition
Organisational sociology	Studying the organisational processes and routines that underpin the provision of interpreting services	To improve service efficiency	Organisation	Ideally, ethnography	Extent to which an effective and efficient process exists for providing an interpreter whenever a patient needs one	Greenhalgh (UK)[82]
Healthcare organisation and management	Estimating the quality of care provided with and without interpreters when these are needed	To maximise quality of care and minimise error	Multiple levels in the healthcare system	Various measures of quality of care	Process of care (e.g. necessary tests completed), biomedical outcomes (e.g. cure), satisfaction, medical errors or adverse events	Green (USA),[81,83] Flores (systematic review of mainly US literature)[84]
Education/professional development	Identifying and addressing training needs of interpreters and clinicians	To ensure trained professionals who work well together	Professional group	Learner profiling, training needs analysis	Match between what is formally taught and what is needed for the job. Hence, fitness-for-purpose of competency frameworks and course curricula	Tebble (Australia),[78] Harmsen (Netherlands),[85] Kalet (USA)[86]

patient and interpreter. Celia Roberts' team from King's College London, for example, studied videotaped consultations between London GPs and limited English-speaking patients, as well as consultations without a language barrier. They undertook detailed sociolinguistic analysis (see Section 6.2) of the transcripts of the consultations and supplemented this with an analysis of the 'body language' seen on the videotape.[76] In one study from this large dataset, they focused on the opening sequences in the discourse – the moments during which the patients have to report on why they have come. They found that English-speaking patients typically presented three things during the opening moments of the consultation: a description of symptoms, the context in which the symptoms occurred and an affective or epistemic stance (e.g. a comment on how much the symptoms mattered). These 'micro discourse routines' were framed in a particular way and associated with the presentation of a 'moral self' (e.g. a conscientious patient who had taken the medication as directed or a caring and concerned parent). Whilst some patients from non-English-speaking backgrounds used similar micro discourse routines, the majority configured the relationship between symptoms, context and the moral self in different and apparently less 'orderly' ways. With these patients, the opening moments of the consultation were typically protracted, frustrating and harder work interactionally for both sides. These findings suggest that the 'accurate translation of what is said' will not enable the consultation to proceed in the same manner that typically occurs in the absence of cultural and linguistic diversity. Rather, clinicians may need to be trained to expect, and respond to, a seemingly 'disorderly' presentation of self and symptoms in patients from certain cultural backgrounds.

My own team interviewed people (GPs, nurses, patients, professional interpreters and family member interpreters) who had been involved in interpreted consultations in inner London GP surgeries. We asked them to tell us some stories about recent interpreted consultations that had gone well and some about consultations that had gone less well.[77,78] We analysed these narratives for insights into the different social roles and relationships as viewed by the particular party we were interviewing. Our most striking finding was how difficult (and unusual) it was to achieve what Habermas called open communicative action (see Section 6.2). Very commonly, the constraints of the consultation – especially pressure of time and profound power imbalances – appeared to drive all parties towards a more strategic form of communication. For example, rather than giving the doctor an honest account of their symptoms and expecting to receive a possible diagnosis and a suggestion for next steps, patients typically entered the consulting room with a particular goal in mind (prescription, referral, sick note) and attempted (with more or less success) to draw the interpreter into this strategic action. More commonly, however, the interpreter 'sided' with the clinician and appeared to collude in professionally led efforts to limit the patient's agenda and get him or her out of the consulting room within the time allocated. A study by Leanza and colleagues in France produced very similar findings.[79]

An interesting finding from this research, which was also found independently by Judith Green's team in a study of child interpreters,[80] was the very positive light in which the lay and family member interpreter was usually depicted. Whereas the professional interpreter tended to align with the 'voice of the system' (e.g. 'editing out' when a patient mentioned using alternative remedies), friends and family member interpreters aligned strongly with the 'voice of the lifeworld' (see Section 6.3). They described an advocacy role – using their power in the consultation to ensure that the patient's concerns were voiced and addressed, and articulating important lifeworld issues such as the impact of pain and disability even when the patient herself had not raised these.[77] Children who interpreted for relatives in healthcare consultations were generally proud of their role and saw it as an integral part of their bilingual identity[80]; patients who brought their children to interpret claimed they did it partly because they could control what the child said more effectively than they could control the input of a professional interpreter![78]

The growing body of research that draws on sociological and sociolinguistic theories adds richness to the study of the interpreted consultation and offers scope for defining new dimensions of quality in healthcare interpreting. The interpreted consultation is a key quality issue in the 'globalised' world of the twenty-first century and can be studied at multiple levels of analysis. Table 6.2 gives examples of researchers who have used epidemiological techniques to measure language need, organisational sociological techniques to study the administrative procedures and routines that support the provision of interpreters and economic techniques to weigh the costs and benefits of different service models of interpreting.

References

1 McWhinney IR. *A Textbook of Family Medicine.* 2nd edn. Oxford: Oxford University Press; 1997.
2 Covington H. Caring presence. Delineation of a concept for holistic nursing. J Holist Nurs 2003;21:301–317.
3 Sappington JY. Nurturance. The spirit of holistic nursing. J Holist Nurs 2003;21:8–19.
4 Meehan TC. Therapeutic touch as a nursing intervention. J Adv Nurs 1998;28:117–125.
5 Rogers C. *Client-Centered Therapy: Its Practice, Implications and Theory* (Originally published, 1956). Philadelphia: Trans-Atlantic Publications; 1995.
6 Frank A. Just Listening: narrative and deep illness. Fam Syst Health 1998;16:197–216.
7 Miller WL. The clinical hand: a curricular map for relationship-centered care. Fam Med 2004;36:330–335.
8 White J, Levinson W, Roter D. 'Oh, by the way....': the closing moments of the medical visit. J Gen Intern Med 1994;9:24–28.
9 Levinson W, Roter DL, Mullooly JP, Dull VT, Frankel RM. Physician–patient communication. The relationship with malpractice claims among primary care physicians and surgeons. JAMA 1997;277:553–559.
10 Kruijver IP, Kerkstra A, Bensing JM, van de Wiel HB. Communication skills of nurses during interactions with simulated cancer patients. J Adv Nurs 2001;34:772–779.

11 Deveugele M, Derese A, De BD, van dB-M, Bensing J, De MJ. Is the communicative behavior of GPs during the consultation related to the diagnosis? A cross-sectional study in six European countries. Patient Educ Couns 2004;54:283–289.

12 Ishikawa H, Hashimoto H, Roter DL, Yamazaki Y, Takayama T, Yano E. Patient contribution to the medical dialogue and perceived patient-centeredness. An observational study in Japanese geriatric consultations. J Gen Intern Med 2005;20:906–910.

13 Ishikawa H, Roter DL, Yamazaki Y, Hashimoto H, Yano E. Patients' perceptions of visit companions' helpfulness during Japanese geriatric medical visits. Patient Educ Couns 2006;61:80–86.

14 Schouten BC, Meeuwesen L, Harmsen HA. The impact of an intervention in intercultural communication on doctor–patient interaction in the Netherlands. Patient Educ Couns 2005;58:288–295.

15 Innes M, Skelton J, Greenfield S. A profile of communication in primary care physician telephone consultations: application of the Roter interaction analysis system. Br J Gen Pract 2006;56:363–368.

16 Margalit RS, Roter D, Dunevant MA, Larson S, Reis S. Electronic medical record use and physician–patient communication: an observational study of Israeli primary care encounters. Patient Educ Couns 2006;61:134–141.

17 Henbest RJ, Stewart MA. Patient-centredness in the consultation. 1: A method for measurement. Fam Pract 1989;6:249–253.

18 Henbest RJ, Stewart M. Patient-centredness in the consultation. 2: Does it really make a difference? Fam Pract 1990;7:28–33.

19 Roter D, Larson S. The Roter interaction analysis system (RIAS): utility and flexibility for analysis of medical interactions. Patient Educ Couns 2002;46:243–251.

20 Del PL, Mazzi M, Saltini A, Zimmermann C. Inter and intra individual variations in physicians' verbal behaviour during primary care consultations. Soc Sci Med 2002;55:1871–1885.

21 Gallagher TJ, Hartung PJ, Gerzina H, Gregory SW, Jr, Merolla D. Further analysis of a doctor–patient nonverbal communication instrument. Patient Educ Couns 2005;57:262–271.

22 Krupat E, Frankel R, Stein T, Irish J. The four habits coding scheme: validation of an instrument to assess clinicians' communication behavior. Patient Educ Couns 2006;62:38–45.

23 Elwyn G, Edwards A, Wensing M, Hood K, Atwell C, Grol R. Shared decision making: developing the OPTION scale for measuring patient involvement. Qual Saf Health Care 2003;12:93–99.

24 Edwards A, Elwyn G. *Evidence Based Patient Choice.* Oxford: Oxford University Press; 2001.

25 Ong LM, de Haes JC, Hoos AM, Lammes FB. Doctor–patient communication: a review of the literature. Soc Sci Med 1995;40:903–918.

26 Teutsch C. Patient–doctor communication. Med Clin North Am 2003;87:1115–1145.

27 Kinnersley P, Stott N, Peters T, Harvey I, Hackett P. A comparison of methods for measuring patient satisfaction with consultations in primary care. Fam Pract 1996;13:41–51.

28 Howie JG, Heaney DJ, Maxwell M, Walker JJ. A comparison of a patient enablement instrument (PEI) against two established satisfaction scales as an outcome measure of primary care consultations. Fam Pract 1998;15:165–171.

29 Ramsay J, Campbell JL, Schroter S, Green J, Roland M. The general practice assessment survey (GPAS): tests of data quality and measurement properties. Fam Pract 2000;17:372–379.

30 Sandvik M, Eide H, Lind M, Graugaard PK, Torper J, Finset A. Analyzing medical dialogues: strength and weakness of Roter's interaction analysis system (RIAS). Patient Educ Couns 2002;46:235–241.

31 Scambler G, Britten N. System, lifeworld, and doctor–patient interaction. In: Scambler G, ed. *Habermas, Critical Theory and Health*. London: Routledge; 2001.

32 Blumer H. *Symbolic Interaction: Perspective and Method*. Berkeley, CA: University of California Press; 1969.

33 Scambler G. *Habermas, Critical Theory and Health*. London: Routledge; 2001.

34 Mishler EG. *The Discourse of Medicine: Dialectics of Medical Interviews*. Norwood, NJ: Ablex; 1984.

35 Barry CA, Bradley CP, Britten N, Stevenson FA, Barber N. Patients' unvoiced agendas in general practice consultations: qualitative study. BMJ 2000;320:1246–1250.

36 Mishler EG. Representing discourse: the rhetoric of transcription. J Narrative Life Hist 1991;1:255–280.

37 Barry CA, Stevenson FA, Britten N, Barber N, Bradley CP. Giving voice to the lifeworld. More humane, more effective medical care? A qualitative study of doctor–patient communication in general practice. Soc Sci Med 2001;53:487–505.

38 Elwyn G, Gwyn R. Stories we hear, and stories we tell – analysing talk and text in the clinical encounter. In: Greenhalgh T, Hurwitz B, eds. *Narrative Based Medicine: Dialogue and Discourse in Clinical Practice*. London: BMJ Publications; 1998.

39 Maynard DW, Heritage J. Conversation analysis, doctor–patient interaction and medical communication. Med Educ 2005;39:428–435.

40 Balint M. *The Doctor, His Patient and the Illness*. London: Routledge; 1956.

41 Freud S. *The Four Fundamental Concepts of Psychoanalysis*. London: Penguin; 1973.

42 Freud S. *Group Psychology and the Development of the Ego*. London: Penguin; 1973.

43 Freud S. *Civilisation and Its Discontents*. London: Penguin; 1973.

44 Osborne T. Mobilizing psychoanalysis: Michael Balint and the general practitioners. Soc Stud Sci 1993;23:175–200.

45 Balint E, Norrell J. *Six Minutes for the Patient: Interaction in General Practice Consultations*. London: Tavistock; 1983.

46 Launer J. *Narrative Based Primary Care: A Practical Guide*. Oxford: Radcliffe; 2002.

47 Sanders K. *Emotional Problems in Primary Care – A Psychoanalytic View*. London: Karnac Books; 2006.

48 Groves JE. Taking care of the hateful patient. N Engl J Med 1978;298:883–887.

49 McDonald PS, O'Dowd TC. The heartsink patient: a preliminary study. Fam Pract 1991;8:112–116.

50 O'Dowd TC. Five years of heartsink patients in general practice. BMJ 1988;297:528–530.

51 Ellis CG. Chronic unhappiness. Investigating the phenomenon in family practice. Can Fam Physician 1996;42:645–651.

52 Mathers N, Jones N, Hannay D. Heartsink patients: a study of their general practitioners. Br J Gen Pract 1995;45:293–296.

53 Mathers NJ, Gask L. Surviving the 'heartsink' experience. Fam Pract 1995;12:176–183.

54 Smucker DR, Zink T, Susman JL, Crabtree BF. A framework for understanding visits by frequent attenders in family practice. J Fam Pract 2001;50:847–852.

55 Butler CC, Evans M. The 'heartsink' patient revisited. The Welsh Philosophy and General Practice Discussion Group. Br J Gen Pract 1999;49:230–233.

56 Undeland M, Malterud K. Diagnostic work in general practice: more than naming a disease. Scand J Prim Health Care 2002;20:145–150.

57 Greenhalgh T. *'What Seems to Be the Trouble?': Stories in Illness and Health Care*. Oxford: Radcliffe; 2006.

58 Jewkes R. Preventing domestic violence. BMJ 2002;324:253–254.

59 Bakhtin M. *Problems of Dostoevsky's Poetics*. Manchester: Manchester University Press; 1984.

60 Kleinmann A. *The Illness Narratives: Suffering, Healing and the Human Condition*. New York: Basic Books; 1988.

61 Charon R. Narrative medicine: form, function, and ethics. Ann Intern Med 2001;134: 83–87.

62 Royal Pharmaceutical Society of Great Britain. From Compliance to Concordance. *Achieving Shared Goals in Medicine Taking*. London: RPSGB; 1997.

63 Towle A, Godolphin W. Framework for teaching and learning informed shared decision making. BMJ 1999;319:766–771.

64 Heath I. *The Mystery of General Practice*. London: Nuffield Provincial Hospital Trust; 1997.

65 Marinker M. The chameleon, the judas goat, and the cuckoo. J R Coll Gen Pract 1978;28:199–206.

66 Klevens J, Sadowski L. Domestic violence towards women. Clin Evid 2005;2293–2302.

67 Aristotle. *Rhetoric* (Translated by Hugh Lawson Tancred). London: Penguin; 2005.

68 Baker P, Eversley J. Multilingual Capital. *The Languages of London's Schoolchildren and Their Relevance to Economic, Social and Educational Policies*. London: Battlebridge Publications; 2000.

69 McPake J. *Translating, Interpreting and Communication Support Services Across the Public Sector in Scotland. A Literature Review*. Edinburgh: Scottish Executive Central Research Unit; 2002.

70 Cambridge J. Information loss in bilingual medical interviews through an untrained interpreter. Translator 1999;5:201–219.

71 Pöchhacker F, Kadric M. The hospital cleaner as healthcare interpreter. A case study. Translator 1999;5:161–178.

72 Elderkin-Thompson V, Silver RC, Waitzkin H. When nurses double as interpreters: a study of Spanish-speaking patients in a US primary care setting. Soc Sci Med 2001;52:1343–1358.

73 Angellelli C. *Interpreting and Cross-Cultural Communication*. Cambridge: Cambridge University Press; 2005.

74 Schouten BC, Meeuwesen L. Cultural differences in medical communication: a review of the literature. Patient Educ Couns 2006;64:21–34.

75 Meeuwesen L, Harmsen JA, Bernsen RM, Bruijnzeels MA. Do Dutch doctors communicate differently with immigrant patients than with Dutch patients? Soc Sci Med 2006;63:2407–2417.

76 Roberts C, Sarangi S, Moss B. Presentation of self and symptoms in primary care consultations involving patients from non-English speaking backgrounds. Commun Med 2004;1:159–169.

77 Greenhalgh T, Robb N, Scambler G. Communicative and strategic action in interpreted consultations in primary health care: a Habermasian perspective. Soc Sci Med 2006;63:1170–1187.

78 Robb N, Greenhalgh T. 'You have to cover up the words of the doctor': the mediation of trust in interpreted consultations in primary care. J Health Organ Manag 2006;20:434–455.

79 Leanza Y. Roles of community interpreters in pediatrics as seen by interpreters, physicians and researchers. Interpreting 2005;7:167–192.

80 Green J, Free C, Bhavnani V, Newman T. Translators and mediators: bilingual young people's accounts of their interpreting work in health care. Soc Sci Med 2005;60:2097–2110.

81 Jacobs EA, Shepard DS, Suaya JA, Stone EL. Overcoming language barriers in health care: costs and benefits of interpreter services. Am J Public Health 2004;94:866–869.

82 Greenhalgh T, Voisey C, Robb N. Interpreted consultations as 'business as usual'? A study of organisational routines in primary care. In: *Ethnicity, Health and Health Care: Understanding Diversity, Tackling Disadvantage*. Sociology of Health and Illness Monograph 13, in press.

83 Green AR, Ngo-Metzger Q, Legedza AT, Massagli MP, Phillips RS, Iezzoni LI. Interpreter services, language concordance, and health care quality. Experiences of Asian Americans with limited English proficiency. J Gen Intern Med 2005;20:1050–1056.

84 Flores G. The impact of medical interpreter services on the quality of health care: a systematic review. MCRR 2005;62:255–299.

85 Harmsen H, Bernsen R, Meeuwesen L, et al. The effect of educational intervention on intercultural communication: results of a randomised controlled trial. Br J Gen Pract 2005;55:343–350.

86 Kalet AL, Mukherjee D, Felix K, et al. Can a web-based curriculum improve students' knowledge of, and attitudes about, the interpreted medical interview? J Gen Intern Med 2005;20:929–934.

CHAPTER 7

The family – or lack of one

Summary points

1 British general practice has traditionally been strongly linked with the family unit, and many other primary care systems worldwide seek to develop 'family medicine'. This makes sense since illness both profoundly affects and is profoundly affected by the structure and the relationships within the family.

2 In Britain, as in many other developed and developing countries, family structure is changing rapidly, with fewer couples making a lifelong commitment and children living in a variety of structures including single parent, stepparents and same-sex parents. Few non-nuclear family structures have been consistently associated with increased health risks to the children, but poverty (which often follows divorce) is strongly associated with poor health outcomes in children.

3 More people are living alone, especially elderly women. Informal social support (e.g. from neighbours) occurs more rarely than it did in the past.

4 Adolescents are, at least on the face of it, less strongly influenced by their family of origin than used to be the case a generation ago and have greater potential to follow different life paths than those mapped out for them by parents. However, the social determinants of health remain powerful and inequalities still recur in successive generations.

5 Love, nurturance and emotionally responsive care from a consistent primary caregiver are essential for the healthy development of the young child. If these are not present consistently and in high quality, problems of attachment may occur which can lead to antisocial behaviour and/or mental health problems later in life. Non-traditional family structures do not in and of themselves appear to lead to attachment disorders, but research evidence is sparse.

6 Most illnesses, even those that have a clear 'genetic' basis, arise from a complex combination of genetic predisposition, the opportunities and constraints (physical and psychological) provided by the environment and the cultural significance of symptoms and experiences. New research approaches, particularly techniques for studying the offspring of twins, are helping to unpack the complex interaction between genetic and environmental influences.

7 Homelessness is increasing in prevalence in many societies. Risk factors for homelessness include the dual diagnosis of mental illness and drug dependency. Both physical and mental health problems, and comorbidity, are

(Continued)

175

(*Summary points continued*)

> common in the homeless and require (but rarely receive) a coordinated response from primary care. Various approaches to supporting the homeless and reducing adverse outcomes have had moderate success in a research setting, but do not provide easy or universal answers to this challenging problem.

7.1 Family structure in the late modern world

My mother, who is old enough to recall when the UK National Health Service (NHS) began in 1948, still refers to her general practitioner (GP) as her 'family doctor'. The start of the NHS marks the time in the history of Britain's Welfare State when free medical care came to be offered not just to working men (as part of an employer's insurance package) but to the whole family. This change was a landmark event, producing almost overnight improvements in antenatal care, developmental surveillance of babies and young children and care of the vulnerable elderly.[1] Looking after the whole family from 'cradle to grave' has been a defining characteristic of British general practice for over 60 years, and it is a feature of which we are justifiably proud.[2] Developing countries, and those in transition (e.g. the former Eastern Europe), rightly place high emphasis on developing a programme of family medicine based in primary care that promotes maternal and child health, family planning and comprehensive (if basic) medical care for the retired, out-of-work and uninsured.[3] Such provision is the least a civilised society can offer its most vulnerable citizens. Research by epidemiologists and economists has shown that investments in the health of mothers and young children and in the prevention of unwanted pregnancy are two of the most cost-effective ways of spending a limited healthcare budget.[4]

All textbooks of general practice rightly emphasise the importance of the family in both the generation of illness (we catch infections from our nearest and dearest, and our relationships with them account for a good deal of our neuroses too) and in the support of the sick person (informal carers within the family help us get better and enable us to cope effectively with disability, disfigurement, loss of function, loss of independence and dying). Box 7.1 shows some examples from my own practice of the impact of the family relationships on the origin and course of illness.

The first example in Box 7.1, Brian, was unlucky to develop a severe form of multiple sclerosis but very fortunate to spend his 25 years of disability cared for by a loving family who readily made compromises in their own lives to accommodate their sick member. Note that Brian's family – white, middle-class, educated and well-connected – were able to tap into a range of available resources such as government-subsidised modifications to their home, a 'dial-a-ride' service paid for by the local council, trained carers and various state benefits such as Incapacity Benefit (paid to someone who is unable to work), Attendance Allowance (paid to an individual who needs 24-hour care) and Mobility Allowance (paid to people who cannot get about without special

Box 7.1 **Examples of the importance of the family in the illness experience.**

These cases, based on real patients, have been fictionalised to protect confidentiality.

The story of Brian

Brian was a university lecturer who had a wife Jane and three grown-up children. When he was 45, he developed progressive neurological symptoms which were subsequently diagnosed as multiple sclerosis. By the time he was 55, he was wheelchair bound and required assistance with every aspect of daily living. The family rallied round. Jane changed her job so that she could provide 2 hours' input to help Brian get ready every morning and put him in the taxi that took him to work, where he continued to teach students until his retirement. The children organised their lives so that they visited their parents every week or so, and friends also dropped in regularly as they knew that Brian and Jane found it more difficult to go out than other couples. Eventually, Brian's condition deteriorated to the point where he could only move one finger, but this was enough to operate the entry phone to the door to let helpers in and an emergency alarm. This arrangement allowed Jane to continue her part-time job, gaining respite from her work as a carer and bringing in much-needed income. Brian occasionally went through periods of low mood, and wondered 'why me?', but benefited from the support of his family until he died after a brief stay in hospital at the age of 69.

The story of John

John developed Type 1 diabetes when he was 7. At the time, he lived with his parents and younger brother Stuart in a semi-detached house on an estate close to his primary school. John developed a close relationship with the diabetes specialist nurse at the local hospital, and the family attended weekend 'camps' organised through the charity Diabetes UK, where he met other children with diabetes. At these camps, John's parents discussed the challenges of bringing up a diabetic child with other parents in the same situation. On Wednesday evenings and Saturday mornings, John's father took him to play football at the local club and made sure he adjusted his food and insulin according to the instructions given by the nurse. When John was 11, his parents got divorced. His mother, who had worked part time from home, took on a full-time job in a local supermarket where she was required to work shifts, including some evenings and weekends. His father moved to a small flat in a town 40 miles away to live with his new fiancée. After a difficult few months, a routine was established where John and Stuart spent alternate weekends with their father. John was dropped from the football team after 'missing too many training sessions', and became increasingly interested in Play Station games. John's mother was unable to make the Diabetes UK weekends because of her shift work, and his father was preoccupied by the impending arrival of a new baby. As John entered adolescence, he spent more time going out with his peer group and worked out how to 'run high' to avoid the risk of hypoglycaemic attacks. Neither of his parents seemed to mind that he was controlling his diabetes without asking for help. At his annual check-up soon after his 16th birthday, John was found to have diabetes control in the 'very poor' range and early retinopathy.

The story of Nermal

Nermal is a 24-year-old Kurdish asylum seeker, originally from Afghanistan. She lives in north London with her three children aged 5, 3 and 2, in a refuge for women who have suffered domestic violence. Her immigration status is insecure because the British government have not yet decided whether to allow her permanent residence in the UK. She has consulted her GP 19 times in the past year, with complaints that might be broadly categorised as 'medically unexplained symptoms'.[5] These include headaches (for which she has had a neurological referral, CT brain scan and a course of cognitive behaviour therapy), upper abdominal pain (for which she has had a gastro-enterological referral, upper GI endoscopy, a course of treatment for *H. Pylori* that had no impact on her symptoms, and five different antacid drugs), non-specific skin rash (for which she has had 12 different skin creams and a dermatological referral at which no diagnosis was made despite a skin biopsy) and depression (for which she has had counselling, three different antidepressants and a psychiatric referral, though she failed to attend her appointment). A thorough assessment undertaken 2 years ago by the UK charity, the Medical Foundation for the Care of Victims of Torture (http://www.torturecare.org.uk/), via an interpreter trained to deal with people with complex needs, established that Nermal's husband is a drug trafficker who was physically and sexually violent towards her and 'put her on the streets' in Pakistan where they lived for 2 years. Her husband is now living in mainland Europe but visits the UK regularly – illegally, since he is wanted by the police. He is the father of the oldest child but the fathers of the other two children are unknown. Nermal lives in fear that she will be sent back to Afghanistan and that her husband will discover where she lives and return to rape her. The two youngest children are being monitored by the health visitor for underweight and 'poor bonding' with their mother.

means)* Brian was also eligible for a modest supplementary pension from his employer that added to his state benefits. He owned his house, so there

---

*Please do not use this book as a reference text on the UK benefits system, which, like that of many other countries, is complex and constantly changing. The point about benefits is that it takes someone who knows the system to identify which benefits the person is eligible for and how to apply for them. In Brian's case, he and his wife were able to access the relevant information and act on it – but consider how much more difficult this would have been for Nermal (case 3 in Box 7.1).

were no clauses from a landlord prohibiting him from making the necessary modifications. And so on. You can probably see how 'the family' in Brian's case was not only supportive at an emotional level but was also nested in a particular social situation that allowed them to operationalise that support at a practical level.

Now consider John. At the beginning of the story he enjoyed a comparable package of family support, with the various family members doing their bit to help him live with his illness. Diabetes, especially in a child, is a family challenge rather than an individual one. Parents can learn the theory of healthy eating, safe exercising and striking a balance between 'protecting the child' and 'promoting independence' in the clinic, but making that theory work in reality needs a different kind of learning – the informal learning gleaned from the personal stories and practical tips of other parents, and from seeing other families actually enacting these worthy principles (see Section 2.8). John's parents' divorce, a distressing enough event for any child, had a particularly devastating impact on his illness experience. The shift from a two-parent to a one-parent family requires the children to manage with much less parental attention (and less money), and whole-family events such as the Diabetes UK weekend camps become more difficult to organise. Like many children who pick up on the signals that parents have other issues to attend to, John got on with managing his diabetes – but the limited support and reduced family cohesion contributed to an inexorable drift towards poor control and complications.[6]

The saddest case in Box 7.1, Nermal, is (somewhat ironically) the individual who has no formally diagnosed disease. Even the 'depression' for which she was treated was not diagnosed on ICD10 criteria (see Section 5.2) but assumed to be present because no physical cause was identified for her multiple symptoms. The problem here is not merely that the family is fragmented, but the social context in which it became fragmented. Despite her young age, Nermal carries the scars of living under the Taliban regime in Afghanistan in which women were not allowed to be educated and had to remain behind the most restrictive of veils; a brutal war that killed many of her relatives; 2 years in a refugee camp and a further spell, living illegally while her husband drifted into criminal behaviour; and (a common solution to abject poverty in times of civil unrest) a period of enforced prostitution. Two of Nermal's children are the products of sexual encounters with strangers in the absence of true consent (and where she was powerless to negotiate contraception), so it is small wonder that she has problems relating to them.

How can we begin to get an academic perspective on the family when the term means so many different things? How can we design primary care systems that recognise the different levels of family support available in the real world, for which Brian, John and Nermal illustrate the contemporary extremes? The 'ologies' set out in Chapter 2 offer several important ways into this complex territory.

Let's start with epidemiology – or at least, applying the tools of epidemiology to provide demographic data on the family at a population level. The mapping of population statistics and trends is explained in more detail in Section 8.1. The latest data from the UK Office of National Statistics, based on survey data from 2005 (see www.statistics.gov.uk),[7] plus a research report based on this and other data sources[8] show that:

• The proportion of one-person households in Great Britain continues to increase – from 17% in 1971 to 29% in 2005.

• Older people are more likely to live alone than younger ones. The overall solo living rate of 30% in the people over 60s masks some important subgroup differences. For example, nearly 60% of women aged 75 and over now live alone.

• Men who live alone have often never married, whereas women who live alone often do so after the break-up of a relationship or the death of a partner.

• People living alone are less likely to own their home, more likely to smoke and to drink more than the recommended alcohol limits and have a lower income than those living with others. However, people living alone tend to have similar numbers of friends and social contacts than people living with others, so the idea that solo living is linked to loneliness is largely unfounded.

• People are marrying later. In 1971 the average age at first marriage was 25 for men and 23 for women; in 2003 it was 31 for men and 29 for women. Many people now go through a temporary period of solo living before marrying or cohabiting.

• The divorce rate is high (one couple in two who marry subsequently get divorced), but has been stable for 20 years and has recently fallen slightly, especially amongst the under 40s – perhaps because an increasing proportion of this group cohabit rather than marry. Divorces in people over 50, though still relatively uncommon, are rising.

• Fewer women are having children (one woman in five now remains childless all her life), and more than two-thirds of 25-year-old women today are childless.

• Children are living in an increasing variety of family structures. In 2005, 42% of children born in Britain were born out of wedlock, compared to 12% in 1980 (see Figure 7.1); one in four dependent children lived in a single-parent family; and one in ten lived with a stepfamily (i.e. with father's or mother's new partner).

• Multiple births are becoming commoner, especially in older women: 21% of all births to women over 35 in 2005 were a twin pregnancy.

• The teenage pregnancy rate in Britain is the highest in Europe. In 2005, 6% of young women aged 16–19 became pregnant and 2.5% had a live birth.

• An increasing proportion of people were born abroad (Table 7.1); of these, almost all will have important personal ties to family outside the UK, whom they may never see again.

These quantitative data are interesting for three reasons. Firstly, they have important implications for the organisation and delivery of healthcare. Imagine an epidemic of severe influenza (flu), for example. In previous epidemics (1918, 1957, 1968, 1975 and 1988), most people who developed flu, especially the frail elderly, were living in households where someone could care for them. If a flu

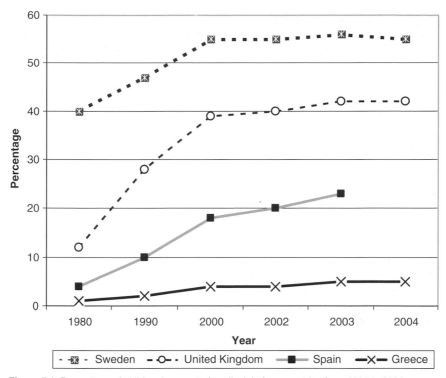

Figure 7.1 Percentage of children born out of wedlock in four countries from 1980 to 2004.

epidemic broke out tomorrow, the health care system (and society in general) would have to consider how to deliver the kind of care in the community that was hitherto provided by families, and on an unprecedented scale.

Secondly, changes in family structure may lead to changes in patterns of illness, disease and risk, as well as to important economic changes that have a crucial indirect impact on health. The dramatic changes in family structure

Table 7.1 UK population and proportion of people living in UK who were born abroad.

	People living in Britain			
	1971	*1981*	*1991*	*2001*
All people	52,559,260	53,550,270	54,888,744	57,103,331
People born abroad	2,390,759	2,751,130	3,153,375	4,301,280
People born abroad as percentage of total	4.55%	5.14%	5.75%	7.53%

Source: UK Office of National Statistics (www.ons.org).

seen in China over the past 25 years as a result of the one-child policy have, arguably, lifted hundreds of millions of people out of abject poverty and underpinned China's dramatic economic growth,[9] but they have also left China in danger of not being able to look after its expanding elderly population in the medium-term future.[10] The loss of large numbers of parents to AIDS has created a highly unstable family structure in many African countries, where AIDS orphans are now looked after by grandparents or simply left to walk the streets. An infant born to an HIV-positive mother in Africa has a virtually 100% chance of being orphaned by the age of 10.[11] Furthermore, because AIDS affects the working generation more than the extremes of age, the impact on both family and national economies may be devastating.[12] These somewhat dramatic examples highlight a more general principle – that family structure affects illness and illness affects family structure. The examples also illustrate how family structure is linked to family income and, as we shall see in Section 9.1, income is closely linked to health outcomes.

Interestingly, whilst numerous variations on the nuclear family model are prevalent in today's society, relatively few structural variables are consistently associated with poor health outcomes in epidemiological studies (Box 7.2).[13] Immigrant families (after controlling for poverty), families headed by a grandparent, families with multiple adults who share childcare and families with gay or lesbian partnerships have not been consistently associated with any adverse health outcome.[13,14] The impact of divorce per se on children's health and development is difficult to disentangle from the impact of having a lone parent – which in turn may be confounded by the impact of poverty. There is some (but not much) evidence that even when parents divorce amicably and then remarry quickly into a new family of comparable or higher income, there is still an impact on children's cognitive performance, behaviour and social adjustment. However, the effect, if present, is small relative to the impact of poverty. The impact of working mothers on children's health is discussed in the next section.

Thirdly, the numerical data referred to above raise questions about qualitative changes in the nature of society. Two more 'ologies' have an important

---

Box 7.2 Family structures that have been consistently associated with ill health and disadvantage in epidemiological studies.[13]

• Lone parents with children, especially those headed by a single unmarried mother and/or a teenage mother (the effect is still present, though much diminished, after controlling for poverty)
• Unemployed parents, especially those experiencing long-term (>1 year) unemployment
• Families with only one wage earner, and that a low earner
• Large families (i.e. with three or more children)

bearing on the structure of the family and its changing role in modern society: sociology (Section 2.4) and anthropology (Section 2.5). In Table 7.2, I have summarised and adapted a theory of social evolution originally proposed by the anthropologist Margaret Mead and developed further by sociologist James Coté.[15,16] I am grateful to Nadia Robb for originally drawing my attention to these sources, whose main points can be summarised as follows. In traditional or pre-modern (e.g. feudal, tribal) societies, social roles are generally fixed and inherited; there is little or no choice for individuals about their present or future roles or social positions; and rigid rules of etiquette are passed on from older to younger generations within the extended family. As society moves into the industrial period, social roles are determined more by the job one does than by kinship links (e.g. whose brother-in-law you are); the predominant family structure is nuclear; the developing child has some choice about his or her future destiny; and both social rules and parental authority can be challenged. In order for a parent to ensure that their child retains the family's social position, it is necessary to invest in him or her and encourage the acquisition of particular attitudes, behaviours and knowledge (an important package known as 'cultural capital' – see Section 9.2), and for the child to conform (more or less) to the identity expected of him or her. As the industrial period gives way to the post-industrial (late modern) period in which we now live, social roles and family structure become more variable and may change over time; opportunities for the developing child are diverse; and there are multiple opportunities for investing in oneself (e.g. a wide range of educational opportunities). Success and social mobility depend on the ability to recognize, prioritise and seize the available opportunities. Parents may play an important role in this process, but their input is, arguably, less crucial than it was in the industrial era.

Sociologist Anthony Giddens has identified late modernity as an important phase in social evolution in which the continuity of cultural tradition and the influence of the family on the individual have both been substantially weakened.[17] People are in charge of their destinies through a process he termed 'individualization' – the purposeful construction of a coherent identity from the myriad of choices available. To a much greater extent than in the past, we can become who we want to become rather than who our parents and grandparents expected us to become. Since people have more choice, they may take more risks – and they are also potentially able to seize unprecedented opportunities, resulting, at least potentially, in dramatic upward (and perhaps downward) social mobility.[18]

Other sociologists, however, have strongly challenged this picture of a fragmented and confused society in which family influence is of minor significance and individuals continually 'reinvent themselves' to capture the opportunities of the moment. Professor Ken Roberts, for example, argues that a child's prospects remain heavily constrained by what he calls 'opportunity structures' – that is over-arching social structures that shape and constrain what the individual sees as a menu of rational choices.[19] People can only choose

Table 7.2 Cultural evolution and the nature of identity.

	Pre-modern	Modern	Late modern
Social structure	Traditional or 'folk' society in which social roles are determined by kinship links	Industrial society characterised by the rise of capitalism, in which production is a key defining feature of social relations	Post-industrial society in which technology supplants labour and creates surpluses, and consumption supplants production as the defining feature of social relations
Family structure	Multiple generations of the same family coexist under one roof	The nuclear family predominates and is seen as the norm, with traditional gender roles and only two generations under the same roof	Multiple family structures exist and these change over time. Single parents, mixed-ethnicity marriages, gay partnerships and second marriages are all accepted as 'normal'; multiple options are available for producing and relating to children. Childlessness is an accepted choice
Predominant culture within the family	Social norms change little from one generation to the next and are beyond questioning by either parents or children. The family is a place of intensive socialization where children learn rigid rules of behaviour from past generations	Social norms are more changeable and intergenerational links more tenuous. Rules of behaviour can still be identified but these (and parental authority) can be questioned. Children and parents learn from their peers	Social norms change rapidly and the knowledge, life experiences and behavioural norms of parents may be seen as irrelevant and little attempt is made to pass these on. Children learn from a wide range of sources and parents may learn from their children
'Social class' best conceptualised as	Inherited social position and role	Relationship to the means of production (Marx) *or* mental sophistication as demonstrated by 'high' culture (Bourdieu)	Resources available to the individual
Implications for children and adolescents	The future adult identity of any child is fixed at birth. Success in developing this identity is more or less guaranteed because no choices are available	A child's future identity can be predicted but not be taken for granted. Parents must shape the development of a hoped-for identity for their child, and the child must invest in this process. Success depends on the child choosing to conform to parental (and others') expectations	There is less certainty of what the future holds for a child, and many more possible choices available. Success in identity development is highly contingent on how well the child appraises, and responds to, emerging opportunities and challenges. Identity construction is thus a lifelong project rather than a phase of adolescence

Adapted from Mead and Coté.[15,16]

between what they see as available and meaningful to them. This may explain why – in an era of apparently unprecedented choice – the sons and daughters of smokers are twice as likely to become smokers as the offspring of non-smokers[20] and the daughters of teenage mothers are significantly more likely to become teenage mothers themselves.[21] If Roberts is correct, the dramatic inequalities in health, educational achievement, and socio-economic status between the children of rich and poor families will continue pretty much unchanged despite the *appearance* that the family is less influential and constraining than it was in the past.

7.2   The mother–child relationship (or will any significant other do these days?)

One of the biggest changes in families in the last 40 years is the role of the mother. The traditional nuclear family, with a male breadwinner and mum keeping house, is now the exception rather than the rule in almost all developed countries. This book, like many academic textbooks these days, was written by a working mother. As a GP, I increasingly see babies and young children brought to me by dads, grandparents, nannies, older siblings and 'au pairs' (some of whom are actually illegal immigrants working as low-paid maids, who have no common language with either the child or its parents). Is this a worrying trend in terms of the health of the next generation – and how might we research such a question?

Epidemiological research by (among others) the Joseph Rowntree Foundation (see www.jrf.org.uk) has shown that in the UK, 70% of adult women of working age are in paid employment and that their income often contributes significantly to the family budget. Indeed, in many countries, the only way for a family with young children to avoid poverty is for both partners to work.[13] The most rapidly growing demographic group of wage earners in the UK is mothers of children under 5, with 60% now in paid employment (see www.statistics.gov.uk). In such families, one of a number of different childcare arrangements may be in place – including state-registered childminders, playgroups, nursery care and informal care by relatives or friends.

Kamerman et al.'s review (see previous section) includes a number of different large-scale cross-sectional surveys in different countries that sought to link the nature and extent of maternal employment with a host of health, educational and social outcomes in children.[13] The results are not easy to interpret, but it would appear that the children of mothers who worked during their first year of life (especially if they worked long hours) showed some developmental delay, notably later reading and more behavioural problems than the children of mothers who looked after their child full-time. The children of mothers who commenced paid work after their child's first birthday appeared to have a small but significant developmental *advantage*, but for adolescents specifically, the impact of mother working full-time was again negative, with lower educational attainment and more social problems compared to the adolescent children of mothers who did not work. Very few of these cohorts of children were followed-up long-term, so it is not known whether these effects are permanent.

Neither is it known whether the relationship between maternal employment and child health is causal (see Section 8.2). Even a 'statistically significant' relationship might be due to ecological fallacy – that is, the *apparent* finding that one variable (A) has caused another (B), but which is actually due to a third, unmeasured (confounding) variable (C). Two obvious potential confounding variables in the data described in the previous paragraph are poverty and maternal education. The mother of a young baby may work because she has no financial choice – and such a mother is also more likely to be uneducated. So if her baby grows up with developmental delay, this delay may not have been *caused* by her working (it would have happened anyway). Conversely, the mother of a 2-year-old who goes out to work may bring in sufficient income to send him or her to a stimulating private nursery. Again, it may not be the mother's working that has *caused* an acceleration in the child's cognitive development, but the nursery place bought with the additional income. Adolescents may have adverse outcomes not because of maternal working but because of a general lack of supervision at an age when they are vulnerable to distractions. And so on.

Because of the impossibility of proving causality from survey-based research designs, the meaning of such studies is often hotly debated. Nevertheless, findings such as 'for every hour a parent works between 6 and 9 p.m., their child has a 16% increase in being in the bottom quartile on maths tests' and 'children whose parents work at night have a 2.7-fold increased risk of being suspended from school, even after controlling for income and education'[22] must be contrasted with UNICEF's finding that low parental income is the largest single contributor to child poverty and poverty is the largest single variable accounting for ill health in children[23] and that parental unemployment is, statistically, strongly associated with child abuse and neglect.[13]

The type and quality of care is crucial to the impact of any childcare or enrichment programme. High-quality early childhood education and care from age 2–3 generally seems to improve cognitive and emotional development compared to home care, and these differences are most marked in children from socio-economically deprived homes.[13,24] 'High-quality' pre-school education is very different from simply keeping the child clean, fed and safe (Box 7.3). Programmes such as Head Start in the USA (http://www.acf.dhhs.gov/programs/hsb/index.htm) and Sure Start in the UK (www.surestart.gov.uk) are based on epidemiological evidence that such programmes produce important long-term benefits for the most disadvantaged children. But formal support programmes may not be available or accessible in all areas, or local myths and misconceptions may deter families from engaging with them. The mother in a poor family today, especially if she is a single parent, may still face an unenviable choice: go out to work (and your child may develop cognitive delay and behavioural problems as a result of low-quality childcare) or stay

---

Box 7.3 Aspects of pre-school education and care that have been shown to improve children's cognitive, linguistic, emotional and social development.[13,24,25]

- High adult–child ratio; small group size
- High levels of provider training
- Classroom environment, including
  - care routines (feeding, changing, sleeping)
  - furnishings and surroundings
  - appropriateness and supervision of activities for language development
  - appropriateness and supervision of activities for fine and gross motor development
  - appropriateness and supervision of creative activities
  - provision for social development (e.g. space for both group work and quiet time alone)
- Quality of the teacher–child relationship
- Teacher sensitivity and responsiveness to child

In most but not all empirical studies cited in the above reviews, these factors have had greatest impact on children whose home environment was classified in some way as 'deprived'

---

at home (and be unable to afford basic food, shelter and education for your child).

Another research tradition that has studied the mother–child (and carer–child) relationship is the application of attachment theory. In one classic experiment (which these days would no doubt be challenged by anti-vivisectionists), baby monkeys were separated at a young age from their biological mothers and offered two different 'mothers': a basic wire mesh frame with a milk supply and a soft, cuddly frame without a milk supply. The baby monkeys spent almost all their time clinging to the cuddly mother, only visiting the wire mesh mother for milk. The authors concluded that there is more to the mother–child relationship than 'cupboard love'.[26] Fifty years of social psychology research have added considerable detail to this important (though somewhat unsurprising) finding.

Developmental psychologist John Bowlby defined attachment as the affective bond that develops between an infant and a primary caregiver, particularly in the context of the infant's bids for attention and comfort.[27,28] Bowlby believed that, like animals, human infants are biologically predisposed to use the caregiver as a haven of safety or a secure base while exploring the environment and that when the infant feels threatened he or she will turn to the caregiver for protection and comfort. Importantly, the caregiver's response to such bids helps mould the attachment relationship into a pattern that allows the infant to begin to anticipate the caregiver's response to subsequent bids. The young infant initially knows no bounds to his or her emotions, and must learn what emotions, and what demands for response, are appropriate (i.e. what the care-giver will accept as reasonable). Bowlby believed that all subsequent emotional relationships (including husband–wife, clinician–patient and the parent–child bond in the next generation) are patterned by this early experience with the mother.

Careful observation of the interactions between human mother–child pairs has produced a taxonomy of attachment behaviours comprising four types[27,28]:

• Secure attachment: The child explores a new environment freely when the mother is present, returning to the mother periodically for reassurance; en-gages with strangers; becomes visibly upset when the mother departs and is happy to see the mother return. Around 65% of children show this pattern of attachment.

• Anxious-resistant insecure attachment: The child is anxious of exploration and of strangers, even when the mother is present; becomes extremely dis-tressed when the mother departs but displays ambivalent behaviour when she returns (e.g. resists when the mother initiates attention). Around 15% show this pattern.

• Anxious-avoidant insecure attachment: The child avoids or ignores the mother and shows little emotion when she departs or returns; does not ex-plore a new environment much, regardless of who is there; displays a narrow range of emotion. Around 15% show this pattern.

• Disorganised attachment: The child does not display a consistent style for coping with new situations or mother's departure – perhaps as a result of confusing experiences with multiple and/or inconsistent caregivers. Up to 10% of children show this pattern.

If you are a clinician, you may recognise some of these behaviour patterns from children you have observed yourself in the clinic or during home vis-its. The consistent empirical finding that a securely attached child (in, say, a laboratory play situation) uses the mother as a 'secure base' from which to explore happily in ever-increasing circles, returning to her in times of novelty and uncertainty, has formed the basis of a detailed theory of the healthy tension between attachment and exploration,[27] which has entered the vernacular (as in 'she smothered him rather than mothered him' or 'if you wrap your child in cotton wool she'll never become independent') and which is widely drawn upon in the intuitive suggestions that primary care clinicians offer to parents who seek their advice.

Attachment theory remains the dominant theory underpinning the manage-ment of emotional and behaviour disorders in children and of child and adoles-cent mental health problems.[27] In studies based on psychological approaches (typically, a series of questionnaire surveys undertaken longitudinally through time as children develop), it is those with secure attachment relationships who are found to take better advantage of their opportunities in life, are better liked by their peers, have superior leadership and social skills, have better conflict management skills (hence 'fly off the handle' less) and are more confident than other children.[29] Boys with anxious-avoidant attachments are at greatly increased risk of developing violent and antisocial behaviour, and girls with this pattern are at risk of depression.[30] In one longitudinal study of a large cohort of US children, the quality of attachments in early childhood and the levels of early childhood support predicted with 77% accuracy the children who subsequently became high-school drop-outs.[30] Mel Bartley has recently shown in the large Whitehall II study (see Section 8.4) that middle-aged men who did not have anxious or avoidant attachment styles were more likely to overcome the disadvantage of a lower level of educational attainment and progress up the professional career ladder, raising the enticing hypothesis that attachment style may be one of the 'missing variables' accounting for socio-economic differentials in health, once behaviour choices such as smoking, diet and exercise were accounted for.[31] Problems with parent–child attachments are increasingly recognised as recurring in successive generations, as people who were insecurely attached themselves become parents and repeat the cycle with their own children.[29]

What causes attachment disorder? The most consistent factor associated with insecure and disorganized attachment patterns is neglect or abuse in infancy and early childhood. Children who have emotionally barren family lives or are raised in large institutions such as orphanages have a high risk of developing insecure attachments.[29,32] Even in children who have had secure attachments in early infancy, a shift to an insecure attachment pattern is more likely following (a) loss of a parent, (b) parental divorce, (c) life-threatening illness in a parent or the child (e.g. diabetes, cancer, heart attack), (d) parental psychiatric disorder and (e) physical or sexual abuse by a family member.[32]

As the mothers of young children spend more time at work, the role of the father in the development of the child is becoming increasingly critical.[33,34] A growing body of research demonstrates that in contemporary society, a child's closest attachment may be with the father rather than the mother, or indeed with multiple attachment figures, and that such attachments are, all other things being equal, just as likely to be secure.[35,36] Indeed, Bowlby has been heavily criticized by feminists for assuming rather than demonstrating that it was the mother rather than the 'primary caregiver' on whom the child's emotional security necessarily rested.[37,38] It has even been suggested that Bowlby's first book advising mothers of young children not to go out to work, published in 1950, was a politically motivated conspiracy, since men had returned from the war a few years earlier to find women doing their jobs with an unexpected degree of competence! Others have suggested that the four 'types' of attachment observed in mother–child dyads in western societies do not transfer to non-western cultures and this taxonomy should not be used uncritically to pathologise ethnic minority families.[39]

Whilst there is much we do not yet know about attachment behaviour, a number of things are now very clear. Insecure and disorganised attachment behaviours are common; they generally arise in infancy; and they can lead to profound and long-lasting emotional and social problems that may recur in subsequent generations. Given the strength of this evidence and the importance of the issue, surely we (as parents, clinicians, teachers and childcare professionals, and taxpayers) should do all we can to prevent attachment pathologies from developing. Most of us would wish on every newborn child two parents (or other caregivers) who love one another and who welcome, love and nurture their child. But many infants are born into a less than perfect emotional world played out in less than perfect physical surroundings. What then?

The UK (along with the USA and Canada) has made it a policy priority to implement programmes to promote and enrich the parent–child (especially mother–child but also father–child) bond, teach and support appropriate parenting behaviour and provide role models for parents who did not themselves receive high-quality nurturing as children. Many such programmes have been targeted largely or exclusively at teenage parents or those otherwise considered at high risk of producing children with emotional and behavioural problems. Two main approaches are used: formal training in parenting (perhaps in a group setting) and home visiting by a mentor who develops a relationship with the family and supports them in their home environment. Whilst both such approaches are 'evidence based' in that the interventions have been derived from sound psychological principles and shown to have significant impact in research trials,[40–44] most such programmes have relatively little impact when replicated in real-world (non-research) settings.[45] The reasons for this research-practice gap are complex, and relate partly to the complex and largely unpredictable interactions between different levels (individual, interpersonal, family, community, society – see Section 3.9) and to the likely presence of multiple unmeasured variables that compound the negative experiences of the victims of multiple deprivation (see Section 8.2).

On a less dramatic note, it is worth acknowledging the growth industry of books, websites and life-coaching programmes that plays on the middle-class parent's anxieties about the quality of their child's upbringing. The 'quality time' package, for example (in which busy working parents are encouraged to compensate for time away from home by providing short periods of positive emotional contact with their young children), has been neither formally defined nor empirically tested, though websites abound telling parents that if they hug their child in a particular way or whisper special words at bedtime, their mutual bond will be duly reinforced! What should we advise such parents? Certainly, that love, nurturance and emotionally responsive care from a consistent primary caregiver are essential for healthy development and that these inputs are complex and unlikely to be fully captured in a 'ten tips for easy parenting' guide. We can also tell them that emotional neglect is by no means the exclusive terrain of the poor or the socially excluded. Parenting is one of life's biggest responsibilities, and it requires compromises. The research literature is largely silent on how many corners may be safely cut by the busy parents without compromising the secure attachment with their child that should surely be every parent's goal.

7.3 Illness in the family – nature, nurture and culture

The three examples in Box 7.1 show how illness is often (perhaps usually) a family affair. The more detail that is added to the knowledge base arising from the human genome project, the more diseases are recognised to have an inherited (genetic) component. A generation ago, conditions such as eczema, heart disease, type 2 diabetes and bipolar affective disorder ('manic depression'), though known to run in families, were not thought of primarily as genetic diseases because they showed neither visible abnormalities in chromosomes (as in Down syndrome or Fragile X) nor the kind of Mendelian single-gene inheritance characteristic of sickle cell anaemia (autosomal recessive), achondroplasia (autosomal dominant) or haemophilia (X-lined recessive). Increasingly, however, the title 'genetic' is used to refer not only to these classic genetic diseases but also to conditions with polygenic inheritance (in which multiple gene loci contribute to the phenotype).

Whilst the detail of the new genetics is beyond the scope of this book, it is worth pointing out that even in single gene disorders like sickle cell anaemia, and especially in polygenic disorders like type 2 diabetes, a person's phenotype (the visible characteristics of that person) is the best his or her genotype can do, given the environment (physical, psychological, emotional) that he or she grows up in. Every child with uncomplicated sickle cell anaemia, for example, possesses two copies of the gene for abnormal haemoglobin and will be predisposed to agonising sickling crises in which sickle-shaped red blood cells physically clog key blood vessels. But epidemiological studies (of who gets sickle cell crises and when) reveal a very skewed pattern: Around 90% of all sickle cell crises occur in 10% of people with the disease. Around one-third of all people with sickle cell anaemia never have a full-blown sickling crisis, whereas a small minority have recurrent hospital admissions with such crises and live the life of an invalid. If the genetic defect is identical in both these extremes, what makes the difference in the phenotype?

The answer is, as the title of this section suggests, a combination of 'nature', 'nurture' and 'culture'. Even a 'pure' single-gene abnormality such as the one that underlies sickle cell disease still interacts extensively with the rest of the person's genetic material. In some people, for example, it is 'normal' for 45% of their blood volume to be made up of serum (the fluid part); in others, the normal haematocrit level is nearer 55%; this is likely to make a huge difference since sickle crises are precipitated by dehydration. But another crucial factor differentiating between the 'recurrently sick' and the 'essentially well' person with sickle cell anaemia is socio-behavioural dimension.[46] To what extent does the family of a child with sickle cell anaemia understand, and follow, the advice to maintain hydration? To what extent are family activities and holidays planned, and minor illnesses such as colds managed, with meticulous attention to the need to avoid dehydration? Furthermore, what is the symbolic meaning to this child (and in this family) of a hospital admission with a sickle cell crisis? Does the child welcome such an experience as temporary respite from an emotionally strained home environment? Is he or she punished – or rewarded – by parents? Whose 'fault' is the crisis seen as? To what extent is the incident seen as a learning opportunity and are measures taken to prevent a similar episode occurring in the future? I hope you can see from this example that whilst an acute illness may be traced back to a rock-solid genetic basis and a clear 'objective' precipitant, the family environment may be all-important in determining both the onset and severity of the episode and the likelihood of recurrence.

As with sickle cell crisis, so (even more so) with the bread-and-butter illnesses of primary health care. The infant with croup, the child with recurrent constipation, the teenager with dysmenorrhoea, the housewife with tiredness, the middle-aged man with high blood pressure and the grandparent with 'memory problems' (to cite a few examples out of the many hundreds we deal with in our surgeries every day) are all attributable partly to nature (genetic predisposition), partly to nurture (the physical environment in which we find ourselves or choose to place ourselves – including our food and shelter arrangements, lifestyle choices such as smoking and exercise, and the quality of our social networks) and partly to culture (the symbolic meaning of particularly symptoms and physical states in particular groups and communities – see Section 2.5). The dominance of the biomedical paradigm in much of healthcare (i.e. the fact that the biological origins of illness are given more space and credence than their social and environmental origins) means that the primary care clinician is often subtly driven towards investigating and managing illness on narrowly biomedical terms rather than in more holistic terms – and, perhaps, to assuming that because an illness is 'inherited', there is little that can be done about it by either patient or clinician. In many cases, this unnecessarily fatalistic attitude has no true scientific basis and does the patient a great disservice.

Let us consider the example of alcohol dependence – a condition that has been officially confirmed as 'polygenically inherited' (i.e. the tendency to become dependent on alcohol is due to a combination of several 'bad genes').[47] An alcohol-dependent father and an alcohol-dependent mother might produce several children, each with a different genetic propensity to become alcohol dependent themselves. But it is also recognised that there is a strong environmental component and that the children who actually became alcohol dependent might not be the ones with greatest genetic propensity but those with a fairly strong propensity who also found themselves in social situations and jobs where alcohol was available and affordable. But what is the relative contribution of 'nature' and 'nurture' here?

Epidemiological studies that have followed twin pairs – both monozygotic ('identical', who share all their genetic material) and dizygotic (who share half) – from childhood to adulthood have suggested that around 50% of the propensity to alcohol dependence is carried in the genes.[47] But studies of identical twins are problematic, since such individuals tend to have a very similar environment right into adulthood. In extreme cases identical twins share a bedroom (perhaps even a bed), are dressed alike, go to the same school and college and eat the same food at almost every meal for the first 15 years of their lives. Non-identical twins are more likely to be treated by parents, teachers and friends (and one another) as two separate individuals rather than a matching pair. In other words, non-identical twins have greater differences in environment as well as greater differences in their genes. For this reason, twin registry studies tend to over-estimate the heritability of complex polygenic traits such as alcoholism, schizophrenia and antisocial personality disorder.[48]

A new variant of the twin registry study is the offspring-of-twins study, in which the children of identical twin pairs are compared. Imagine identical twins Bill (who has a son called Bob) and Fred (who has a son called Frank). Bill has alcohol dependence, but as it happens, Fred shows no sign of the condition. Bob, who has inherited a high genetic propensity for alcohol dependence *and* has been raised in an adverse environment (poor role model, alcohol readily available, etc.), is many times more likely than average to develop alcoholism. But it was recently shown that Frank, who has inherited exactly the same level of *genetic* propensity to alcoholism as Bob but has been raised in a more favourable environment, is no more likely than anyone in the general population to develop alcohol dependence.[49]

Where does all this leave us? The answer is that the inheritance of alcohol dependence appears to be closer to nurture and farther from nature, than was thought to be the case 5 years ago. But interestingly, offspring-of-twins studies in schizophrenia have demonstrated the opposite – that the children of people with schizophrenia have almost exactly the same risk of developing schizophrenia themselves (17%) as the offspring of their non-schizophrenic monozygotic twins.[50] It would appear that there is a strong genetic predisposition which may lie 'dormant' in one generation because of lack of environmental trigger, but which is nevertheless passed on to the next generation just as strongly as if the parent had suffered from the condition himself or herself. This, of course, begs the question of what the environmental trigger in schizophrenia is and how we might prevent susceptible individuals from being exposed to it – for which there are no simple answers, but you may find a recent review helpful.[51]

The evidence on caregiver–child attachment (see previous section) suggests that the emotional environment is an especially critical aspect of nurture in the genesis of mental health problems – even those with an established genetic basis. As I emphasised previously, attachment disorders tend to repeat themselves down the generations. Repetti and her colleagues have introduced the notion of 'risky families' – characterised by conflict and aggression and by relationships that are cold, unsupportive and neglectful.[52] Such families do not 'cause' mental health problems by some simple linear connection, nor do they cause chronic physical diseases such as high blood pressure or ischaemic heart disease by (always and predictably) raising serum cortisol levels and otherwise generating a physiological stress response. But as Repetti et al. demonstrate, risky families are statistically linked with chronic mental health problems, chronic physical illness (especially heart disease) and substance abuse (smoking, alcohol and illegal drugs).

7.4 Homelessness

When I am not writing textbooks, teaching students or doing research, I still work as a GP, seeing patients in a north London practice. An increasing proportion of the patients I see have nowhere they can really call home. Like Nermal (Box 7.1), they may be temporarily housed in a refuge or other place of safety. Or they may be staying temporarily, and sequentially, with different friends and acquaintances ('couch surfing'). Or they may be genuinely sleeping in subways and on park benches, and given a false address to gain access to the services offered at my surgery. An often-quoted statistic, whose origins I cannot verify, says that 8% of the patients registered with a GP practice makes up 50% of the clinical workload and 2% makes up 25% of the workload. If this is true, I suspect that most of the homeless lie in that 2%.

Numerous systematic reviews on the problems of the homeless have been undertaken.[53–58] These summarise dozens of surveys across the world which have consistently documented higher mortality rates, higher rates of acute and chronic illness and higher risks of being exposed to violence and injuries in the homeless (Box 7.4). Whilst the exact prevalence of each condition varies with country and region (and also with the definition of homelessness used in the research study), morbidity in the homeless is phenomenally high. One review found that the overall prevalence of mental disorders among homeless individuals varied from 80–95% in the USA, Australia, Canada, Norway and Germany to 25–33% in Ireland and Spain, and a relative risk of mortality amongst the homeless between 3.7 and 8.5 compared to non-homeless people of the same age and gender; their rate of hospital admission is around five times that of the general population, and they stay in hospital longer.[57] The reasons why so many people with physical and mental health problems slide into homelessness are complex and multifaceted (Box 7.4); one group of researchers has applied social ecology theory (see Section 3.9) to explain the interplay of genetic risk factors, psychological resources (or, sometimes, lack of these), adverse physical and emotional environment and unfavourable social, political and economic structures in the trajectory into homelessness.[63]

The studies cited in Box 7.4 also document the significantly lower ability of the homeless to access services for health and social care, because of lack of personal documentation, inability to make appointments, low literacy and ignorance of what is available. Probably for this reason, the homeless are traditionally much more likely to seek (and receive) their care in accident and emergency departments, to present late in the course of illness and to fail to receive the continuity of care required for optimum management of conditions like diabetes, mental illness or HIV/AIDS.[53,59,60,64]

How should primary care respond to the growing problem of homelessness? In some ways, this question is not as difficult as it appears to be. The

Box 7.4 Homelessness: a summary.

Risk factors for becoming homeless

Individual

   Poverty
   Non-white ethnicity
   Low educational attainment
   Low health literacy
   Low psychological resilience and resourcefulness
   Foster care or abuse as a child
   Parental drug dependence
   Limited social networks (see Section 9.2)
   Major mental illness
   Alcohol or drug abuse, *especially* concurrent mental illness and substance
      abuse

Environmental/Societal

   Housing cost and availability
   Labour market conditions
   Extent of social services 'safety net'
   Social attitudes and the nature and extent of social exclusion (e.g. racism)
   High prevalence of crime and illegal drug use locally

Conditions that are significantly more common in the homeless

Addiction problems, e.g. drug dependency, alcohol dependency and related
   conditions
Other mental health problems, e.g. depression, affective disorders, psychotic
   disorders, schizophrenia and personality disorders
Infections diseases, e.g. tuberculosis, HIV/AIDS, other sexually transmitted
   infections
Diseases linked to exposure, e.g. hypothermia, sunstroke
Diseases linked to environmental pollution and smoking, e.g. asthma,
   bronchitis
Diseases linked to trauma and prolonged walking, e.g. cellulitis, foot ulcers,
   'trench foot'.
Diseases linked to poor diet, e.g. diabetes, coronary heart disease
Conditions linked to social problems, e.g. domestic violence
Developmental and emotional problems in children, e.g. attachment disorders
   (see Section 7.2)

Compiled from various sources.[53–62]

other sections in this book present a wealth of evidence that the core values and principles of primary care set out in Section 1.1 (such as continuity of care; a strong and trusting clinician–patient relationship; coordinated, multi-professional evidence-based management of chronic disease; holistic care and so on) are associated with better outcomes for patients. In no group is this more true than in the homeless. But what is less clear is the best service model for delivering primary care services to this challenging group. GPs are traditionally reluctant to take on patients who require maintenance for drug addition, and may use the lack of fixed address as a reason not to take on the patient. As I will explain in Section 10.4, one organisational response of GP practices to rising external pressure is to turn away patients who are perceived as being 'high maintenance' and/or who are perceived as threatening the social ambience of the 'family' practice.[65] The response of homeless people to a lack of welcome in traditional general practice is to circumvent the family doctor system entirely, ignore preventive care and minor symptoms, and go directly to hospital when their symptoms become intolerable. Here, par excellence, is an example of Tudor Hart's inverse care law: People most in need of health care are least likely to seek it or receive it.[66]

Because of the complex (and, often, multiple) problems of the homeless and because of ethical and practical issues to do with access (i.e. gaining access to research participants and their informed consent to do the research), research on homelessness is relatively sparse. A comprehensive review of this research is beyond the scope of this book, but I will briefly describe four very different research studies that illustrate how a clear grounding in theory can inform creative and illuminative research in this challenging area.

One important task for researchers into homelessness is to document the contribution of different putative risk factors to the onset of homelessness. In one such study on homeless young people, Craig and colleagues used a case-control design (see Section 3.3 and Figure 3.5, page 69).[67] Their 'cases' were 161 homeless people recruited from the streets and their controls were 107 individuals of the same age and gender recruited from GP lists. Each participant was interviewed using a questionnaire and asked about demographic data (e.g. years of education) and about a range of experiences in early childhood, as well as some questions designed to diagnose formal psychiatric illness. The questionnaire data were entered into a computer program, and the authors used regression analysis to determine the likely contribution of different factors to the outcome of homelessness. Sixty-nine per cent of homeless and a third of controls reported a childhood lacking in affection, with indifferent and often violent carers. The responses suggested formal psychiatric illness in 62% of the homeless respondents and a quarter of the controls. Multivariate analysis of this data set suggested that adverse emotional environment in childhood, low educational attainment and the presence of psychiatric disorder all independently increased the likelihood of homelessness in this population. Findings such as this are intuitively plausible but raise the 'chicken and egg' question (which caused which – the homelessness or the psychiatric disorder); for more on the question of causality see Section 8.2.

A very different type of research study into homelessness aims to describe and document the nature of continuity of care (or absence of such continuity). Fortney et al. used a multimethod design to unpack the notion of 'continuity of care' and see how well a particular health system measured up in providing this to its homeless population.[68] In the first phase of their study, they used a quasi-systematic literature review to identify five dimensions of continuity of care: timeliness, intensity, comprehensiveness, stability and coordination. They developed questionnaire items to measure each of these dimensions. In the second phase, they recruited homeless participants from various sources (shelters, streets and public mental health clinics) and administered a questionnaire to assess continuity of care according to their new scale. They also looked retrospectively at the health care records of participants to add to data on continuity. Unsurprisingly, they found that the homeless had much lower scores on all the dimensions of continuity of care. The main contribution of this particular study was not to document what we already know about lack of continuity, but to provide an easily administered measure of this continuity, which might be used in subsequent studies of interventions to improve such continuity.

My third example of an approach to researching homelessness comes from social science. In Section 9.2, I will discuss the important concept of social networks and their contribution to individual health. A number of studies have sought to measure social networks and social support in homeless people. Twelve of these were summarised in a systematic review by Meadows-Oliver and colleagues, a team of nursing researchers who focused on social support for homeless women.[56] The basic technique in social network studies is to ask people who they know (quantitative network analysis) and/or what they get out of the friendship or contact (qualitative network analysis). In keeping with what one would expect from what we know about social networks and deprivation (see Section 9.2), homeless women perceived themselves as having lower overall social support than housed women. Statistical analysis showed that this difference was attributable to four deficiencies in their social networks: size (homeless women knew fewer people), composition (the sort of people they knew were less resourceful than the sort of people known by housed women), frequency of contacts (homeless women saw their contacts less often) and the nature of support (when they did see their contacts, less support was given). The authors conclude that nurses who work with homeless families may be in a position to help develop ways for these families to cultivate and maintain their social support networks while homeless, as well as offering direct support themselves in relation to accessing health services.

A final example of research into homelessness is the randomised controlled trial of a complex intervention, usually designed to provide an integrated ('holistic') package of health and social care services specifically for the needs of the homeless, in which (for example) drug dependency (including opioid replacement), mental health, sexually transmitted infections and social problems such as domestic violence and home seeking are all addressed. Numerous such packages have been developed and tested; see two systematic reviews for examples.[54,55] In an early study in the UK by Marshall and colleagues, case management of homeless drug users was compared with usual care in a randomised controlled trial design.[69] The basic principle of the 'case management' approach is that a designated case manager takes responsibility for a client and arranges an assessment of need, a comprehensive service plan, delivery of suitable services and monitoring and assessment of services delivered. At 14-month follow-up, outcome was assessed by standardised interviews. Perhaps surprisingly, there were no significant differences between groups in number of needs, quality of life, employment status, quality of accommodation, social behaviour or severity of psychiatric symptoms, though the case-management group showed significantly less 'deviant behaviour'. The authors concluded that 'It is unfortunate, in view of the limited effectiveness we have shown, that social services case-management was not evaluated in randomised controlled trials before its implementation in the UK'.

Overall, the research literature on homelessness suggests what every primary care clinician knows intuitively – that the needs of the homeless, especially in our increasingly diverse and fragmented society, are multiple and complex, and that there is no simple model of care that will alleviate these needs and be transferable across different contexts and systems of care. Whilst the principles of effective primary health care apply equally to those with and without homes to go to, the high prevalence of substance abuse and mental health problems makes delivering patient-centred, coordinated, evidence-based care a major challenge for primary care teams. But primary care should aspire to do more than 'muddle through'. Further research is undoubtedly needed to develop theory-driven interventions and should ideally be based on a multi-level theoretical framework in which individual, family and societal influences are all considered and addressed.

References

1 Porter R. *The Greatest Benefit to Mankind: A Medical History of Humanity*. London: Fontana Press; 1999.
2 Portillo M. The Bevan legacy. BMJ 1998;317:37–40.
3 Mash B. *Handbook of Family Medicine*. 2nd edn. Cape Town: Oxford University Press; 2006.
4 Starfield B. *Primary Care: Balancing Health Needs, Services and Technology*. New York: Oxford University Press; 1992.
5 Kirmayer LJ, Groleau D, Looper KJ, Dao MD. Explaining medically unexplained symptoms. Can J Psychiatry 2004;49:663–672.
6 Amer KS. Children's adaptation to insulin dependent diabetes mellitus: a critical review of the literature. J Pediatr Nurs 1999;25:627–641.
7 Anonymous. Households and families. *Social Trends No. 36*. London: Office of National Statistics; 2006.

8 Smith A, Wasoff F, Jamieson L. *Solo Living Across the Adult Lifecourse*. Edinburgh: University of Edinburgh, Centre for Research on Families and Relationships; 2004.

9 Potts M. China's one child policy. BMJ 2006;333:361–362.

10 Jiang L. Changing kinhsip structure and its implications for old-age support in urban and rural China. Population Stud 1995;49:127–145.

11 Whiteside A. The real challenges: the orphan generation and employment creation. AIDS Anal Afr 2000;10:14–15.

12 Naidu V, Harris G. The impact of HIV/AIDS morbidity and mortality on households – a review of household studies. S Afr J Econ 2005;73(suppl):533–544.

13 Kamerman SB, Neuman M, Waldfogel J, Brooks-Gunn J. *Social Policies, Family Types, and Child Outcomes in Selected OECD Countries*. OECD Social, Employment and Migration Working Papers No. 6. Paris: OECD; 2003.

14 Bos HM, van BF, van dB. Lesbian families and family functioning: an overview. Patient Educ Couns 2005;59:263–275.

15 Coté JE. Sociological perspectives on identity formation: the culture-identity link and identity capital. J Adolesc 1996;19:417–428.

16 Mead M. *Culture and Commitment. A Study of the Generation Gap*. Gardin City: Doubleday; 1970.

17 Giddens A. *The Consequences of Modernity*. Cambridge, UK: Polity Press; 1990.

18 Beck U. *Risk Society: Towards a New Modernity*. London: Sage; 1992.

19 Roberts K. *Youth and Employment in Modern Britain*. Oxford: Oxford University Press; 1995.

20 Lloyd-Richardson EE, Papandonatos G, Kazura A, Stanton C, Niaura R. Differentiating stages of smoking intensity among adolescents: stage-specific psychological and social influences. J Consult Clin Psychol 2002;70:998–1009.

21 Kahn JR, Anderson KE. Intergenerational patterns of teenage fertility. Demography 1992;29:39–57.

22 Heyman SJ. *The Widening Gap: Why American Families Are in Jeopardy and What Can Be Done About It*. New York: Basic Books; 2000.

23 UNICEF. *Child Poverty in Rich Countries 2005*. UNICEF Innocenti Report Card No 6. Florence: United Nations Children's Fund; 2006.

24 Peisner-Feinberg ES, Burchinal MR, Clifford RM, et al. The relation of preschool child-care quality to children's cognitive and social developmental trajectories through second grade. Child Dev 2001;72:1534–1553.

25 Waldfogel J. Child care, women's employment, and family types. J Population Econ 2002;15:527–548.

26 Harlow HF, Harlow MK. Effects of various mother–infant relationships on rhesus monkey behaviors. In: Foss BM, ed. *Determinants of Infant Behavior*. Vol. 4. London: Methuen; 1969.

27 Bretherton I. Bowlby's legacy to developmental psychology. Child Psychiatry Hum Dev 1997;28:33–43.

28 Bowlby J. *Attachment and Loss*. London: Tavistock Publications; 1969.

29 Levy TM, Orlans M. *Attachment, Trauma, and Healing*. Washington, DC: Child Welfare League of America Press; 1998.

30 Sroufe A, Duggal S, Weinfeld N, Carlson E. Relationships, development and psychopathology. In: Sameroff A, Lewis M, Miller S, eds. *Handbook of Developmental Psychopathology*. 2nd edn. New York: Plenum Publishers; 2000.

31 Bartley M, Head J, Stansfeld S. Is attachment style a source of resilience against health inequalities at work? Soc Sci Med 2007;64(4):765–775.

32 Waters E, Merrick S, Treboux D, Crowell J, Albersheim L. Attachment security in infancy and early adulthood: a twenty-year longitudinal study. Child Dev 2000;71:684–689.

33 Cabrera NJ, Tamis-LeMonda CS, Bradley RH, Hofferth S, Lamb ME. Fatherhood in the twenty-first century. Child Dev 2000;71:127–136.

34 Tiedje LB, rling-Fisher C. Fatherhood reconsidered: a critical review. Res Nurs Health 1996;19:471–484.

35 Schaffer HR. *Social Development*. Oxford: Blackwell; 1996.

36 Rutter M. *Maternal Deprivation Reassessed*. Harmondsworth: Penguin; 1981.

37 Williams F. Troubled masculinities in social policy discourses: fatherhood. In: Popay J, Hearn J, Edwards J, eds. *Men, Gender Divisions and Welfare*. London: Routledge; 1998.

38 Taylor J, Daniel B. The rhetoric vs. the reality in child care and protection: ideology and practice in working with fathers. J Adv Nurs 2000;31:12–19.

39 Minuchin P. Cross-cultural perspectives: implications for attachment theory and family therapy. Fam Process 2002;41:546–550.

40 Barlow J, Parsons J. Group-based parent-training programmes for improving emotional and behavioural adjustment in 0–3 years old children. Cochrane Database Syst Rev 2003;(1):CD003680.

41 Barlow J, Coren E. Parent-training programmes for improving maternal psychosocial health. Cochrane Database Syst Rev 2001;(2):CD002020.

42 Cameron G, Cadell S. Fostering empowering participation in prevention programs for disadvantaged children and families: lessons from ten demonstration sites. Can J Commun Ment Health 1999;18:105–121.

43 Kendrick D, Elkan R, Hewitt M, et al. Does home visiting improve parenting and the quality of the home environment? A systematic review and meta analysis. Arch Dis Child 2000;82:443–451.

44 Hoyer PJ. Prenatal and parenting programs for adolescent mothers. Annu Rev Nurs Res 1998;16:221–249.

45 Tucker S, Klotzbach L, Olsen G, et al. Lessons learned in translating research evidence on early intervention programs into clinical care. MCN Am J Matern Child Nurs 2006;31:325–331.

46 Edwards CL, Scales MT, Loughlin C, et al. A brief review of the pathophysiology, associated pain, and psychosocial issues in sickle cell disease. Int J Behav Med 2005;12:171–179.

47 Hines LM, Ray L, Hutchison K, Tabakoff B. Alcoholism: the dissection for endophenotypes. Dialogues Clin Neurosci 2005;7:153–163.

48 Joseph J. Twin studies in psychiatry and psychology: science or pseudoscience? Psychiatr Q 2002;73:71–82.

49 Jacob T, Waterman B, Heath A, et al. Genetic and environmental effects on offspring alcoholism: new insights using an offspring-of-twins design. Arch Gen Psychiatry 2003;60:1265–1272.

50 Gottesman II, Bertelsen A. Confirming unexpressed genotypes for schizophrenia. Risks in the offspring of Fischer's Danish identical and fraternal discordant twins. Arch Gen Psychiatry 1989;46:867–872.

51 Walker E, Kestler L, Bollini A, Hochman KM. Schizophrenia: etiology and course. Annu Rev Psychol 2004;55:401–430.

52 Repetti RL, Taylor SE, Seeman TE. Risky families: family social environments and the mental and physical health of offspring. Psychol Bull 2002;128:330–366.

53 Wright NM, Tompkins CN. How can health services effectively meet the health needs of homeless people? Br J Gen Pract 2006;56:286–293.

54 Hwang SW, Tolomiczenko G, Kouyoumdjian FG, Garner RE. Interventions to improve the health of the homeless: a systematic review. Am J Prev Med 2005;29:311–319.

55 Frankish CJ, Hwang SW, Quantz D. Homelessness and health in Canada: research lessons and priorities. Can J Public Health 2005;96(suppl 2):S23–S29.

56 Meadows-Oliver M. Social support among homeless and housed mothers: an integrative review. J Psychosoc Nurs Ment Health Serv 2005;43:40–47.

57 Martens WH. A review of physical and mental health in homeless persons. Public Health Rev 2001;29:13–33.

58 Crane M, Warnes AM, Fu R. Developing homelessness prevention practice: combining research evidence and professional knowledge. Health Soc Care Community 2006;14:156–166.

59 Douaihy AB, Stowell KR, Bui T, Daley D, Salloum I. HIV/AIDS and homelessness, Part 1: background and barriers to care. AIDS Read 2005;15:516–520, 527.

60 Douaihy AB, Stowell KR, Bui T, Daley D, Salloum I. HIV/AIDS and homelessness, Part 2: treatment issues. AIDS Read 2005;15:603–604, 618.

61 Rees CA. Thinking about children's attachments. Arch Dis Child 2005;90:1058–1065.

62 March JC, Oviedo-Joekes E, Romero M. Drugs and social exclusion in ten European cities. Eur Addict Res 2006;12(1):33–41.

63 Haber MG, Toro PA. Homelessness among families, children, and adolescents: an ecological-developmental perspective. Clin Child Fam Psychol Rev 2004;7:123–164.

64 Gallagher TC, Andersen RM, Koegel P, Gelberg L. Determinants of regular source of care among homeless adults in Los Angeles. Med Care 1997;35:814–830.

65 Charles-Jones H, Latimer J, May C. Transforming general practice: the redistribution of medical work in primary care. Sociol Health Illn 2003;25:71–92.

66 Hart JT. *A New Kind of Doctor*. London: Merlin Press; 1988.

67 Craig TK, Hodson S. Homeless youth in London: I. Childhood antecedents and psychiatric disorder. Psychol Med 1998;28:1379–1388.

68 Fortney J, Sullivan G, Williams K, Jackson C, Morton SC, Koegel P. Measuring continuity of care for clients of public mental health systems. Health Serv Res 2003;38:1157–1175.

69 Marshall M, Lockwood A, Gath D. Social services case-management for long-term mental disorders: a randomised controlled trial. Lancet 1995;345:409–412.

CHAPTER 8

The population

Summary points

1 Data collected on individual patients in the primary care setting can contribute to population-level analysis of burden of disease and trends in disease patterns. Such data enable health services to be designed according to need and preventive initiatives planned and targeted. But these data are only as reliable as the accuracy and completeness of the recording of individual data by the primary care team.

2 Primary care clinicians increasingly deal with people's anxiety about the causation of disease. An association between a potentially harmful exposure (e.g. measles, mumps and rubella (MMR) vaccine) and a disease (e.g. autism) does not necessarily mean that the exposure has caused the disease.

3 Disease in a population may be detected by screening programmes delivered or coordinated in primary care. But screening programmes, even when based on accurate tests, are not always workable, acceptable or cost-effective. There is no point screening for a disease that is untreatable or in which early treatment holds no long-term advantage. False positive and false negative tests lead to unnecessary anxiety and false reassurance respectively.

4 Certain sectors in a population (notably the poor) are at greater risk of disease and death than others. Some but not all of this increased risk can be explained by behavioural risk factors such as smoking, physical inactivity and poor diet. Even risk factors that are apparently under individual choice are socially patterned: we all make the choices that seem realistic and available to us.

8.1 Describing disease in populations

I explained in Section 2.2 that epidemiology is the study of patterns of disease, and in Section 3.3 that the key research methods for elucidating these patterns are the cross-sectional survey (which detects prevalence, the total number of cases in a population); the longitudinal survey (which detects incidence, the number of new cases arising in a given time period); and the case-control study (which compares people with and without a disease to explore differences in past exposure to possible harmful influences. This is not a textbook of epidemiology (if you're looking for one, try Coggon/Rose[1] or Starfield[2]), but as Box 8.1 illustrates, primary care (and general practice in particular) has traditionally been an important source of data for epidemiologists.[3] Ensuring the accuracy,

Box 8.1 The UK General Practice Research Database (GPRD).

The GPRD is the world's largest computerised database of anonymised longitudinal medical records from primary health care. Data are currently being collected on over 3.4 million active patients from around 450 general practices throughout the UK. The GPRD is used worldwide for research by the pharmaceutical industry, clinical research organisations, regulators, government departments and academic institutions. Data from the GPRD supports research in a variety of areas including:

• clinical epidemiology (tracking the incidence and prevalence of diseases in particular populations and subgroups);

• health service planning (predicting what services will be necessary in the future based on trends in patterns of disease);

• studies of treatment (monitoring what treatments are currently offered to people with a particular disease or symptom);

• clinical research planning (identifying priorities for future research investment);

• drug utilisation (monitoring who is prescribed what drugs and what happens to them);

• drug safety (identifying adverse drug reactions and drug interactions);

• health outcomes (e.g. monitoring the natural history of disease when detected at an early stage);

• pharmacoeconomics (monitoring the costs of drug treatments).

The GPRD is available to researchers via a secure Internet connection or via datasets on CD-ROM. See Table 8.1 for examples of how it has been used in research.

This information was taken from the official website of the GP Research Database http://www.gprd.com/home/.

completeness and consistency of such data is an important responsibility of the primary care team (see Section 5.2 for further discussion on standardised disease taxonomies).

Good primary health care requires a population perspective, for a number of reasons. First, the planning and delivery of primary care services in any locality should reflect patterns of actual need rather than, say, historical tradition ('we've always had a dermatology service here' or 'we've never provided drug rehabilitation in this locality in the past'). Second, much disease is subclinical – that is, people have the condition but have not consulted a doctor, nurse, pharmacist or other health professional, either because they don't yet feel ill or because they are ignoring their symptoms for one reason or other. Some of these people would benefit from earlier diagnosis, and I address the options for this in Section 8.2. Third, a population perspective will attune us to the natural history of illness and disease over time and provide substance to clinical impressions such as 'mild to moderate depression seems to get better over time whatever treatment is given' or 'babies who appear to be "happy wheezers" tend to develop full-blown asthma in later childhood'.

Table 8.1 shows some examples of how large primary care databases such as the UK GP Research Database (GPRD, Box 8.1) can help epidemiologists answer a wide range of research questions relating to the incidence, prevalence, natural history and treatment options of different diseases and pre-disease states. Note, however, what I said in Section 2.2 – that epidemiological evidence is only as good as the representativeness of the samples, the quality of the data collected and the appropriateness of the statistical analyses. In relation to the GPRD, there may be systematic biases in the recording of data (e.g. a person with known diabetes may be more likely to have his smoking status and blood pressure recorded than someone without known diabetes), and there may be systematic inaccuracies in the data recorded (e.g. smokers may claim to have given up when they haven't; men with sexual dysfunction may not declare this even if asked). Because of these potential (and partly irredeemable) flaws in the data recorded on primary care databases, we should interpret research studies based on them with some level of scepticism. Of course, that is true of any research, but the sheer size of these databases sometimes induces an unjustified faith in the accuracy and robustness of the data they hold!

The GPRD is the largest, and also the most accurate and reliable, database in UK primary care, since GP practices that have opted into using it are also signed up to its use for epidemiological research (not least by the pharmaceutical industry, whose payments for the use of data subsidise the maintenance of the database and a range of non-commercial research). But many other similar databases exist and are used increasingly at local level to plan and monitor services in primary care. For example, almost all UK general practices are now computerised and are able to produce aggregated data (i.e. individual data summed to produce a picture of the whole population) on practice demographics (how many patients, how old, what gender, etc.) and – increasingly – on patterns of disease and treatment. Most UK general practitioners will be able to tell you, for example, what proportion of their adult female patients have had a cervical smear in the last 3 years, and estimate the level of glycaemic control of their patients with diabetes (percentage with HbA1c level below 7%, between 7 and 9%, or above 9%). These practice-based aggregates are used not only to plan and audit services (perhaps to target further training to practices who have not achieved 'targets'), but also to reward or punish practitioners for their performance and, hopefully, induce clinicians to raise the overall quality of care (see Sections 5.5 and 11.2 for more discussion on influencing clinical performance).

8.2   Explaining the 'causes' of disease

In these days of near-universal access to information, people increasingly attend their primary care clinician with a belief that some external factor (an

Table 8.1 Examples of research studies that have used the UK GP research database.

Author/year	Research question	Type of study and sample size	Main findings
Ashworth 2006[4]	Are patients with coughs and sneezes consulting more or less than they used to – and are clinicians prescribing more or fewer antibiotics?	Longitudinal cohort study* of 108 GP practices (650,000 registered patients) between 1995 and 2000	Consultation rates for 'all respiratory infections', 'sore throat', 'ear infection', 'bronchitis' and 'chest infection' declined in all age groups, more so in children. Antibiotic prescribing also declined
Smeeth 2004[5]	Does MMR vaccine cause autism?	Case-control study† (1294 cases, 4469 controls)	Children with autism were no more likely to have received MMR vaccine than children without autism
Clifford 2000[6]	What happens to men with lower urinary tract symptoms and/or benign prostatic hyperplasia?	Longitudinal cohort study* (61,364 men with lower urinary tract symptoms but no diagnosis of cancer)	As time goes on, fewer men with these symptoms are being treated with surgery, and surgery is happening later. More men are taking medical treatment (e.g. alpha blocker drugs); many remain on no medication for years. Taking medication appears to delay the need for surgery
Hernandez-Diaz 2001[7]	What is the risk of side effects with non-steroidal anti-inflammatory drugs (NSAIDs)? What factors make these side effects more or less likely?	Case-control study† nested within a longitudinal cohort study* (1899 patients taking NSAIDs, 10,000 controls not taking these drugs)	NSAIDs were associated with increased incidence of upper gastrointestinal bleeding and perforation (UGIB), acute liver injury, acute renal injury, heart failure and adverse reproductive outcomes. Dose, duration of treatment, patient age and history of ulcer all increased incidence
Farmer 1999[8]	What is the risk of a woman developing thrombo-embolic disease on the oral contraceptive pill, and is any class of this drug safer than any other?	Case-control study† nested within a longitudinal cohort study* (384 cases, 1464 controls), plus a review of previous epidemiological studies	The incidence of venous thrombo-embolism (VTE) in women on the contraceptive pill is around 4 per 10,000 exposed woman-years. Overweight women and those who smoke are at much greater risk of VTE. Second generation contraceptives are significantly safer than newer third-generation ones

*Figure 3.4, page 68, shows the design of a longitudinal cohort study.
†Figure 3.5, page 69, shows the design of a case-control study.

environmental exposure, something a health professional has done or plans to do, an individual behaviour choice and so on) will cause disease. In the last year, my patients have asked me to comment on whether:
- Fasting during the Muslim holy month of Ramadan causes peptic ulcer;
- Measles, mumps and rubella (MMR) vaccine causes autism;
- Early weaning of infants causes eczema;
- Mobile phones cause infertility;
- Telephone masts cause leukaemia;
- Eating eggs causes high cholesterol levels;
- Smoking marijuana causes psychosis;
- Breast feeding causes higher intelligence in babies.

You can probably add to this list with examples from your own clinical practice. In the remainder of this section, I want to talk a little about what we mean by *causality* in this context. Many patients (and almost as many clinicians) are confused about the difference between association and causation. In Section 7.2, when considering whether mothers going out to work had adverse effects on babies' cognitive and social development, I introduced the ecological fallacy – the apparent finding that one variable (A) has caused another (B), but which is actually due to a third, unmeasured ('confounding') variable (C). The number of unemployed people in a town may bear a close relationship to the number of crimes, but that doesn't mean that the unemployed are committing the crimes – both unemployment and crime may be due to economic recession! In order to demonstrate causality (e.g. that A causes B), a study must do more than show that when A increases, so does B. It must also fulfil the famous criteria developed by Sir Austin Bradford Hill (Box 8.2).

Box 8.2 Bradford Hill criteria for establishing disease causation.[9]

1 *Temporal relationship.* Exposure always precedes outcome, so the putative cause must happen before the occurrence of any disease. This is the only essential criterion.

2 *Strength of relationship* as measured by appropriate statistical tests. The stronger the association, the more likely it is that the relation is causal. For example, the more highly correlated hypertension is with a high sodium diet, the more likely it is that such a diet causes hypertension.

3 *Dose–response effect.* If more of the putative cause is associated with more disease, the relationship is more likely to be causal. Conversely, if a specific factor is the cause of a disease, the incidence of the disease should decline when exposure to the factor is reduced or eliminated. But absence of a dose-response relationship does not mean the relationship is not causal, since there may be a threshold above which a dose-response relationship could be demonstrated.

4 *Consistency.* Results are replicated in studies in different settings using different methods. For example, the link between smoking and lung cancer has been consistently demonstrated in thousands of studies in different countries, ethnic groups, and both genders.

5 *Plausibility.* The association can be explained using currently accepted models of pathological processes. However, studies that disagree with current 'normal science' may force a re-evaluation of accepted mechanisms of disease. This criterion is especially important in studies when numerous variables are measured and correlated with one another using computer software packages such as SPSS (Statistical Package for Social Sciences). 'Significant' correlations between two variables that lack a plausible explanation are very often due to chance or confounding.

6 *Consideration of alternative explanations.* In judging whether a reported association is causal, it is necessary to determine the extent to which researchers have taken other possible explanations into account and have effectively ruled out these alternatives.

7 *Coherence.* The proposed causal explanation should be compatible with existing theory and knowledge. For example, in the 1970s, peptic ulcer was seen as 'caused' by stress, but in the light of new knowledge that the bacterium *Helicobacter pylori* is strongly associated with peptic ulcer, new theories about a bacterial cause were introduced in the 1990s. However, as with plausibility, a possible causal association that goes against established theory and knowledge is not automatically false – it may force a reconsideration of accepted beliefs and principles.

8 *Experiment.* The condition can be altered (prevented or ameliorated) by an appropriate experimental regimen. For example, the treatment of peptic ulcer with antibiotics rather than 'stress reduction' added considerable weight to the hypothesis that bacteria *cause* peptic ulcer.

9 *Specificity.* This is established when a single putative cause produces a specific effect. This is not an especially strong criterion (e.g. lung cancer can occur in the absence of cigarette smoking), but if present, it strengthens the overall case for causality.

To take one example of a causality question from the ones I listed in the bullet points above, let us consider whether the MMR vaccine causes autism. In February 1998, the *Lancet* published a small research study by Dr Andrew Wakefield and colleagues which claimed to have demonstrated (provisionally, the authors admitted) a causal link between MMR triple vaccine and autism, with a putative explanation that involved the induction of inflammation of the bowel (hence: MMR vaccine → bowel inflammation → [perhaps] absorption of poisons → autism).[10] The study was a report on 12 children who had been referred to a paediatric gastroenterology clinic with both bowel symptoms (diarrhoea, abdominal pain, bloating and food intolerance) and pervasive developmental disorder characterised by loss of skills that had been previously acquired. Various blood tests, gastrointestinal biopsies and a sample of cerebrospinal fluid were taken from the children. The samples were examined to explore the extent of inflammatory reaction in the bowel and to exclude other diseases (such as thyroid disease, inherited metabolic syndromes and so on). Of dozens of tests done on each child, a number were abnormal, though no test was consistently abnormal in all the children. Eleven of the 12 children had microscopic evidence of inflammatory reaction in their bowel. The parents were asked to remember back and identify if and when MMR vaccine had been given. In 8 of the 12 children, the onset of developmental delay was said to have occurred within 2 weeks of having the MMR vaccine, and in 3 it was said to have occurred within 48 hours.

The first (and the only essential) Bradford Hill criterion is impossible to establish in the Wakefield study. Parental recall of whether their child has been vaccinated against MMR has been shown to be poor (in particular, most parents of unvaccinated children report that the vaccine was given).[11,12] Furthermore, parents of children who were showing signs of autism might have made a closer temporal link between the vaccination and the onset of symptoms than had actually been the case – an example of recall bias (see Section 3.7). The strength of the relationship is impossible to assess from the study design used by Wakefield et al. Indeed, this design is probably the best example of sampling bias ever published in the *Lancet* – as its editor later ruefully admitted.[13] The authors deliberately picked out the tiny number of children who had been referred to a major specialist centre because they had both bowel symptoms and an autism-like syndrome. So the fact that these rare conditions occurred together proves nothing at all. The fact that children with diarrhoea or other chronic gastrointestinal symptoms have microscopic evidence of inflamed bowels is also, in itself, unsurprising. The Wakefield study also falls down on plausibility, consideration of alternative explanations and consistency. No other research group has replicated the association demonstrated by Wakefield's team – and numerous much larger and better-designed studies (notably Liam Smeeth's excellent case-control study using the GP Research Database and listed in Table 8.1[5]) have shown no link whatsoever between MMR vaccine and either bowel disease or autism.

One of the most tragic spin-offs from the 1998 Wakefield paper was the widespread uptake by lay people and the media of the scientifically implausible hypothesis that MMR vaccine given in a single 'triple' dose posed a risk of autism, but that children could be safely given the three vaccines separately (at the same time, using three different needles). Again, there was no evidence from high-quality clinical trials that single vaccines were safer than the triple MMR. But the refusal of large numbers of parents to accept triple vaccine led some clinicians to take the line that it is better to 'play along' with their misconceptions and administer single vaccines than leave children unimmunised. Others (the majority) stuck to their guns and continued to offer only triple vaccine. This conundrum raises the interesting question of how much we should base our practice on patients' beliefs and fears whether well-founded or not, and how much we should adopt a 'doctor knows best' stance – a question that probably requires humanism, situational judgment and a dash of intuition (see Section 5.3).

8.3 Detecting disease in populations

To what extent should we bother people who don't feel ill in order to detect disease at an early (treatable) stage? We might do this by:
• screening (testing an entire population subgroup for early signs of a disease – for example, checking the hips of all newborn babies for congenital dislocation);
• opportunistic testing (offering a test when someone attends for another reason – e.g. taking the blood pressure of a middle-aged person who attends his or her GP for something else); or
• health promotion (raising awareness of disease in targeted high-risk groups so that people come forward – e.g. putting notices up in mosques attended by people of Asian ethnicity listing the symptoms of diabetes, or leafleting university students about the early symptoms of meningitis).

All these approaches may, overall, improve the health of the population, but they are also somewhat intrusive and may be interpreted as unwelcome 'nanny state' interventions. In this section, I consider the pros and cons of screening and opportunistic testing. Health promotion is a huge area which, purely because of space constraints, I have covered only tangentially in this book (see Section 9.5); if you are interested in health promotion I recommend one of the specialist textbooks in this area.[14,15]

In my own GP practice, we have active screening programmes for cervical pre-cancer (women aged 21–64 are offered a cervical smear test every 3 years), breast cancer (women aged 50–69 are offered a mammogram every 3 years) and various congenital abnormalities and developmental delays in children (especially congenital dislocation of the hip and deafness). Our community midwives and health visitors screen newborn babies for phenylketonuria (an enzyme abnormality that leads to mental retardation unless certain foods are avoided in the diet), hypothyroidism, cystic fibrosis and haemoglobinopathies (sickle cell anaemia and thalassaemia) if these tests have not already been done in hospital. Pregnant women are routinely offered various blood tests and ultrasound scans during pregnancy to detect (or hopefully, exclude) a range of abnormalities in the fetus. In addition, we take the blood pressure opportunistically of just about every adult who enters the building, and often tick extra boxes on blood test request forms (e.g. glucose or cholesterol) even when patients have no relevant symptoms. Are all these tests a good idea – and should we be sending for even more people who feel fine and subjecting them to blood tests, X-rays, questionnaires, vaginal swabs or analysis of their urine and stools?

Box 8.3 gives some definitions of the properties of a good screening test, and Box 8.4 shows the famous criteria developed 40 years ago by Wilson and Jungner for a good screening programme.[16] Note that a poor test (e.g. not

---

Box 8.3 Properties of a good screening test.[16,17]

• *Reliable.* Consistent results are obtained from the same individual by different observers on different occasions.
• *Practicable.* The test is easy to perform and interpret.
• *Acceptable.* People are happy to have the test performed on them.
• *Sensitive.* It correctly identifies people who have the disease.
• *Specific.* It correctly excludes people who do not have the disease.
• *High positive predictive value.* A positive result on the test means that it is very likely that the person has the disease.
• *High negative predictive value.* A negative result on the test means that it is very likely that the person does not have the disease.

---

sufficiently sensitive or specific) will never support a good screening programme, but the converse is not necessarily true – a good screening *test* does not automatically give you a good screening *programme*, since good tests might do no more than pick up diseases that are untreatable or not detect them until they have become symptomatic anyway!

I want to illustrate the principles of screening tests using two examples: breast cancer screening in women over 50 (or, as some have suggested, over 40[18,19]) and screening pregnant women for Down syndrome in the fetus.

The value of breast cancer screening, even in countries where it is highly prevalent, is hotly debated. As Table 8.2 shows, experts are divided on whether the standard screening test (one-view mammography) fulfils the criteria for a good test (Box 8.3) and whether the UK's National Breast Screening Programme (http://www.cancerscreening.nhs.uk/breastscreen/), in which women aged 50–69 are recalled three-yearly and those over 70 may request to remain in the programme, fulfils the criteria for a good programme (Box 8.4). The controversy cuts to the core of how epidemiological data should be generated and the extent to which they can be trusted. Seven large randomised trials

---

Box 8.4 Criteria for a good screening programme (Wilson and Jungner).[16]

• The screening test fulfils the criteria in Box 8.3.
• The condition should be an important health problem.
• The natural history of the condition should be understood.
• There should be a recognisable latent or early symptomatic stage.
• There should be an accepted treatment recognised for the disease.
• Treatment should be more effective if started early.
• There should be a policy on who should be treated.
• Diagnosis and treatment should be cost-effective.
• Case-finding should be a continuous process (i.e. the programme should not be a 'one-off').

Table 8.2 Characteristics of mammography test and screening programme for breast cancer.

Characteristic	Extent fulfilled	Comment
The disease		
Importance of problem	● ● ● ● ●	In Western countries, breast cancer is the commonest cancer in women and one of the commonest causes of death. It is much less common in Eastern countries such as China but the incidence is increasing rapidly
Known natural history with treatable latent or early symptomatic phase	● ●	The pathophysiology of breast cancer is highly controversial, with many authorities claming that by the time a breast cancer is detectable on mammogram there are often micro-metastases throughout the body, reducing the plausibility of mammographic screening as a method of prolonging life
Recognised treatment that is more effective if started early	● ●	Radical surgery is of limited or no value. Efficacy of drug therapy differs with tumour cell type. New 'designer' treatments are emerging that can potentially be tailored to biochemical properties of the tumour ('receptor status')
The test		
Reliability	● ● ●	The standard test, 1-view mammography, is less reliable but cheaper than 2-view mammography. The ability to interpret mammograms varies with professional background, training and supervision, and not all centres achieve the best standards
Practicability and acceptability	● ●	Mammography can be undignified, sometimes experienced as painful, and difficult in the obese. White middle class women find the test more acceptable than minority ethnic and lower socio-economic groups
Sensitivity and specificity	● ●	One woman in 10 is recalled with an 'abnormal' mammogram but only one in 2000 has cancer diagnosed and effectively treated. One cancer in 3 is missed since some histological types are radioneutral
Predictive value	● ● ●	Depends on prevalence, hence varies considerably with age (see Figure 2.1, page 29)
The programme		
Overall efficacy	● ● ●	Experts disagree. Depends partly on how efficiently diagnosis is linked to prompt and effective treatment. See text for discussion

(Continued)

Table 8.2 (*Continued*)

Characteristic	Extent fulfilled	Comment
Clear policy on who should be treated	● ● ●	UK offers 3-yearly screening for women aged 50–69
Diagnosis and treatment should be cost-effective	● ● ●	Disputed and constantly changing since new 'designer' anti-cancer drugs are constantly being developed; whilst these may offer benefit to some subgroups, they dramatically alter the overall cost-effectiveness of screening. Screening is 3–5 times as cost-effective in women aged 50–70 as in those aged 40–50 because of higher prevalence, but cost-effectiveness in over-70s is lower because of competing causes of death
Case finding is continuous rather than one-off	● ● ●	Repeated testing is built into programme design in UK, but in some studies women have failed to return for subsequent screening rounds, leading to attrition of the cohort at the age of highest vulnerability

Compiled from various sources.[20,21–27]

(in which women were randomised to either routine screening or no screening) have shown a 20–30% *relative* risk reduction in breast cancer mortality in the screened group, depending on age. But *absolute* risk reduction for overall mortality in randomised trials was much less (0.5%), and anxiety and unnecessary tests due to false positives were often high. Epidemiologists disagree on whether RCT evidence should over-ride the findings of cohort studies suggesting greater overall benefit of screening – for example, the official report from the UK Breast Cancer Screening Programme that it is now 'saving 1400 lives a year'.[28] In stark contrast to this, a Cochrane review by the internationally renowned epidemiologist and systematic reviewer Peter Goetsche has concluded that *'for every 2000 women invited for screening over 10 years, one will have her life prolonged. In addition, 10 healthy women . . . will be diagnosed as breast cancer patients [ductal carcinoma-in-situ and indolent lesions] and treated unnecessarily'*.[20]

In the face of this ongoing controversy in the pages of academic journals, what should we advise our patients about breast cancer screening? I think there are three key messages on the basis of current evidence. First, that whilst much scientific evidence *points towards* a worthwhile benefit from being screened regularly from age 50, not all experts are agreed on this interpretation and that we do not know 100% that breast screening is 'worth it'. Every woman must make up her own mind about attending for screening, based on how much value *she personally* places on early detection of cancer versus the anxiety of false positive and non-life-threatening findings. Second, that the commonest 'abnormal' result in a woman who attends for screening is a false alarm, so

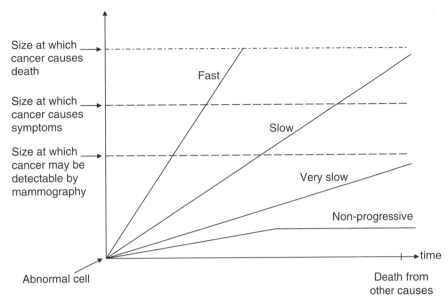

Figure 8.1 Schematic diagram of four breast cancers with different growth rates, showing how detection by mammographic screening offer potential for improved outcome in only some.

our patients should not fear the worst if they get recalled for further tests. And third, as Figure 8.1 shows, breast cancer is a heterogeneous condition; whilst it is still a major killer in many women, many others die with cancer rather than of it. Women who attend for screening should understand that much hangs on the 'staging and grading' tests that will follow the diagnosis of malignancy. If women have grasped all these points, they will be in a better position to make an informed decision about participating in the screening programme even in the face of the residual scientific uncertainty discussed above.

Antenatal screening for Down syndrome is an interesting example of how systematic research can improve the quality of screening programmes. Down syndrome (Trisomy 21) is almost always associated with severe mental retardation and very often with physical abnormalities too (congenital atresia of the small bowel, heart defects, as well as short stature and characteristic facial appearance). Whilst many children (and some adults) with Down syndrome have a good quality of life, the condition places a huge burden on families, with considerably higher rates of mental illness in primary caregivers, divorce in parents and illness in siblings.[29,30] Detecting (with a view to aborting) affected fetuses is, arguably, justified on ethical as well as clinical grounds. But any screening test takes its toll on anxiety levels and inevitably medicalises a normal pregnancy.[31] A few years ago, I spent a number of sleepless nights myself waiting for the outcome of antenatal screening tests that were described as 'borderline'.

Until recently, risk of Down syndrome was estimated by the 'triple' blood test taken at 16 weeks (alpha fetoprotein, unconjugated oestriol and total human chorionic gonadotrophin). This replaced the previous 'double' test, which lacked the oestriol component. Importantly, none of these blood markers, singly or in combination, could distinguish a Down syndrome fetus from a normal one with 100% accuracy, because whatever cut-off was used for the different values, some normal fetuses were associated with 'abnormal' levels and vice versa (see Table 3.3, page 71, for an illustration of the false positive and false negative phenomenon in a screening test). Statistical algorithms were used to predict the chance of Down syndrome (e.g. '1 in 145'), given a particular value on each of the blood tests. Women in a statistically high-risk category were advised to have a more definitive test – amniocentesis (a needle inserted directly into the womb) for alpha fetoprotein. Because the incidence of Down syndrome increases dramatically with maternal age (from 1 in 1500 at age 20 to 1 in 200 at age 38 and in 6 at age 50), older mothers often found themselves in the amniocentesis queue. But amniocentesis was not without risks: one fetus in 200 spontaneously aborted, leaving the parents having to come to terms not merely with losing a much longed-for baby late in gestation, but also with the idea that had they turned down the screening test, their child would probably have survived.

The triple test for Down syndrome scores well on some of the criteria in Boxes 8.3 and 8.4 (the problem is common, important and well understood; prenatal diagnosis is possible) but poorly on others. Most notably, this combination of tests has a very high false negative rate (i.e. a low sensitivity) – some 40% of fetuses with Down syndrome were being missed by the screening programme, and most of these were occurring in women who had been told by well-meaning professionals (who did not understand the statistics) that the baby they were expecting was 'normal'. This was an unacceptable situation all round. In about 1995, a new test became available for women who had presented early enough in pregnancy: an ultrasound scan at around 11 weeks to look for translucency of the nuchal fold at the back of the neck. But again, some fetuses were misclassified and women still had to opt for amniocentesis to be sure of their diagnosis.

Nick Wald and his colleagues at St Barts Hospital, London, have been working to develop a new test for Down syndrome that avoids the need for amniocentesis and which, where possible, detects affected fetuses early in pregnancy so that a termination of pregnancy, if this option is chosen, is less traumatic. They recently published their final report on what is known as the Serum Urine and Ultrasound Screening Study (SURUSS).[32] In this huge longitudinal survey, they recruited over 47,000 women with singleton pregnancy (of whom 101 turned out to be expecting a Down syndrome fetus). Each woman provided blood and urine samples in early pregnancy (9–13 weeks), mid pregnancy (14–20 weeks) and also had an ultrasound scan at 11 weeks. From the various specimens, a number of tests and combinations of tests were performed,

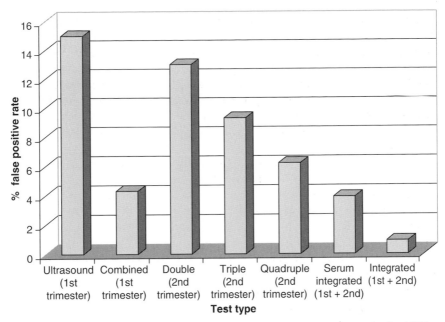

Figure 8.2 % false positive rates for different screening tests for Down syndrome at a fixed 85% detection rate. (Data taken from Wald et al.[32])

resulting in seven different possible tests: the traditional double and triple tests (explained above), the 'quadruple test' (triple test plus one more blood marker, inhibin-A), the 'combined' test (a combination of blood tests for various markers plus first trimester ultrasound, whose result could be available as early as 13 weeks), the 'serum integrated test' (a combination of blood tests at different stages of pregnancy) and the 'integrated test' (the above plus the first trimester ultrasound result).

As Figure 8.2 shows, Wald and colleagues' meticulous epidemiological work has identified a 'screening test' (actually a combination of four blood tests and an ultrasound scan, where the results of tests done at one stage of pregnancy are added in to the results at later stages) – the 'integrated test' – which achieves what no single non-invasive test is able to do: detect 85% of all Down syndrome cases with a less than 1% false positive rate. However, whilst this test scores much higher than the old triple test on accuracy, it involved substantially more blood tests and is more expensive. At the time of writing, the standard test in my own practice is the quadruple test, but things may change rapidly in this field as new blood markers become available.

In the light of changes in family structure (see Section 7.1), specifically the rising maternal age in many countries (which means that increasing numbers of Down fetuses are being conceived), the still imperfect screening tests for this condition, and the fact that different women (and different couples) will have different views on whether termination of pregnancy for this diagnosis is acceptable, there is no simple advice to be offered when a pregnant woman asks 'should I have the test' or 'what will it mean if the test is positive [or negative]?'. Personally, I would make three things clear. First, that the test cannot tell you for sure if you are carrying a Down syndrome fetus; it can tell you how *likely* this diagnosis is. Second, whilst a negative test makes the chance of Down syndrome less likely, it does not eradicate this possibility entirely. And third, if the diagnosis of Down syndrome is made, nobody but the couple themselves can say whether the pregnancy 'should' be terminated. This is a personal, ethical decision and no amount of research evidence or professional knowledge will say what is right or wrong in a particular set of circumstances. As far as possible, couples who enter the screening programme (or who choose not to enter it) should be clear about these three points.

Other screening programmes that have been suggested, but not widely introduced, in primary care because they fail to fulfil Wilson and Jungner's criteria include diabetes (earlier detection may be of marginal benefit in the long term compared to the anxiety and stigma linked to the diagnosis, especially when we remember that the lifestyle advice offered to people with diabetes actually applies to all of us[33–35]), Chlamydia (uncertainty about cost-effectiveness, women's concerns about unpleasantness of test and potential stigma[36,37]), depression (uncertainty as to whether to screen the entire population or target particular groups such as the elderly or institutionalised[38,39]), colorectal cancer (high false positive rate, high cost, low uptake when tests are offered),[40,41] do-it-yourself kits for home HIV testing (likely to be taken up predominantly by the affluent worried well, thereby diverting resources into dealing with their anxieties),[42] domestic violence (reluctance of doctors to ask, so screening programme likely to be poorly operationalised[43]) and visual impairment in the elderly (no evidence of benefit to patients[44]).

In conclusion, no screening test is a panacea, and each comes with its own false positive and false negative rate. Furthermore, different people (and different interest groups) have different views on the acceptability of different screening tests. Understanding the principles behind a 'good screening test' and a 'good screening programme', together with rigorous epidemiological research, can substantially improve the efficacy, cost-effectiveness and overall usefulness of the screening tests we offer in our practice and community.

8.4 'Risk': an epidemiological can of worms?

Risk is defined by the online encyclopaedia Wikipedia as '*a concept that denotes a potential negative impact to an asset or some characteristic of value that may arise from some present process or future event*'. As Ulrich Beck has perceptively observed, we now live in a 'risk society'.[45] People get on in life by taking risks. In healthcare, we are increasingly encouraged to 'target' our efforts at prevention and support towards 'risk groups' of one sort or another. A person might find himself in a risk group simply by virtue of his age, gender or other demographic variable – as my husband discovered a few years ago when we both took out life insurance. His premiums were three times what I was asked to pay, simply because being male placed him 'at risk' of HIV infection (or so the actuaries believed at the time). Lifestyle choices, physiological states and even parts of the body can be designated 'at risk' (as in 'risk behaviour', 'the at-risk pregnancy' or 'the at-risk foot'). Adolescence has been described as a time of 'ritualistic risk-taking'.[46] But being designated 'high risk' can (sometimes) become a self-fulfilling prophecy. Of all the general practice consultations I have had in my career, the one I most regret is when I informed an angry young man that the reason I wanted him to see a counsellor was because he was in a high-risk group for self-harm. Six days later, he took his own life.

Despite that chilling example, risk is not some kind of supernatural force poised above us like Macbeth's dagger. In the epidemiological sense (see Section 2.2), it is simply a statistical association between one population-level variable and another. Statistically, risk is the probability of an event occurring multiplied by the severity of the impact of the event. The task of the epidemiologist is, arguably, to estimate with accuracy and precision the magnitude of risk in particular circumstances (e.g. by surveys or mathematical modelling) and convey this estimate to patients and the public.

In epidemiology, risk has traditionally been studied as linked to discrete variables – as in 'risk factors'. Smoking, for example, is a risk factor for developing lung cancer (people who smoke are 15 times as likely to get lung cancer as those who don't, and most of the cancers in non-smokers are due to passive smoking[47]) and for infant mortality (the infants of mothers who smoke are 1.9 times as likely to die of Sudden Infant Death Syndrome as infants whose mothers do not smoke[48]). Table 8.3 shows the known risk factors for one medical condition (stroke). I have divided these into non-modifiable (things that increase the risk of stroke but which we can't change), modifiable and well established (things that certainly increase the risk of stroke and which we can change – hence the primary targets for preventive action) and modifiable and less well established (things that probably increase the risk of stroke).

Many of the modifiable risk factors in the middle column in Table 8.3 are what epidemiologists refer to as 'behavioural risk factors' – lifestyle choices that have been statistically linked to adverse health outcomes. The US Center for Disease Control runs a massive surveillance project, the Behavioral Risk Factor Surveillance Survey (http://www.cdc.gov/brfss/about.htm), in which some 350,000 people are surveyed every year for such 'factors' – such as tobacco and alcohol intake, not taking physical exercise, not wearing seatbelts, not having

Table 8.3 Risk factors for stroke. The following factors have been shown by epidemiological studies to increase the risk of stroke.

Non-modifiable	Modifiable, well-established link with stroke	Modifiable, less well-established link with stroke
Age Family history of stroke	High blood pressure (risk increased if poorly controlled) Smoking	Geographical origin (incidence of stroke varies with geography even when known risk factors are controlled for)
Ethnicity (commoner in African Caribbeans)	Diabetes (risk increased if poorly controlled)	Socio-economic status (incidence of stroke varies with income even when known risk factors are controlled for)
Gender (commoner in men) Past history of stroke or transient ischaemic attack	Carotid or peripheral artery disease (risk increased if > 75% narrowing of one or both carotid arteries) Atrial fibrillation (risk reduced if taking anticoagulants) Coronary or other heart disease (including cardiomyopathy, valve disease and ischaemic heart disease) Hypercholesterolaemia (risk increased if poorly controlled) Obesity Physical inactivity (mainly via an effect on obesity and blood pressure) Poor diet (via an effect on serum cholesterol levels) Sickle cell anaemia	Alcohol misuse (increased risk of haemorrhagic stroke with excessive alcohol intake) Drug abuse (cocaine, amphetamines and heroin)

a flu jab and failing to turn up when invited for a mammogram. Numerous research studies have been published (and more are ongoing) by this team that document the quantitative contribution of each risk factor to particular adverse outcomes.

Targeting individual behavioural risk factors seems (on the face of it) very reasonable, since who could argue with a strong statistical link between particular behaviours and particular outcomes? The answer is many social epidemiologists and sociologists. That is not to say these people would dispute the associations demonstrated, but they would challenge the privileging of a level of analysis focused on individual behaviour (see Section 3.6). Yes, individuals' behaviour choices are important determinants of their health, but risk can also be analysed at a number of other levels – most notably why people make particular choices in the first place (why, for example, do so many teenage mothers from poor backgrounds choose to smoke and not to breast feed?). I consider the 'upstream' aspects of health behaviour in Section 9.3.

A classic early study of the impact of different risk factors on health was Michael Marmot's Whitehall I study. His team followed 10,000 civil servants for 10 years and demonstrated a strong statistical association between higher job grade and coronary heart disease mortality. While low grade was associated with obesity, smoking, less leisure time physical activity, more baseline illness, higher blood pressure and shorter height, controlling for all of these risk factors accounted for no more than 40% of the difference in chronic heart disease (CHD) mortality with different grade of job.[49,50] After controlling for standard risk factors, the lowest grade of civil servant still had a relative risk of 2.1 for CHD mortality compared to the highest grade.[49]

In other words, it would appear that there is an 'underdog' effect on CHD risk, even after controlling for behavioural choices (such as the fact that lower grade staff take less exercise, smoke more and so on). The precise nature of this underdog effect has occupied Michael Marmot for most of his professional career, and you could do worse than spend a day in the library reading up on his work, including the Whitehall II study (another 10-year study of several thousand civil servants, this time including women and focusing more on psychological stress in the work environment[51]) and some more recent studies on the impact of work stress,[52] why being badly paid is bad for your health[53] and the social structuring of health choices.[54] I will return to the 'unexplained 60%' of socioeconomic differentials in health in the next chapter (especially Sections 9.1–9.3) when I consider what makes a healthy (and an unhealthy) community. Health literacy (Section 4.5) may also explain some of the differential, though (to my knowledge) this was not measured directly in the Whitehall studies.

I want briefly to consider the question of non-modifiable risk factors, especially 'genetic' ones. For example, the 'thrifty genotype' hypothesis – that ethnic groups who have survived periods of famine in their evolutionary past have evolved an economical metabolism that predisposes them to obesity – is often used to explain such phenomena as the massively high prevalence of diabetes (around 50%) in the Pima Indians of the USA. Some purists would say that genetic predisposition is not strictly speaking a risk *factor* at all, since (like age and gender) it cannot be altered nor can an individual be 'exposed' to it, but it can certainly contribute to that person's inherent predisposition to develop disease. Others are comfortable with the notion of 'non-modifiable' risk factors as illustrated in Table 8.3. But as I have argued elsewhere in this book (see Section 7.3), so-called 'genetic' risk factors exert their effect by interacting with environmental influences, and there is a real danger of both racial stereotyping and genetic fatalism (subconsciously thinking that it is the risk itself rather than the person's genetic make-up that is 'non-modifiable') when the genetic element of risk is found to be linked to particular ethnic groups.[55] Arguably, the *main* cause of the huge increase in diabetes in the Pima Indians is not the genotypes carried by individuals but the ubiquitous availability of cheap fast food and high-calorie soft drinks in the USA![56]

One final note on the topic of risk. In addition to the 'objective' measures of risk produced by epidemiologists (e.g. Table 8.3), there is an important *subjective* dimension to risk. We all have our own unconscious perceptions of risk which (even when informed by hard data) are framed by cognitive biases. Some things (such as driving on a busy motorway or lighting up another cigarette) seem less dangerous than they actually are, whereas others (such as nuclear power or a general anaesthetic) seem more dangerous. Box 8.5 shows

---

Box 8.5 Some cognitive biases in the perception of risk.[57,58]

Acceptable risk. Some risks (such as lung cancer from smoking) are subjectively viewed as more acceptable than others (such as vaccine damage), even when the actual probabilities of occurrence are in the other direction. Hazards generally deemed acceptable are familiar, perceived as under the individual's control, have immediate rather than delayed consequences and are linked to perceived benefits. Unacceptable hazards have a 'dread factor' (catastrophic, involuntary, uncontrollable) and an 'unknown' factor (not observable, poorly understood, long term, new) and are thus less acceptable.

Anchoring. In the absence of objective probabilities, people judge risk according to a reference point. This may be arbitrary, for example, the status quo (what is routine and customary) or some perception of what is 'normal'.

Availability bias. Events that are easier to recall are judged as more likely to happen. Ease of recall is influenced by recency, strong emotions and anything that increases memorability (e.g. press coverage, personal experience).

Categorical safety and danger. People may perceive things as either 'good' or 'bad', irrespective of exposure or context. This may make them unreceptive to explanations that introduce complexity into the decision (e.g. balance of benefit and harm).

Framing of information. A glass can be described as either 'half empty' or 'half full' – the problem is the same but it is framed differently. This can have a direct and powerful impact on decisions of lay people and professionals alike. A specific instance is prospect theory: losses loom larger than gains.

Illusory correlation. Prior beliefs and expectations about what correlates with what leads people to perceive correlations that are not in the data.

Inability to distinguish between small probabilities. We cannot meaningfully compare very small risks (e.g. of different adverse effects) such as 1 in 20,000 and 1 in 200,000. Expressing harm as relative rather than absolute risk dramatically shifts the subjective benefit-harm balance because the risk of harm *appears* greater.

Preference for status quo. Most people are reluctant to change current behaviours, such as taking a particular drug, even when the objective evidence of benefit changes. It may be due to persistence of illusory correlation.

some well-documented biases that distort our perception of risk. They go some way to explaining why patients rarely react as predicted when we try to explain risk. A particularly interesting subfield in the risk perception literature is how people perceive 'genetic' risk – both in relation to single gene disorders such as familial breast cancer (e.g. BRCA1) and in more complex inheritance patterns such as premature coronary heart disease. I recommend Teresa Marteau's well-written overview of this topic area.[59] Given the cognitive biases that both we and our patients are likely to hold about estimates of risk (and the fact that few of us are in top shape when in comes to sums), it is small wonder that explaining risk to patients is becoming a major research field in its own right; try these references for an introduction to this fascinating area.[60–62]

References

1 Coggon G, Rose G, Barker DJP. *Epidemiology for the Uninitiated*. 5th edn. London: BMJ Publications; 2003.

2 Starfield B. *Primary Care: Balancing Health Needs, Services and Technology*. New York: Oxford University Press; 1992.

3 Pickles W. *Epidemiology in Country Practice*. Bristol: John Wright; 1939.

4 Ashworth M, Charlton J, Latinovic R, Gulliford M. Age-related changes in consultations and antibiotic prescribing for acute respiratory infections, 1995–2000. Data from the UK general practice research database. J Clin Pharm Ther 2006;31:461–467.

5 Smeeth L, Cook C, Fombonne E, et al. MMR vaccination and pervasive developmental disorders: a case-control study. Lancet 2004;364:963–969.

6 Clifford GM, Logie J, Farmer RD. How do symptoms indicative of BPH progress in real life practice? The UK experience. Eur Urol 2000;38(suppl 1):48–53.

7 Hernandez-Diaz S, Garcia-Rodriguez LA. Epidemiologic assessment of the safety of conventional nonsteroidal anti-inflammatory drugs. Am J Med 2001;110(suppl 3A): 20S–27S.

8 Farmer RD, Lawrenson RA, Todd JC, Williams TJ, MacRae K. Oral contraceptives and venous thromboembolic disease. Analyses of the UK general practice research database and the UK mediplus database. Hum Reprod Update 1999;5:688–706.

9 Bradford Hill A. The environment and disease: association or causation? Proc Roy Soc Med 1965; 58:295–300.

10 Wakefield AJ, Murch SH, Anthony A, et al. Ileal-lymphoid-nodular hyperplasia, non-specific colitis, and pervasive developmental disorder in children. Lancet 1998;351: 637–641.

11 Lyratzopoulos G, Aston R, Bailey K, Flitcroft J, Clarke H. Accuracy of routine data on MMR vaccination coverage and validity of parental recall of vaccination. Commun Dis Public Health 2002;5:305–310.

12 Bolton P, Holt E, Ross A, Hughart N, Guyer B. Estimating vaccination coverage using parental recall, vaccination cards, and medical records. Public Health Rep 1998;113: 521–526.

13 Horton R. A statement by the editors of the Lancet. Lancet 2004;363:820–821.

14 Davies M, Macdowall W, Bonnall C. *Health Promotion Practice*. Milton Keynes: Open University Press; 2006.

15 Davies M. *Health Promotion Theory*. Milton Keynes: Open University Press; 2005.

16 Wilson JMG, Jungner G. Principles and Practice of Screening for Disease. Public Health Papers 134. Geneva: World Health Organisation; 1965. Available from: http://whqlibdoc.who.int/php/WHO_PHP_34.pdf.

17 Greenhalgh T. *How to Read a Paper: The Basics of Evidence Based Medicine*. 3rd edn. Oxford: Blackwells; 2006.

18 Djulbegovic B, Lyman GH. Screening mammography at 40–49 years: regret or no regret? Lancet 2006;368:2035–2037.

19 Moss SM, Cuckle H, Evans A, Johns L, Waller M, Bobrow L. Effect of mammographic screening from age 40 years on breast cancer mortality at 10 years' follow-up: a randomised controlled trial. Lancet 2006;368:2053–2060.

20 Gotzsche PC, Nielsen M. Screening for breast cancer with mammography. Cochrane Database Syst Rev 2006;4:CD001877.

21 Nystrom L, Andersson I, Bjurstam N, Frisell J, Nordenskjold B, Rutqvist LE. Long-term effects of mammography screening: updated overview of the Swedish randomised trials. Lancet 2002;359:909–919.

22 Gelmon KA, Olivotto I. The mammography screening debate: time to move on. Lancet 2002;359:904–905.

23 Blanchard K, Colbert JA, Puri D, et al. Mammographic screening: patterns of use and estimated impact on breast carcinoma survival. Cancer 2004;101:495–507.

24 Colbert JA, Kaine EM, Bigby J, et al. The age at which women begin mammographic screening. Cancer 2004;101:1850–1859.

25 Jones AR, Caplan LS, Davis MK. Racial/ethnic differences in the self-reported use of screening mammography. J Community Health 2003;28:303–316.

26 Smith-Bindman R, Miglioretti DL, Lurie N, et al. Does utilization of screening mammography explain racial and ethnic differences in breast cancer? Ann Intern Med 2006;144: 541–553.

27 Kagay CR, Quale C, Smith-Bindman R. Screening mammography in the American elderly. Am J Prev Med 2006;31:142–149.

28 Advisory Committee on Breast Cancer Screening. *Screening for Breast Cancer in England: Past and Future*. NHSBSP Publication No. 61. London: NHS Breast Screening Programme; 2006.

29 Fisman S, Wolf L. The handicapped child: psychological effects of parental, marital, and sibling relationships. Psychiatr Clin North Am 1991;14:199–217.

30 Hauser-Cram P, Warfield ME, Shonkoff JP, Krauss MW, Sayer A, Upshur CC. Children with disabilities: a longitudinal study of child development and parent well-being. Monogr Soc Res Child Dev 2001; 66(3):114.

31 Marteau TM. Psychological costs of screening. BMJ 1989;299:527–528.

32 Wald NJ, Rodeck C, Hackshaw AK, Rudnicka A. SURUSS in perspective. Semin Perinatol 2005;29:225–235.

33 Harris R, Donahue K, Rathore SS, Frame P, Woolf SH, Lohr KN. Screening adults for type 2 diabetes: a review of the evidence for the U.S. preventive services task force. Ann Intern Med 2003;138:215–229.

34 Hoerger TJ, Harris R, Hicks KA, Donahue K, Sorensen S, Engelgau M. Screening for type 2 diabetes mellitus: a cost-effectiveness analysis. Ann Intern Med 2004;140:689–699.

35 Goyder EC, Irwig LM. Screening for type 2 diabetes mellitus: a decision analytic approach. Diabet Med 2000;17:469–477.

36 Roberts TE, Robinson S, Barton P, Bryan S, Low N. Screening for Chlamydia trachoma-
tis: a systematic review of the economic evaluations and modelling. Sex Transm Infect
2006;82:193–200.

37 Pavlin NL, Gunn JM, Parker R, Fairley CK, Hocking J. Implementing chlamydia screening: what do women think? A systematic review of the literature. BMC Public Health
2006;6:221.

38 Carmin CN, Klocek JW. To screen or not to screen: symptoms identifying primary care
medical patients in need of screening for depression. Int J Psychiatry Med 1998;28:
293–302.

39 Sharp LK, Lipsky MS. Screening for depression across the lifespan: a review of measures
for use in primary care settings. Am Fam Physician 2002;66:1001–1008.

40 Gazelle GS, McMahon PM, Scholz FJ. Screening for colorectal cancer. Radiology
2000;215:327–335.

41 Lieberman D. How to screen for colon cancer. Annu Rev Med 1998;49:163–172.

42 Walensky RP, Paltiel AD. Rapid HIV testing at home: does it solve a problem or create
one? Ann Intern Med 2006;145:459–462.

43 Elliott L, Nerney M, Jones T, Friedmann PD. Barriers to screening for domestic violence.
J Gen Intern Med 2002;17:112–116.

44 Smeeth L, Iliffe S. Community screening for visual impairment in the elderly. Cochrane
Database Syst Rev 2006;3:CD001054.

45 Beck U. *Risk Society: Towards a New Modernity*. London: Sage; 1992.

46 Heath I. *The Mystery of General Practice*. London: Nuffield Provincial Hospital Trust;
1997.

47 Doll R, Peto R, Boreham J, Sutherland I. Mortality from cancer in relation to smoking: 50
years observations on British doctors. Br J Cancer 2005;92:426–429.

48 Anderson M, Johnson D, Batal H. Sudden infant death syndrome and prenatal maternal
smoking: rising attributed risk in the back to sleep era. BMC Med 2005;3(1):4.

49 Marmot M. Work and other factors influencing coronary health and sickness absence.
Work Stress 1994;8:191–201.

50 Marmot MG, Shipley MJ, Rose G. Inequalities in death – specific explanations of a general
pattern? Lancet 1984;1:1003–1006.

51 Marmot M, Brunner E. Cohort profile: the whitehall II study. Int J Epid 2005;34:
251–256.

52 Marmot M, Brunner E. Epidemiological applications of long-term stress in daily life. Adv
Psychosom Med 2001;22:80–90.

53 Marmot M. The influence of income on health: views of an epidemiologist. Health Aff
(Millwood) 2002;21:31–46.

54 Siegrist J, Marmot M. Health inequalities and the psychosocial environment-two scientific
challenges. Soc Sci Med 2004;58:1463–1473.

55 Fee M. Racializing narratives: obesity, diabetes and the 'Aboriginal' thrifty genotype. Soc
Sci Med 2006;62:2988–2997.

56 Bennett PH. Type 2 diabetes among the Pima Indians of Arizona: an epidemic attributable
to environmental change? Nutr Rev 1999;57:S51–54.

57 Slovic P. Perception of risk. Science 1987;236:280–285.

58 Greenhalgh T, Kostopoulou O, Harries C. Public perceptions of the benefit-harm balance
in health care. BMJ 2004;329:47–50.

59 Marteau TM. Communicating genetic risk information. Br Med Bull 1999;55:414–428.

60 Hanne H. Explaining risk factors to patients during a general practice consultation: conveying group-based epidemiological knowledge to individual patients. Scand J Prim Health Care 1999;17:3–5.

61 Dudley T, Nagle J. Explaining risk to patients. Patient Care 2003;3:70–75.

62 Edwards A, Elwyn G, Mulley A. Explaining risks: turning numerical data into meaningful pictures. BMJ 2002;324:827–830.

CHAPTER 9

The community

Summary points

1 Health inequalities are differences in health states or health outcomes between different groups in society. Deprivation (lack of access to resources to meet needs, especially poverty, overcrowding and lack of education) in a community is consistently associated with health inequalities. A number of different indices of deprivation have been developed, some of which are used to reallocate resources to primary care teams working in areas of high need.

2 The effects of deprivation are mediated at least partly via social networks, which (depending on their extent and quality) may bring social support, social influence, social engagement and access to resources. The term 'social capital' is often used to summarise the material and non-material resources to which a well-networked individual has access.

3 A novel way of thinking about community level deprivation is in terms of 'risk regulators' – aspects of social structure and social life that shape and constrain lifestyle choices and health outcomes. Risk regulators include the built environment, crime and fear of crime, workplace stress and oppression, availability of food, the 'walkability' and social connectedness of the neighbourhood, laws and policies and prevailing cultural norms and expectations.

4 Increasingly, primary care clinicians and managers find themselves addressing the health of communities rather than just of individuals. Efforts to develop 'healthy communities' are difficult and do not bear fruit overnight. Whilst short-term success has been described with intensive externally led programmes using the community-oriented primary care model, community development initiatives that place strong emphasis on partnership with local communities may be equally successful, less expensive and more sustainable in the long-term. However, broad-based community partnerships are no bowl of cherries, and the ideology of 'working together' may prove difficult or impossible to operationalise on the ground.

9.1 Unpacking health inequalities I: deprivation

Research on health inequalities (i.e. differences in health states and health outcomes by income, education, ethnic origin, gender and so on) has consistently shown that staying healthy is especially difficult for the 'have-nots' in any population (see, for example, the Whitehall studies discussed in Section 8.4). The first national level report to summarise this evidence in the UK was Sir

225

Douglas Black's politically contentious book, commissioned by the Department of Health and Social Security and printed in its thousands in August
1980. Black showed, using sound epidemiological data, that (a) ill health and
early death were unequally distributed in the UK population (i.e. were much
commoner in the poor and disadvantaged); (b) these inequalities had been
widening since the National Health Service (NHS) was introduced in 1948;
and that (c) widening inequalities were due not primarily (or even at all) to
the failings of the NHS, but to social inequalities including those in income,
education, housing, diet, employment and conditions of work.

The Black report, as it was universally known, was never published. Thousands of copies were famously removed from the printing warehouse and
pulped the evening before publication on the personal orders of Conservative
Prime Minister Margaret Thatcher, who found its message politically unpalat-
able, and original copies of the Black Report remain rare collectors' items.
The Acheson Report, a similar epidemiological analysis undertaken in 1998,
showed similar trends and offered similar explanations.[1] Whilst this report
was endorsed rather than rejected by the Labour government of the time, many
public health specialists believe that its message was not fully understood and
that politicians still see 'health' as the exclusive domain of the health professionals and fail to engage with what are known as the *social* determinants of
health.

Yet in every country in the world, people with higher socio-economic status
live longer, healthier lives than those with lower status. Figure 9.1 shows infant

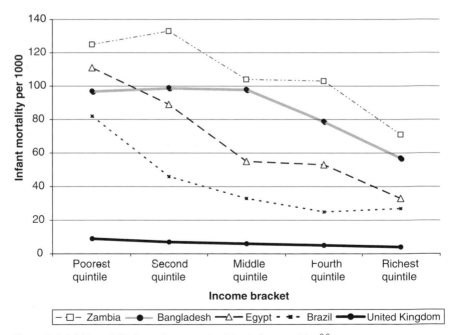

Figure 9.1 Infant mortality by socio-economic status in five countries.[2,3]

mortality rates in five countries.[2,3] Whilst the UK offers its newborns dramatically better chances of survival than most developing countries, the offspring of the richest 20% in society are still 50% more likely to survive their first year than the offspring of the poorest 20%.

If being poor has such consistent and strong links with health outcomes even after controlling for damaging behaviours like smoking, what exactly is it about being poor that is bad for health? In the remainder of this section and in Sections 9.2 and 9.3, I will consider three concepts that are widely used in the study of health inequalities: deprivation, social networks (and the related concept of social capital) and life course epidemiology. Let us consider the first of these now. In the UK, payments to general practitioners are linked to something called a 'deprivation score' of the community they serve, with practices in more 'deprived' areas being paid substantially more per patient than those working in less 'deprived' areas because patients in these areas are known to have more illness. But what is actually being measured when we make these estimates?

The terms 'deprivation' and 'poverty' are often used interchangeably, but they are not synonymous. Officially, 'poverty' means not having enough financial resources to meet needs, whereas 'deprivation' refers to the presence of unmet needs due to lack of resources that are not just financial.[4] Numerous 'deprivation indices' have been developed by academics and policymakers to document unmet need and shortfalls in resources in defined geographical areas. In the UK, most have been derived from the ten-yearly population census (see www.statistics.gov.uk/census) and are calculated for the smallest area on which aggregated data are produced – previously known as the enumeration district and more recently renamed the Super Output Area (SOA), a small geographical area comprising 200–500 dwellings. Aggregate scores based on the sum of scores in such areas are, unsurprisingly, known as 'small area statistics'.

The first census-based deprivation index to be used in UK primary care (and one that is still widely cited) is the Jarman Underpriviledged Area (UPA) Score, which was developed in 1983 by Brian Jarman, a professor of general practice at Imperial College London, with a view to ensuring that general practitioners in deprived areas were appropriately remunerated for their greater workload.[5] In other words, the Jarman Index (as it is universally known) was never intended to be a direct measure of deprivation but a vehicle for remunerating fairly the workload of general practitioners. The Jarman Index used eight census area indicators:

a *Unemployement* – unemployed residents aged over 16 as a proportion of all economically active residents aged over 16.

b *Overcrowding* – persons in households with 1 and more persons per room as a proportion of all residents in households.

c *Lone pensioners* – lone pensioner households as a proportion of all residents in households.

d *Single parents* – lone parents as a proportion of all residents in households.

e *Born in New Commonwealth* – residents born in the New Commonwealth as a proportion of all residents.

f *Children aged under 5* – children aged 0–4 years of age as a proportion of all residents

g *Low social class* – persons in households with economically active head of household in socio-economic group 2 as a proportion of all persons in households.

h *One year migrants* – residents with a different address 1 year before the census as a proportion of all residents.

The Townsend Index, introduced in 1988, is made up of only four variables: (a) unemployment; (b) overcrowding; (c) the proportion of households with no access to a car; and (d) the proportion of households not owning their own home.[6] The Carstairs and Morris Scottish Deprivation Score (known as the Carstairs Index) was developed by Scottish epidemiologists at about the same time.[7,8] It is very similar to the Townsend Index, being a composite of four scores including male unemployment, overcrowding and non-car ownership but replaces the last score (home ownership) with a measure of social class – the proportion of all persons in private households with an economically active head with head of household in social class 4 or 5.

These three indices are all still useful up to a point (wide disparities in the prevalence of certain diseases have been demonstrated by Townsend and Carstairs indices[9,10]), but in many ways have been superseded by the IMD score described below. Many published 'Jarman scores' or 'Townsend scores' are now very out of date as they were calculated on census data collected in 1980 (or sometimes 1990). Although in theory there is no reason why these scores should not be recalculated on more recent data, published papers and book chapters have the effect of setting in stone yesterday's figures. Another criticism commonly levelled at the above scores is that they overemphasise urban deprivation at the expense of rural deprivation. For more on the strengths and weaknesses of these measures of deprivation, I recommend a review by Carstairs herself.[11]

In 2000, the UK Office of National Statistics introduced the Indices of Multiple Deprivation (IMD) as the most robust measure of deprivation in a Super Output Area and for which data are consistently available for the whole of the country and can be updated regularly. The IMD is made up of seven subscores (known as Domain Indices), each with a different weighting that reflects research evidence on the extent to which this particular aspect of deprivation contributes to wider inequalities[4]:

a Income deprivation −22.5%;

b Employment deprivation −22.5%;

c Health deprivation and disability −13.5%;

d Education, skills and training deprivation −13.5%;

e Barriers to housing and services −9.3%;

f Crime −9.3%;

g Living environment deprivation −9.3%.

Box 9.1 Measuring deprivation in England and Wales using the IMD score.

The IMD score is derived from 2001 Census (General Household Survey) data for England and Wales.[4] It reflects the average income (22.5%), employment (22.5%), health and disability (13.5%), education, skills and training (13.5%), barriers to housing and services (9.3%), crime (9.3%), and living environment (9.3%) of an area of 200–500 households. To calculate the IMD score of your home address (if in UK):

1 Go to http://www.gigateway.org.uk/areasearch/default.html and put in your home postcode. When the data table appears, find the 'Lower layer super-output area' row and note the code (e.g. E01000319).

2 Go to the website of the government's 'Communities and Local Government' website http://www.communities.gov.uk/index.asp?id=1128440 and open the Excel database 'SOA level ID'.

3 Using the 'find' function, find the SOA code you noted above, and read off (a) the absolute IMD score and (b) the ranking of that SOA against all other SOAs in England and Wales (where 1 = most deprived). A ranking of 8121 or lower places the SOA in the most deprived 25% of all communities in England and Wales.

Compared to the traditional deprivation indices described above, the IMD score is more up-to-date, more statistically robust and is calculable from data publicly available on the Internet. The IMD score is also more highly correlated with ill health than the other three scores reviewed above, but this is hardly surprising since one of the measures making up the IMD score is a direct question about ill health![12] Only a handful research papers in which this was the chief measure of neighbourhood deprivation have appeared in the literature at the time of writing,[13–16] but this is likely to change rapidly now that IMD is the official measure of deprivation used by the Office of National Statistics. If you live in England or Wales and plan to do research around deprivation yourself, you should generally use the IMD score unless you can justify using one of the older indices. Box 9.1 shows how you can calculate the IMD score of a household from their home postcode using information that is publicly available on the Internet.

9.2 Unpacking health inequalities II: social networks and social capital

The best article I have read on social network theory and its place in health is by Lisa Berkman and colleagues,[17] who explain how the concept of social networks arose historically. Up until the 1950s, anthropologists had tended to study human behaviour and meaning systems in relation to traditional groups such as families ('kinship groups'), physically delineated communities (e.g. a village) or class-based ones (e.g. 'the working class'). But as society became more fluid and heterogeneous, these groups offered decreasing scope for explaining behaviour and social phenomena. Anthropologists discovered that another useful unit of analysis (see Section 3.6) was the social network – broadly defined as social ties that cut across traditional kinship or other easily identified social groups. A social network might be studied 'egocentrically' (i.e. starting with one index person and exploring the people that that individual interacts with) or 'multicentrically' (i.e. defining a network such as a professional community and mapping the multiple interactions of multiple people).

Social networks can be large or small, with clear or fuzzy boundaries, richly or weakly interconnected (i.e. more or fewer people in the network have multiple ties within it) and more or less homogeneous (people share many or few characteristics with one another). Numerous studies have demonstrated clear and consistent links between the strength of people's social networks and just about any cause of mortality.[18–21] The more people you interact with, the less likely you are to die of any cause. But whilst the importance of social networks has been well established for decades, the mechanism by which social network membership (measured by asking people to enumerate their social contacts) affects health outcomes remains a subject of debate. Four mechanisms have been proposed: (a) social support (being able to call on people for help and advice); (b) social influence (e.g. learning healthy behaviours from one another); (c) social engagement (everyone feeling that they are a member of a community and participating in its activities); and (d) access to resources and material goods.[17]

The 'stuff' that gets exchanged via social networks and which protects against health inequalities is sometimes referred to as social capital. Social capital theory was first put forward by Lyda Judson Hanifan, an educational sociologist who studied school communities in the USA in the early twentieth century. He defined social capital as *'those tangible substances [that] count for most in the daily lives of people'*.[22] Hanifan was particularly concerned with the cultivation of goodwill, fellowship, sympathy and social interaction among those that make up a social unit (in this case, a school). The concept of social capital was extended and placed on both the policy, research and health agendas, by (among others) Robert Putnam, who defined it as follows:

> *Whereas physical capital refers to physical objects and human capital refers to the properties of individuals, social capital refers to connections among individuals – social networks and the norms of reciprocity and trustworthiness that arise from them. In that sense social capital is closely related to what some have called 'civic virtue'. The difference is that 'social capital' calls attention to the fact that civic virtue is most powerful when embedded in a sense network of reciprocal social relations. A society of many virtuous but isolated individuals is not necessarily rich in social capital.*[23, p.19]

Much of the research on social capital has been around the economic development of communities and societies. The World Bank, for example, sees social capital as a key mechanism through which health inequalities are mediated and its development as a means to bring people out of poverty. The theory is that (after differences in inherited characteristics, access to health care and lifestyle choices are controlled for), the poor are less active as citizens (hence often live in less cohesive and supportive communities); they also have fewer people they can trust and whose support they can call on when unwell or at risk. This means (so the theory goes) that they are less able to cope with physical or mental stress, more vulnerable to a range of diseases from coronary heart disease to depression and to take longer to recover when they become ill.[24] To put it another way, whilst low social capital does not itself cause ill health, social capital can act as a 'buffer' that reduces the adverse effect of socio-economic deprivation. The latest research on social capital has focused on exploring the interaction between individual characteristics (personality, metabolism, physical and psychological vulnerability to stress) and the stuff of social capital, producing hypotheses about what sort of person is especially vulnerable to the impact of deprivation.[25,26]

Whilst social capital is intuitively plausible as the 'missing variable' in the health inequalities equation, it has been extensively criticised as an ill-defined construct, which often boils down to the simpler notion of social support. It has also been somewhat politicised, being seen as aligned with the 'third way' agenda (see next section). As one group of critics put it, social capital theory presents *'an appealing common sense idealist social psychology to which everyone can relate (e.g. good relations within your community are good for your health)'* and offers a convenient excuse to ignore *'both state centred economic redistribution (e.g. living wage, full employment, and universal health insurance) and party politics'.*[27] The measurement of social capital (usually via quantitative surveys of the extent of social networks rather than qualitative studies of the quality of these relationships or the resources or support exchanged) is fraught with controversy.[24] These limitations notwithstanding, both social network theory and social capital theory remain extensively used in research studies on health inequalities.[26]

A closely related concept to social networks and social capital is social exclusion, which might be defined as limitations in an individual's opportunity to find good work, decent housing, adequate health care, quality education, safe and secure living conditions and fair treatment by the legal and criminal justice systems. In other words, social exclusion is a combination of economic disadvantage, lack of access to resources (or the ability to make use of them) and social prejudice and discrimination. 'The socially excluded' are a heterogeneous and ill-defined group who may include the homeless, those with stigmatising conditions (e.g. HIV positive, mental health problems), those with disabilities, single parents, low-income groups and (in some societies) certain ethnic or religious minorities. Unsurprisingly, social exclusion of any kind tends to be strongly linked to poor health outcomes. Conversely, reducing social exclusion is essential to reducing health inequalities – and requires both political will and (usually) fundamental social and cultural change.[28]

In Section 7.4, I briefly describe a research study into the social networks of homeless women. For additional examples of development projects in primary care that take a (predominantly) social capital perspective, see Joe Kai and Chris Drinkwater's excellent compilation.[29]

9.3 Unpacking health inequalities III: life course epidemiology and 'risk regulators'

Other sections in this book have considered individual-level risk factors (such as behaviour choices – see Section 8.4) and the social support that occurs to a greater or lesser extent in a community (see Section 9.2) as determinants of health inequalities. At another level of analysis, there is considerable evidence that the wider structure of society – living conditions (including the built environment, transport, communications and the provision of health and social care), laws (such as on where people may smoke, when they may drink or what sort of foods may be advertised to children), policies (economic, social, crime, food and agriculture and so on) – puts some groups more at risk of adverse health outcomes than others.[26,30,31] If all this is becoming confusing, let's break down the inherent complexity of the social determinants of health in three ways:

a They are *multifactorial* – that is, many different influences interact to produce socio-economic differences in health outcomes;

b They are *multi-level* – that is, as Figure 9.2 (explained below) shows, they operate at individual, interpersonal, family, community and societal levels, and an influence at any of these levels impacts on other levels (e.g. stress in the workplace may exert its impact partly via a change in hormone levels[32]; lack of social integration may exert its impact via a change in individual risk behaviour[26,30]);

c Their influence *changes over time* – that is, different influences have a different impact at different stages in a person's life (e.g. nutritional stress in utero programmes the body's metabolism to make it more susceptible to heart disease in later life[33]; workplace stress has greater effect in mid career than it does at the extremes of the working life[34]; the effect of adverse social conditions is cumulative, hence often has particular impact on the elderly[35]).

An epidemiologist whose work you should check out if you are interested in the multifactorial, multi-level determinants of health and how their impact changes over time is George Davey Smith. Of his prodigious output of fascinating publications, the one I particularly recommend is his book *Health Inequalities: Lifecourse Approaches*.[31] Life course epidemiology moves beyond the study of 'risk factors' as independent variables to the study of how different influences interact with one another and how this influence changes at different stages in a person's life.

An excellent paper that takes lifecourse epidemiology almost to an art form is Glass and McAttee's 'Behavioral science at the crossroads'.[32] They introduce a metaphor for the life course – that of a flowing stream (Figure 9.2). They

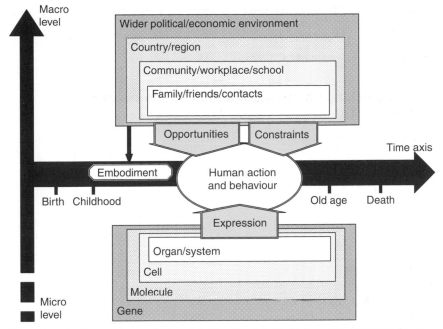

Figure 9.2 The 'stream of causation' model of health-related behaviour. (Simplified from Glass and McAtee.[32])

add a vertical dimension to this metaphor, with the 'river bed' being the micro influences on behaviour and function (genetic make-up, hormonal influences and other biological expression, individual personality and predispositions), and the higher points on this vertical axis being mezzo-level social structure (the family, the school or workplace), the macro level of the nation state, and even the world economy! Rather than seeing all these as a confusing 'soup' of overall influence, Glass and McAtee suggest that each level influences, and is influenced by, the other levels in a complex, dynamic and to some extent unpredictable way as the individual follows his or her life course. You might like to compare this model with the biopsychosocial model developed by Engel (and popularised by McWhinney and team), illustrated in Figure 5.1, page 131. Whilst both models see a nested hierarchy of influence on individual health outcomes, social epidemiologists such as Glass and McAtee have tradition-ally majored on studying the community and environmental levels whereas clinicians like Engels and McWhinney have majored on individual illness and behaviour.

Glass and McAtee use the term 'risk regulators' to refer to conditions in the social environment which, while not deterministic of individual behaviour, create the preconditions for adverse lifestyle choices. Table 9.1 shows some risk regulators, which may mediate the complex link between low socio-economic status and self-destructive behaviours such as smoking, overeating,

Table 9.1 Examples of risk regulators.

Risk regulators a: the level of community and society are the 'macro' conditions in which adverse health choices become more likely. Examples include:

Material conditions	Laws, policies and regulations	Area deprivation	Cultural norms and expectations	Community ethos	Conditions of work
Availability of fresh healthy food	National (taxes on cigarettes	Poverty	Diet	Crime and fear of crime	Control over nature and pace of job
Presence of fast food outlets	Local (traffic calming measures)	Unemployment	Exercise	Neighbourliness	Discrimination/ oppression at work
Availability of sports and leisure facilities		Overcrowding	Smoking/alcohol	Local support networks	
Built environment (e.g. walkability, connectivity)			Religious observance		

Adapted from Glass and McAtee.[32]

drug-taking, sexual promiscuity and so on. As you can see from Figure 9.2, whilst the model pulls together numerous intuitively plausible influences on health inequalities, it gives us no easy formula for predicting precisely who will get ill at what stage in their life. Nor (as I will explain in Chapter 10) should we expect such easy answers from a complex system!

Embedded within Glass and McAttee's model is an acknowledgement of structural theory, which proposes that the structure of society is a very powerful influence on individual behaviour and health outcome. According to this viewpoint, even 'free' choices (such as whether to smoke, or whether to apply to university) are strongly socially patterned. We only choose from a limited range of options (the ones that match our identity, which make us feel included, which seem achievable and realistic, which others like us are making and so on).

As I implied in Section 9.2 in relation to social capital theory, aligning oneself with the position that individual health is (or, alternatively, is not) strongly and unavoidably influenced by social structure is a political statement.[27] Margaret Thatcher's most famous quote illustrates one extreme of this continuum:

> 'I think we've been through a period where too many people have been given to understand that if they have a problem, it's the government's job to cope with it. 'I have a problem, I'll get a grant'. 'I'm homeless, the government must house me'. They're casting their problem on society. And, you know, there is no such thing as society. There are individual men and women, and there are families. And no government can do anything except through people, and people must look to themselves first.'
>
> Margaret Thatcher in Woman's Own Magazine, 31 October 1987.

At the other extreme, traditionally left-wing politicians and organisations, such as the UK's Socialist Health Association (www.sochealth.org.uk/), take the view that social structure is critical to individual health and that radical changes to social structure are a prerequisite for reducing health inequalities (Box 9.1). Without such changes, 'choice' is a vacuous concept that is used by self-serving political groups to absolve themselves of their responsibilities towards the less fortunate. This viewpoint has come to be seen as somewhat outdated in the UK, given the considerable evidence that structural changes alone (better buildings, more police on the streets, more or different primary care services, plus see the examples in Box 9.2) have limited impact on the health of a community in the absence of engagement of both the community and front-line staff in health and social care; the development of learning organisations (see Section 11.6); increases in the social capital of vulnerable individuals; and so on.[29]

An alternative view, widely referred to as the 'third way', states that whilst society surely exists and provides structure for our personal choices, individuals are not dupes. They can (and should) take responsibility for their choices and by doing so, they cannot only overcome disadvantage but also begin to change the nature of society. This perspective is based on an important theory

> **Box 9.2 Example of a strongly structuralist perspective on health inequalities.**
>
> At its 2005 annual conference, the Socialist Health Association (www.sochealth .org/) passed a resolution calling on the government of England and Wales to adopt a much bolder and more radical approach to public health including:
> • a complete ban on smoking in all public places with NO exemptions as is proposed in Scotland;
> • a comprehensive transport policy which both encourages physical exercise and reduces environmental pollution by promoting accessible and affordable public transport and by discouraging private motor car use by measures such as road use charges;
> • substantial improvements in the diet of children through a complete ban on advertising of processed foods except at point of sale and through provision of free healthy school meals to all;
> • effective measures to ensure that the obstruction of breastfeeding mothers is a criminal offence as it is in Scotland.

developed by sociologist Anthony Giddens, called structuration theory. Giddens proposed that social life is more than random individual acts, but is not merely determined by social forces.[36] The 'micro' of human agency and the 'macro' of social structure are related to each other such that the repetition of acts of individual agents reproduces the structure. The traditions, institutions, moral codes, technologies and established ways of doing things that make up our social structure strongly influence our behaviour, but they can be changed when we start to ignore them, replace them or reproduce them differently.

Here's an example of structuration. In the 1960s, single mothers were so socially ostracised that most babies born out of wedlock were given up for adoption. Nowadays, single motherhood remains a tough choice, but individuals finding themselves in this position meet with far more understanding and less discrimination than they would have received 40 years ago (though, arguably, we still have some way to go). What caused the change in attitudes? The answer is (at least partly) individual mothers, who stubbornly and courageously refused to bow to social pressures and persevered with their choice to raise their own son or daughter rather than hand them over to a more 'suitable' set of parents. Eventually, the actions of these individual women led to changes in the social norms and expectations within which the choices of contemporary women (and men) are nested.

Structuration theory (and, perhaps, third-way politics) implicitly underpins the far-reaching Wanless Report,[37] in which a highly regarded economist recently considered three different scenarios for the future of public health. The first scenario was 'slow uptake', in which the public continued (as now) to be largely disengaged with their own health and that of their community, and took little if any individual action oriented to staying healthy and making sensible and equitable use of healthcare services. The second scenario was 'solid progress', in which the level of individual engagement steadily increased, leading to healthier lifestyle choices, more effective and equitable use of health services and measurable increases in life expectancy. Finally (and not considered very likely), there was 'full engagement' in which people were interested and committed to make positive lifestyle choices, used health services in a highly efficient way and contributed to community initiatives that promoted health. In this last scenario, overall health status and life expectancy would increase dramatically and the public would enthusiastically help shape the design and delivery of services.

Despite a change in UK government from Conservative to Labour in 1997 and the subsequent espousal of 'third way' values, much government policy in this country (and elsewhere) remains built on the assumption that the level of intervention for improving the health of a community should be individual risk behaviour (exhorting people to give up smoking) rather than, say, legislation (e.g. food labelling, opening hours of supermarkets and pubs, smoking in public places), the design of public spaces (provision of pedestrian precincts, well-lit parks and cycle tracks), social organisation (e.g. providing a more comprehensive social care system for frail elderly people living alone) or – most controversial of all – the power relations in society and the fact that some people are in much greater control of their lives and destinies than others.

Some would argue that 'third way' health policies (encouraging informed individuals to exercise good citizenship and choice, thereby improving their own and others' prospects, for example, encouraging individuals not to smoke) are too often used as an excuse for political inaction (such as not bothering to make laws banning smoking in public places).[27] A more politically radical public health agenda would directly and emphatically address structural influences on health inequalities (such as unequal distribution of income, poor housing, unsafe streets and discrimination). Vincent Navarro, one of the world's most widely respected epidemiologists, has demonstrated that countries with broadly social democratic policies (redistribution of income from rich to poor, and high investment in public services) have lower gradients in health inequalities than those with more conservative policies.[38] But the relationship is not a simple or universally consistent one, and you must read the original article and the ensuing correspondence to make up your own mind on the politics of redressing health inequalities!

9.4 Developing healthy communities I: community oriented primary care

'Developing healthy communities' covers a multitude of sins both theoretically (what is meant by 'health' and 'community'; what is the assumed mechanism of change; what are the critical success factors, and so on) and in terms of the practicalities of achieving the goal. I will make no attempt to cover this topic comprehensively. Rather, I will offer two contrasting examples of approaches to developing a 'healthy community' from two very different theoretical traditions (though as it turns out, with some overlap in terms of what happens on the ground). In this section I will discuss community oriented primary care (broadly, a biomedical theory adapted to a community development setting); and in the next section I will give some examples of participatory approaches (broadly, variants of community development theory adapted to address health issues).

The community oriented primary care (COPC) model was originally developed in South Africa, but has since been applied in a variety of settings including the USA and UK.[39,40] Its origins lie firmly in the field of biomedicine, with explicit principles derived from epidemiology, primary care, preventive medicine and health promotion. The essential model, which requires a definable community and an established primary health care team providing at least basic services to the local population, is in some ways the medical consultation writ large. In the first stage, the development team does the community equivalent of getting to know the 'patient' – that is, they undertake *community profiling*, setting out the physical boundaries of the community, its demographics, socio-economic characteristics, key cultural practices and so on. The next stage is a detailed epidemiological assessment with a view to making a *community diagnosis* – that is, mapping and quantifying the different health problems. Next, a *primary care programme* is developed, based on systematic prioritisation of which problems should take precedence (e.g. nature, seriousness and prevalence of diseases, their natural history, prognosis, therapy and evidence on the efficacy of preventive measures). This programme is then implemented and its efficacy *evaluated* using appropriate measures of process and outcome.

The COPC model bears remarkable resemblance to the approach described by one of the all-time great names in British general practice, William Pickles, who extolled the need for the GP to apply epidemiology to the community as long ago as 1939.[41] But the term 'community oriented primary care' was not used until the 1950s, when physician Sydney Kark took a systematic approach to improving the health status of the population of Pholela, South Africa, using the four-stage COPC model. Whilst Kark was a passionate advocate of the biomedical basis of ill health (he required his multi-disciplinary team of nurses and local health workers to take lessons in physiology and basic pharmacology, as well as in the research techniques necessary for mapping the epidemiology of local disease), he was not tied to conventional biomedical 'treatments' for his target community. His initial priorities in the first phase of the COPC cycle were syphilis and tuberculosis, but when the measures implemented made relatively little overall impact on the health of the community, Kark soon moved to consider more 'upstream' causes of ill health. The following is quoted from his original paper published in the *South African Medical Journal* in 1952 and reproduced recently as a 'classic' paper in the *American Journal of Public Health* (available in full text online and worth looking up)[42]:

'Soil erosion and migrant labour have resulted in:
a Failure to produce sufficient food for the needs of the community, with evidence of gross malnutrition in plant and animal life as well as in the people;
b An instability in family life and maladjustment in family relationships, associated with a high incidence of emotional disturbances . . . ;
c The continuous introduction of fresh foci of infection by these returning from work in the towns. A high incidence of tuberculosis and syphilis is maintained by this process'.

Kark's recommendation for the next COPC 'cycle' was to improve basic sanitation, prevent soil erosion (thereby reducing the need for the men to travel in search of work), and urgently address the nutritional status of the population. The interventions were so successful (e.g. infant mortality fell from 27.5% to 10%) that Kark was awarded all the grant money he could wish for by the South African government to repeat his success in other deprived communities![39] If that sounds like a fairy story, there is a serious moral which Longlett et al. draw out in their historical account of COPC programmes across the world. COPC programmes have been most successful when large amounts of external funding have been provided to a project and when the work has been led by a well-trained external team based in an academic unit. Having said that, training for local community health workers and amicable partnerships with community leaders are also critical to success. Failed COPC initiatives (of which there are many examples) tend to be characterised by lack of dedicated funding, lack of training of front line staff, lack of vision and drive by programme directors, and occasionally, changes in the direction of the political wind, as in the dark years of National Party rule in South Africa (1948–1994) when funding for community projects was systematically withdrawn and academic departments of primary care closed down.[39,43]

Because successful COPC initiatives have historically required considerable external funding, often from philanthropic sources, controversy exists about the feasibility of using the COPC model in 'everyday' primary care practice. Few, if any, institutions have successfully implemented training in COPC within a traditional medical school curriculum or integrated it with the postgraduate training of primary care clinicians. Many published stories of small-scale COPC successes state unashamedly that the COPC cycle was applied by the personal dedication of the primary health care team with no additional remuneration from a healthcare system designed to reward reactive rather than proactive care.[44] A recent commentary concluded that

'COPC's contribution to current health practice [in South Africa] remains more symbolic than substantive. Despite a policy framework that favors the widespread introduction of COPC, various political, structural, managerial, and human resource obstacles constrain its effective implementation'.[45]

What can we conclude about this enticing model of building a healthy community? Perhaps, that when appropriately trained experts and willing community partners find the right chemistry between them, as well as political will and generous funding, the COPC programme offers potentially huge advantages in the health status of the population, but the spread and sustainability of such projects is likely to be limited. Perhaps this is why the World Health Organisation's peak phase of enthusiasm for this model was in the 1970s and 1980s, and interest has now moved on to more participatory, 'home grown' solutions as described in the next section.

9.5   Developing healthy communities II: participatory approaches

Sidney Kark (see previous section) recognised the importance of community consultation and involvement, but he certainly didn't major on it, nor did he (as far as we know) apply a theoretical perspective to this aspect of his work. One of the first people who did was Sherry Arnstein, a US community activist in the 1960s. She recognised that there were different ways of 'involving' a community in any development initiative, and that these could be ranked on a 'ladder' from manipulation to full citizen control (Figure 9.3).

Whilst Arnstein's model is a great place to start thinking about how to involve communities in developing their health services, a recent article has challenged the continuing use of this model.[47] Tritter and McCallum claim that it is static and unidimensional, based on a simplistic notion of power (and the extent to which that power is shared).[47] They call for a more sophisticated model that reflects different aspects of healthcare planning in many contemporary communities:

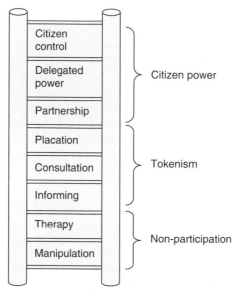

Figure 9.3 Arnstein's ladder of participation.[46]

• The complex nature of power (distributed between many different individuals and groups and not amenable to a simple 'zero-sum' redistribution as implied by the 'ladder' analogy);
• The heterogeneous nature of communities (composed of multiple diverse groups each with different priorities and values) and of health service users (who represent a range of different illnesses and risk groups, and different stages in the illness journey);
• The agency of users (some keen to be involved, others not, or wanting different types and levels of input in different circumstances); and
• The dynamic and evolving nature of policymaking.

These authors argue against any particular 'preferred' model of user involvement and advocate a mixed economy of schemes, negotiated with user groups and appropriately integrated with one another, which reflect the inherent complexity of planning and delivering healthcare.

One example of a (rare) initiative led by primary care doctors that sits high on Arnstein's ladder of participation and which also addresses some of the complexities raised by Tritter and McCallum is Ann Macaulay's team's participatory action research with the Ojibwa-Cree indigenous community in Kanawauke, Canada.[48–50] They used an approach called participatory action research (see Section 3.5 for an explanation and Figure 3.7, page 75, for a diagram of this approach). They worked closely with community leaders to develop a school-based diabetes prevention programme, taking a 'whole systems' approach including raising community awareness of diabetes and its potential complications, promotion of exercise within and outside school, education about weight and diet, challenging schools' policies on soft drink vending machines and so on. The research team put in considerable ground work not merely to form partnerships with members of the target community but to address the community's priorities (as defined by that community) in ways seen as appropriate by that community. In other words, the 'diagnosis' was developed *with* the community, nor offered to the community by visiting experts. Incidentally, if you are convinced that taking a lay perspective on health needs is necessarily a compromise compared to what a 'professional' team would produce, you should read Jennie Popay and Gareth Williams' article, which suggests that 'lay knowledge' has as many advantages as limitations in the context of community development.[51] Macaulay's team successfully implemented their complex project despite a funding hiatus midway through and attributed this success to four interrelated factors:

1 Integration of community people with researchers as equal partners at every phase, including (for example) co-authorship on reports and academic publications.
2 The structural and functional integration of the intervention and evaluation components of the initiative – in other words, 'evaluation' was not seen as an add-on component undertaken at the end of the project but as part and parcel of the work itself.

3 A flexible, responsive agenda in which changes of pace and direction were possible to meet local contingencies (as opposed to developing an 'evidence-based' master-plan and driving it through).

4 The recognition and valuing of the learning opportunities offered by the project to all stakeholders.

Whilst these authors placed partnership with service users at the top of their list of critical success factors, it was by no means easy to achieve. The process of creating and sustaining shared meanings, goals and success criteria across multiple agencies and subcultures was demanding of time, energy and diplomacy, and required an entirely new infrastructure to be set up. Progress on the ground was considerably slower than the researchers initially anticipated, and interim results were relatively unimpressive (the prevalence of obesity amongst teenagers, for example, did not fall overnight). However, after more than 10 years of community partnership, real progress has now been made on the main risk factors for diabetes in this high-risk population, and the project has sufficient critical mass that it has continued despite changes in both community leaders and key research staff.[50]

In reality, participatory action research projects like the one described here are often undertaken on small (or even non-existent) budgets and may be periodically rebranded to capture small-scale local funding streams. Whilst this may appear to the purists to be no way to run an important community health initiative, there is some evidence that locally owned, home-grown initiatives are more successful the *less* dedicated funding they receive! In another Canadian health promotion programme, the Ontario Heart Health Promotion Project (comprising a total of 189 interventions on risk factor screening, courses for smoking cessation, healthy eating or physical activity, support groups to promote healthy lifestyles, environmental modification, dissemination of information), a survey of the success and sustainability of each of the 189 primary projects showed that a positive response to the question 'the intervention used no paid staff' was associated with a 3.7-fold greater chance that the initiative continued beyond the life of the funding period![52] The success of action research initiatives in building health communities is not guaranteed, but because local ownership is inherent to the action research design, such initiatives are less likely to lose momentum if the funding stream dwindles (and more likely to take responsibility for seeking further funds).

The principle of participation features heavily in the rhetoric of numerous community health initiatives around the world, in which 'partnership' and 'community involvement' is a prerequisite for the allocation of funding, but where 'top down' planning also features strongly. As Roussos and Fawcett point out in their excellent review of community partnerships for health, many such initiatives include an element of 'top down' (i.e. social planning led by experts, see previous section) *and* 'bottom up' (i.e. grassroots community organising) features. In other words, the distinction between community-oriented primary care (Section 9.4) and participatory approaches (this section) is something

---

Box 9.3 The WHO Healthy Cities programme (see www.euro.who.int/healthy-cities).[57]

The WHO Healthy Cities programme engages local governments in health development through a process of political commitment, institutional change, capacity building, partnership-based planning and innovative projects. It promotes comprehensive and systematic policy and planning with a special emphasis on health inequalities and urban poverty, the needs of vulnerable groups, participatory governance and the social, economic and environmental determinants of health. It also strives to include health considerations in economic, regeneration and urban development efforts.

Over 1200 cities and towns from more than 30 countries in the WHO European Region are healthy cities. These are linked through national, regional, metropolitan and thematic Healthy Cities networks, as well as the WHO Healthy Cities network for more advanced cities.

At the time of writing, the WHO Healthy Cities programme is in its fourth phase (2003–2008). Cities currently involved in the Phase IV Network are working on three core themes: healthy ageing, healthy urban planning and health impact assessment. In addition, all participating cities focus on the topic of physical activity/active living.

---

of a false dichotomy.[53] National and international-level examples of what might be called hybrid development initiatives (i.e. which have an element of both top down strategy, perhaps centrally driven, and local grass-roots emergence) that you may have heard of include Sure Start (USA),[54] Health Action Zones (UK)[55,56] and the WHO Healthy Cities Programme which was implemented in many cities across the world (Box 9.3).[58] Examples of more local hybrid initiatives include the Healthy Communities Initiatives (USA),[59] the 'Partnership' health promotion programme (Northern Ireland),[60] the Highfield Community Enrichment Project (Canada),[61] and the Dumbiedykes primary care programme in Scotland.[62] Two more sources of good examples are Fran Baum's book from Australia, entitled *The New Public Health*,[63] and Joe Kai and Chris Drinkwater's compilation of stories from an urban deprived community in the north of England.[29]

Whilst case studies of 'healthy cities' and 'healthy communities' projects abound and often make inspiring reading, a critical appraisal of these publications (see Section 3.7) often raises questions about observer bias (people 'telling it like they wish it had been'), publication bias (only writing up projects that had been at least moderately successful) and the rigour of the methods used to assess 'success' at all – even when the authors promise a 'warts and all' account (but especially when they don't).[64] There is now beginning to emerge a scholarly literature that takes a critical view of the notion of 'partnership' and which analyses successes and failures (as well as initiatives that are difficult to classify on this axis) through a political science lens.* Back in 2000, Roussos and Fawcett lamented the dearth of evidence either for or against particular approaches to community partnerships in relation to public health, and argued that the model in general rested on three untested assumptions:

a involving lots of organisations and stakeholders will (implicitly, always) allow a community development goal to be reached more easily or fully than could occur if one individual or group worked alone towards the same goal;

b it is best to include a range of individuals and groups who represent the full diversity of the population in terms of demographics, background and perspective on the issue; and

c shared interests will make consensus among the prospective partners possible.[53]

Interestingly, while all these principles chime with 'new public health' ideology (and were among the critical success factors listed by Ann Macaulay's team in the project discussed above[50]), there is some evidence emerging which challenges the universality of these principles. Dina Berkeley and colleagues, for example, recently reviewed the evaluations of the European Healthy City projects and English Health Action Zones and considered a number of barriers to their success.[65] They distinguish between cultural barriers (which stem from different philosophical, organisational, and professional/experiential cultures), and political barriers (which stem from both party political and realpolitik concerns). These barriers, they found, often operate together, compounding the individual impact of each of them, with detrimental effects for the wider initiative. They conclude that whilst it is certainly 'politically correct' to promote an alternative, and more appropriate, vision of how health can be maintained and enhanced, entrenched cultural and political barriers effectively function to sustain the hegemony of the status quo which was, and is, based on a different and outdated vision. They offer no easy answers, but warn that acknowledging the persistence of these barriers is an essential first step towards turning the prevailing health-related rhetoric into reality.

Anna Gilmore, in another article subtitled 'rhetoric or reality', takes a hard look at the Social Exclusion Unit, a UK government initiative that was explicitly set up as a 'cross cutting' unit to work across organisational boundaries within central government and between central and local government to address community level contributors to health inequalities.[66] Her findings suggest that the success of the Social Exclusion Unit has been limited, due partly to lack of coordination (cross-boundary initiatives being particularly difficult to coordinate, as Section 10.2 emphasises) and partly to widespread lack of understanding locally about the role public health initiatives can play in tackling health inequalities.

---

*You will probably have spotted that when academic primary care starts to consider community development, it needs to get its head round yet another 'ology' – political science.

In conclusion, whilst partnerships oriented towards healthy communities are currently extremely popular, and various hybrids between 'top down' and 'grass roots' models of community partnership are in operation, no such model is a panacea. It is possible that given the operational difficulty of 'keeping everyone on board' and 'achieving consensus', the pendulum may swing back in future years towards initiatives that are somewhat less comprehensive, less multifaceted, and involve less consultation with stakeholders. Watch this space.

References

1 Acheson D. *Independent Inquiry into Inequalities in Health*. London: Department of Health; 1998.
2 Davidson G, Rutstein S, Johnson K, Pande R, Wagstaff A. *Round I Country Reports on Health, Nutrition, Population Conditions among Poor and Better-Off in 45 Countries*. Geneva: World Bank; 2000.
3 Secretary of State for Health. *Tackling Health Inequalities: 2002 Cross-Cutting Review*. London: Department of Health; 2002.
4 Anonymous. The English Indices of Deprivation 2004 (revised). *Measuring Multiple Deprivation at the small area level: A Conceptual Framework*. London: Office of the Deputy Prime Minister, Neighbourhood Renewal Unit; 2004.
5 Jarman B. Identification of underprivileged areas. BMJ 1983;236:1705–1708.
6 Townsend P. Deprivation. J Soc Policy 1987;16:125–146.
7 Carstairs V, Morris R. Deprivation and health in Scotland. Health Bull 1990;48:162–175.
8 Morris R, Carstairs V. Which deprivation? A comparison of selected deprivation indexes. J Public Health Med 1991;13:318–326.
9 Eachus J, Williams M, Chan P, et al. Deprivation and cause specific morbidity: evidence from the Somerset and Avon survey of health. BMJ 1996;312:287–292.
10 Kreitman N, Carstairs V, Duffy J. Association of age and social class with suicide among men in Great Britain. J Epidemiol Community Health 1991;45:195–202.
11 Carstairs V. Deprivation indices: their interpretation and use in relation to health. J Epidemiol Community Health 1995;49(suppl 2):S3–S8.
12 Jordan H, Roderick P, Martin D. The index of multiple deprivation 2000 and accessibility effects on health. J Epidemiol Community Health 2004;58:250–257.
13 Edwards R, McElduff P, Harrison RA, Watson K, Butler G, Elton P. Pleasure or pain? A profile of smokers in Northern England. Public Health 2006;120:760–768.
14 Stephens MR, Blackshaw GR, Lewis WG, et al. Influence of socio-economic deprivation on outcomes for patients diagnosed with gastric cancer. Scand J Gastroenterol 2005;40:1351–1357.
15 Cooper D, Arnold E, Smith G, et al. The effect of deprivation, age and sex on NHS Direct call rates. Br J Gen Pract 2005;55:287–291.
16 Stafford M, Cummins S, Macintyre S, Ellaway A, Marmot M. Gender differences in the associations between health and neighbourhood environment. Soc Sci Med 2005;60:1681–1692.
17 Berkman LF, Glass T, Brissette I, Seeman TE. From social integration to health: durkheim in the new millennium. Soc Sci Med 2000;51:843–857.
18 Berkman LF. The role of social relations in health promotion. Psychosom Med 1995;57:245–254.

19 Kawachi I, Berkman LF. Social ties and mental health. J Urban Health 2001;78:458–467.

20 Cohen S, Doyle WJ, Skoner DP, Rabin BS, Gwaltney JM, Jr. Social ties and susceptibility to the common cold. JAMA 1997;277:1940–1944.

21 House JS, Robbiins CYNT, Metzner HL. The association of social relationships and activities with mortality: prospective evidence from the Tecumseh Community Health Study. Am J Epidemiol 1982;116:123–140.

22 Hanifan LJ. *The Community Center*. Boston: Silver Burdett; 1920.

23 Putnam RD. Bowling Alone. *The Collapse and Revival of American Community*. New York: Simon and Schuster; 2000.

24 Morgan A, Swann C. *Social Capital for Health: Issues of Definition, Measurement and Links to Health*. London: Health Development Agency; 2004.

25 Moore S, Haines V, Hawe P, Shiell A. Lost in translation: a genealogy of the 'social capital' concept in public health. J Epidemiol Community Health 2006;60:729–734.

26 Siegrist J, Marmot M. *Social Inequalities in Health: New Evidence and Policy Implications*. Oxford: Oxford University Press; 2006.

27 Muntaner C, Lynch J, Smith GD. Social capital, disorganized communities, and the third way: understanding the retreat from structural inequalities in epidemiology and public health. Int J Health Serv 2001;31:213–237.

28 Hills J, Piachaud D, Le Grand J. *Understanding Social Exclusion*. Oxford: Oxford University Press; 2002.

29 Kai J, Drinkwater C. *Primary Care in Urban Disadvantaged Communities*. Oxford: Radcliffe; 2003.

30 Rose G. Sick individuals and sick populations. Int J Epidemiol 1985;14:42–48.

31 Davey Smith G. *Health Inequalities: Lifecourse Approaches*. Bristol: The Policy Press; 2003.

32 Glass TA, McAtee MJ. Behavioral science at the crossroads in public health: extending horizons, envisioning the future. Soc Sci Med 2006;62:1650–1671.

33 Hales CN, Barker DJ. The thrifty phenotype hypothesis. Br Med Bull 2001;60:5–20.

34 Marmot M. Work and other factors influencing coronary health and sickness absence. Work Stress 1994;8:191–201.

35 House JS, Lepkowski JM, Kinney AM, Mero RP, Kessler RC, Herzog AR. The social stratification of aging and health. J Health Soc Behav 1994;35:213–234.

36 Giddens A. *The Constitution of Society*. Berkeley: University of California Press; 1986.

37 Wanless D. *Securing Our Future Health: Taking a Long-Term View*. London: H.M. Treasury; 2002.

38 Navarro V, Shi L. The political context of social inequalities and health. Int J Health Serv 2001;31:1–21.

39 Longlett SK, Kruse JE, Wesley RM. Community-oriented primary care: historical perspective. J Am Board Fam Pract 2001;14:54–63.

40 Iliffe S, Lenihan P. Integrating primary care and public health: learning from the community-oriented primary care model. Int J Health Serv 2003;33:85–98.

41 Pickles W. *Epidemiology in Country Practice*. Bristol: John Wright; 1939.

42 Kark SL, Cassel J. The pholela health centre: a progress report. 1952. Am J Public Health 2002;92:1743–1747.

43 Yach D, Tollman SM. Public health initiatives in South Africa in the 1940s and 1950s: lessons for a post-apartheid era. Am J Public Health 1993;83:1043–1050.

44 Gillam S, Schamroth A. The community-oriented primary care experience in the United Kingdom. Am J Public Health 2002;92:1721–1725.

45 Tollman SM, Pick WM. Roots, shoots, but too little fruit: assessing the contribution of COPC in South Africa. Am J Public Health 2002;92:1725–1728.

46 Arnstein S. A ladder of citizen participation. J Am Inst Plann 1969;35:216–224.

47 Tritter JQ, McCallum A. The snakes and ladders of user involvement: moving beyond Arnstein. Health Policy 2006;76:156–168.

48 Macaulay AC, Ryan JG. Community needs assessment and development using the participatory research model. Ann Fam Med 2003;1:183–184.

49 Cargo M, Levesque L, Macaulay AC, et al. Community governance of the Kahnawake Schools Diabetes Prevention Project, Kahnawake Territory, Mohawk Nation, Canada. Health Promot Int 2003;18:177–187.

50 Potvin L, Cargo M, McComber AM, Delormier T, Macaulay AC. Implementing participatory intervention and research in communities: lessons from the Kahnawake Schools Diabetes Prevention Project in Canada. Soc Sci Med 2003;56:1295–1305.

51 Popay J, Williams G. Public health research and lay knowledge. Soc Sci Med 1996;42:759–768.

52 O'Loughlin J, Renaud L, Richard L, Gomez LS, Paradis G. Correlates of the sustainability of community-based heart health promotion interventions. Prev Med 1998;27:702–712.

53 Roussos ST, Fawcett SB. A review of collaborative partnerships as a strategy for improving community health. Annu Rev Public Health 2000;21:369–402.

54 Roff M. Levelling the playing fields of England: promoting health in deprived communities. J R Soc Health 2003;123:20–22.

55 Powell M, Moon G. Health action zones: the 'third way' of a new area-based policy? Health Soc Care Community 2001;9:43–50.

56 Crawshaw P, Bunton R, Gillen K. Health action zones and the problem of community. Health Soc Care Community 2003;11:36–44.

57 Lafond LJ, Heritage Z, Farrington JL, Tsouros AD. *National Healthy Cities Networks: A Powerful Force for Health and Sustainable Development in Europe.* Geneva: World Health Organisation; 2003.

58 Baum F. *Healthy Cities, Local Agenda 21, and Healthy Settings: The New Public Health.* 2nd edn. Melbourne, Australia: Oxford University Press; 2002.

59 Adams CF. Healthy communities and public policy: four success stories. Public Health Rep 2000;115:212–215.

60 Heenan D. A partnership approach to health promotion: a case study from Northern Ireland. Health Promot Int 2004;19:105–113.

61 Nelson G, Pancer SM, Hayward K, Kelly R. Partnerships and participation of community residents in health promotion and prevention: experiences of the highfield community enrichment project (better beginnings, better futures). J Health Psychol 2004;9:213–227.

62 Murray SA, Tapson J, Turnbull L, McCallum J, Little A. Listening to local voices: adapting rapid appraisal to assess health and social needs in general practice. BMJ 1994;308:698–700.

63 Baum F. *The New Public Health.* 2nd edn. Melbourne, Australia: Oxford University Press; 2002.

64 Van Maanen J. *Tales of the Field: On Writing Ethnography.* Chicago, Illinois: University of Chicago Press; 1986.

65 Berkeley D, Springett J. From rhetoric to reality: barriers faced by health for all initiatives. Soc Sci Med 2006;63:179–188.

66 Gilmore AB. Joint working, reality or rhetoric? J Public Health Med 2001;23:5–6.

CHAPTER 10

Complex problems in a complex system

Summary points

1 The patterns of illness seen in primary care have changed in recent years from mostly acute illness to a predominance of chronic progressive illness, frequently with comorbidity. The changing nature of illness has driven major changes in the roles of all primary care professionals, the division of labour between these professionals and the nature and extent of teamwork.

2 Integrated care pathways (ICPs) are one approach to coordinating the care of complex conditions between multiple professionals. But such pathways alone will not produce smooth coordination between different parts of a complex system. Attention must be paid to the roles and infrastructures that support the essential boundary spanning which underpins 'seamless care'.

3 The electronic patient record (EPR), which offers huge potential for improving and monitoring care, is a social innovation as well as a technical one. It shapes and constrains what we define as illness as well as the nature of our professional roles and the way we work together.

4 The recent epidemiological, organisational and technological changes in primary care have virtually abolished the exclusive and confidential GP–patient relationship and eroded trust in both the clinician and the system. Arguably, the nature of trust must change from being an interpersonal property linked to the personal virtues of the clinician and become a property of the system, linked to robust technical security measures, data protection procedures and governance schemes.

10.1 Illness in the twenty-first century: chronicity, comorbidity and the need for coordination

Most traditional textbooks of general practice include a list of 'common illnesses' (or common diseases, depending on whether the author leans towards a 'subjective' or 'objective' taxonomy). Such lists provide estimates (for example) of the proportion of patients who attend the 'average GP' with upper respiratory tract infection, dyspepsia, skin rash, mental health problems and so on. The data are almost always out of date by the time they are published, and they apply only to the particular sample that was used in the research study cited – a classic example of the spurious objectivity in quantitative data that I described in Section 2.2. For this reason, I have resisted the temptation to tell you what proportion of the patients you yourself see have particular things wrong with them!

More interesting is the broader picture of a changing epidemiology of illness in primary care over time. When our grandfathers (and perhaps one or two of our grandmothers) were practising, a high proportion of the patients they saw were (or believed they were) suffering from an acute infectious disease,[1] though as Michael Balint pointed out, many also had a 'hidden' psychological agenda (see Section 6.3).[2] A generation ago, the picture had changed to include a higher proportion of chronic disease, especially ischaemic heart disease, arthritis, chronic obstructive airways disease (often smoking related) and formally classifiable depression and anxiety.[3] Nowadays, acute infectious illness accounts for a relatively small proportion of consultations in UK general practice, the bulk of which are taken up with reviews (or exacerbations) of chronic disease, screening (e.g. cervical smears, developmental checks on infants) and the surveillance and care of the growing proportion of patients who have survived cancer.[4] Having said that, acute problems are by no means rare: Every surgery still has its quota of sore throats, coughs, urinary tract infections and people who have (or wish to exclude) a sexually transmitted infection. But for the remainder of this section, I want to focus on chronic diseases because they contribute to most of the 'complex problems' that form the focus of this chapter.

Most chronic diseases follow five more or less discrete phases (which I have called disease-free, pre-symptomatic, chronic, deteriorating and terminal, though other authors have used different labels), as shown in Figure 10.1. I first saw a similar diagram used in about 1993 in a workshop by Dr Sue Roberts, then a consultant diabetologist and subsequently the UK's National Clinical Director for Diabetes, who also introduced me to the idea that the provision of care for people with chronic disease can be thought of (broadly speaking) as a 'pyramid' (Figure 10.2):

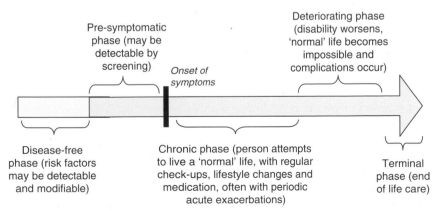

Figure 10.1 Diagrammatic representation of the course of chronic disease.

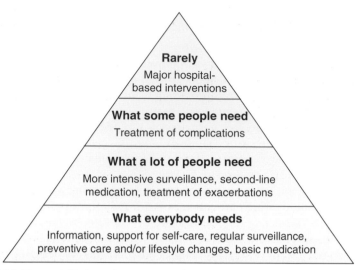

Figure 10.2 The pyramid of care for people with chronic disease.

• Everyone requires a 'standard package' comprising information, support for self-care, surveillance (i.e. regular check-ups and/or self-monitoring), preventive measures and/or lifestyle changes (e.g. in the case of type 2 diabetes, everyone needs to address weight control, food choices, exercise, giving up smoking and so on) and (often) basic first-line medication (oral hypoglycaemic, antiyhpertensive and cholesterol-lowering drugs).

• Many but not all people also need additional tests or procedures, more intensive surveillance (e.g. more frequent visits to the clinician or self-monitoring), second-line medication (e.g. insulin) and treatment of exacerbations (e.g. deterioration of diabetic control during infections).

• A few people need treatment of complications (e.g. people with diabetes may need laser therapy for eye disease or management of diabetic foot ulcer).

• A tiny minority need major hospital-based interventions (e.g. vitreoretinal surgery, amputation).

I have used diabetes as an example, but the diagram in Figure 10.2 applies equally well to almost any chronic disease from progressive kidney failure to multiple sclerosis, and a very similar model has the official stamp of the UK government in its Long Term Conditions strategy (Box 10.1).[5] Note that I have referred to 'people with chronic disease' and not 'patients'. As I argued in Sections 4.1 and 4.4, the 'sick role' in a typical chronic disease is very different from 'passively receiving care from professionals', and few would contest that self-management demands active involvement by the person who is ill. Whilst we are all by definition 'patients' when we present ourselves to the health care system, most chronic disease – at least in its early phases – is managed outside that system, so we should not use the term 'patient' for someone in this situation!

Box 10.1 The UK Department of Health Long Term Conditions Care Model.[5]

The NHS and Social Care Long Term Conditions Model is based on the notion that people at different stages in the illness trajectory (see Figure 10.1) have different needs. Broadly speaking (and with many individual exceptions), there are three levels of care:

Level 1: Supported self-care. The mainstay of care is collaboratively helping individuals and their carers to develop the knowledge, skills and confidence to care for themselves and their condition effectively.

Level 2: Disease-specific care management. This mainly involves providing people with responsive, specialist services using multi-disciplinary teams and disease-specific protocols and pathways, such as the National Service Frameworks and Quality and Outcomes Framework.[6]

Level 3: Case management. This level requires identification of the high-intensity users of unplanned secondary care. Care for these patients should be managed using a community matron of other professional, with a case management approach, with the aim of anticipating, coordinating and joining up health and social care. Local health and social care partners should ensure that self-care and self-management are priorities in local planning and commissioning and should mainstream activities to support self-care.

If we combine Figure 10.1 with Figure 10.2, you should see that the primary health care team will be involved most often at (or before) diagnosis and during the pre-symptomatic and chronic phases of a chronic disease. As I mentioned briefly in Section 1.1, the cornerstone of management in such circumstances is what another of the 'great names' of UK general practice, Julian Tudor Hart, described as 'doing simple things well, for large numbers of people, few of whom feel ill'.[7] In the case of type 2 diabetes, these 'simple things' include[5,8,9]:

• Supporting the persons to monitor their condition and become confident in self-management;

• Having a high index of suspicion and testing opportunistically if a person is at high risk of the condition; encouraging preventive lifestyle changes;

• Confirming and recording the diagnosis of diabetes using standard diagnostic criteria; providing information and education, again using a structured checklist to confirm all topics have been covered;

• Offering structured care (i.e. using a standard checklist of clinical tests and investigations) at recommended intervals;

• Referring promptly to a specialist when complications are present or likely to occur.

The pyramid of care raises issues for the workload of the primary care team, since (numerically speaking) there are a lot more people whose needs lie in the bottom two layers of the pyramid than those who fit into the top two layers. The difference between 'shared care' and 'shifted care' has long been a bone

Table 10.1 Comorbidities described in patients with diabetes.

Hypercholesterolaemia	70%[12]
Obesity	53% (men), 58% (women)[13]
Polycystic ovary syndrome	52% of females[14]
Arthritis	46%[15]
Hypertension	35% (men), 46% (women)[16]
Ischaemic heart disease	34% (men)[17], 29% (women)[15]
Cancer	17%[15]
Depression[†]	10–14%[18]
Heart failure	12%[93]
Eating disorder	6–8% of females[94]

This table does not include the microvascular complications of diabetes, diabetic eye disease (25%), diabetic kidney disease (10%) and diabetic neuropathy (15%).
[†]A large Canadian study entitled 'Diabetes does not increase the risk of depression' demonstrated a low prevalence of depression despite high levels of other comorbidity, but was criticized for excluding patients whose depression began before diabetes was diagnosed.[15]

of contention between primary and secondary care; for a review of some of the issues in the division of labour (and the management of the interface), see Kvamme and colleagues' review.[10]

Let us move now to the challenge of comorbidity (or multimorbidity as some prefer to call it[11]). I recently had a student who wanted to recruit people with type 2 diabetes into a research study. She initially decided that to make the study more 'scientific' she would exclude those with other things wrong with them as well. She began with a list of 250 primary care patients with type 2 diabetes and ended up with only 28! This finding accords with the wider literature: Table 10.1 shows the typical comorbidities found in people with type 2 diabetes. Incidentally, as I explained to my student, it is no longer seen as good research practice only to include 'pure' cases in studies, since the findings would then only apply to the small minority of people with nothing else wrong with them (who would, incidentally, include very few people over the age of 65).[19–21]

The histogram in Figure 10.3 was drawn from data collected in a large study of nearly 61,000 primary care patients by Marjan van den Akker and her colleagues in Maastricht, Netherlands.[22] The prevalence of comorbidity rose sharply with age, such that 60% of people aged 60–79 and 78% of people over 80 had two or more chronic conditions. They also showed that after controlling for age and gender, comorbidity occurred significantly more commonly in patients with fewer years of education and in those in residential homes, but was no commoner in people living alone than in those living with families. Other surveys in different countries and settings have produced even higher estimates of the prevalence of comorbidity.[23–25] In the words of Barbara Starfield, *'There is little doubt that diseases are not randomly distributed in populations, but rather than they cluster in particular individuals and population subgroups'.*[26]

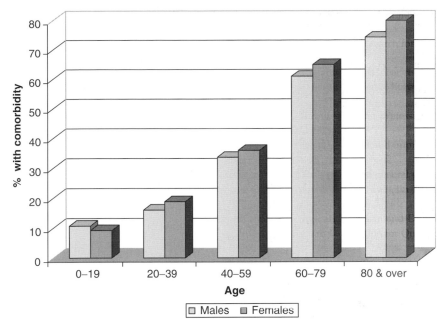

Figure 10.3 Proportion of individuals registered with general practices in Maastricht, Netherlands, who had known comorbidity (two or more chronic diseases concurrently).[22]

Despite the fact that comorbidity is the norm rather than the exception in people older than 55 years, it is relatively under-researched. Martin Fortin and colleagues searched the Medline database and found that for every article on comorbidity or multimorbidity, there are 74 on asthma, 94 on hypertension and 38 on diabetes![27] Of the research that has been done on this topic, most studies have been cross-sectional epidemiological surveys (generating the kind of data shown in Figure 10.3), with one or two cohort studies following the progress of comorbidity over time[28] and validation studies checking the accuracy and consistency of diagnosis and documentation.[29] Only a tiny fraction of all studies on comorbidity (3%) have been undertaken in primary care. There have been very few qualitative studies on the experience of comorbidity, though Fortin's team have developed measures of quality of life (see Section 11.1) that are valid for use in comorbidity studies, and shown that – unsurprisingly perhaps – the more chronic conditions a person suffers from, the lower his or her quality of life.[30] Whilst most researchers (and almost all clinicians) use a simple 'disease count' to measure comorbidity, a more accurate measure of its impact is the Cumulative Illness Rating Scale, which incorporates an estimate of disease severity.[31]

Apart from reminding us that we need to recognise the problem in our clinical practice, why do primary care academics need to be interested in comorbidity? I think there are four main reasons. First, because the study of comorbidity requires a holistic perspective, and primary care (which, as I pointed out in

Section 5.1, is a generalism rather than a specialism) has a much greater potential to provide that perspective than any single clinical specialty. Second, because as I explained in Section 8.1, primary care databases are a powerful tool for studying the epidemiology of chronic disease and offer unique potential for research into what are known as 'cluster profiles' (identifying which chronic diseases occur together and raising hypotheses about whether this is pure coincidence or whether particular diseases may have common causes). For example, Deboarh Saltman and her colleagues in Australia used a large electronic database to identify the 10 most common conditions and the 10 most common drugs prescribed, thereby confirming many intuitive perceptions about the co-occurrence of certain conditions (e.g. hypertension and lipid disorders).[25] Third, as Barbara Starfield has demonstrated, comorbidity is strongly related to organisational issues, in that resource use in any clinic is more closely related to the degree of comorbidity in each patient than the primary diagnosis for which they are being seen.[32] This finding has huge implications for the administration of services (especially for the elderly) and resource planning. Fourth, as the next two sections emphasise, the greater the chronicity and comorbidity, the greater the managerial complexity of healthcare and the need for sophisticated coordination of care (which occurs increasingly through electronic systems).[33] Finally, comorbidity is a wide open topic for qualitative research into the illness experience (see Section 3.2), and if you are a student looking for an MSc or PhD project, you will find many potential avenues to explore here.

Before we move on to consider cross-boundary care, is worth considering what patients themselves see as the priorities for primary care services in this age of complexity, comorbidity and the need for coordination. Angela Coulter, now Chief Executive of the Picker Institute (www.pickereurope.org) which addresses the patient perspective in healthcare, recently reviewed the research literature on people's aspirations for healthcare services, covering both systematic reviews of the research literature and some important 'grey literature' (published outside mainstream research databases, e.g. policy documents).[34] Some key findings are summarised in Box 10.2. Specifically in relation to general practice, Wensing and colleagues found that people's most important priority was 'humaneness', which was ranked highest in 86% of the studies that had included this dimension as an option. This was followed by 'competence/accuracy' (64%), 'patients' involvement in decisions' (63%) and 'time for care' (60%).[35] We should bear these findings in mind when we consider the organisational aspects of care.

10.2   Coordinating care across professional and organisational boundaries

Figure 10.1 suggests that many chronic diseases follow a more or less standard route (though the speed with which the patient progresses along this route may vary considerably). Because of this common course, the management of much chronic (and acute-on-chronic) disease is – or, arguably, should

---

Box 10.2 Aspirations of patients and citizens for healthcare services.

Patients (people seeking or receiving healthcare) would like:
- Fast access to reliable health advice
- Effective treatment delivered by trusted professionals
- Participation in decisions and respect for preferences
- Clear, comprehensible information and support for self-care
- Attention to physical and environmental needs
- Emotional support, empathy and respect
- Involvement of, and support for, family and carers
- Continuity of care and smooth transitions

Citizens (i.e. people, when not patients) would like:
- Affordable treatment and care, free at the point of use
- Safety and quality
- Health protection and disease prevention
- Accessible local services and national centres of excellence
- Universal coverage, geographical and social equity
- Responsiveness, flexibility and choice
- Participation in service developments
- Transparency, accountability and opportunity to influence policy decisions

Summarised from Coulter.[34]

---

be pretty standard wherever care is delivered. But whilst the principles of common clinical management wherever care is delivered and of 'seamless' links between different sectors of care (such as primary and secondary, or public and voluntary) are something almost everyone is signed up to, achieving this is often an operational nightmare – and failure to achieve this accounts for countless examples of medical error, litigation and wasted resources.[10,33,36]

One popular approach to achieving 'seamless care' is integrated care pathways (ICPs, also known as patient pathways or care protocols), defined as predefined management plans for a particular symptom cluster, diagnosis or intervention that aim to make care more structured, consistent and efficient.[37–39] ICPs incorporate specific standards, protocols and processes developed either as part of the pathway itself or (more usually) taken 'off the peg' from separate evidence-based guidelines (see Section 2.2). An ICP typically contains recommendations for investigations, drugs or therapies and includes checklists (with named roles assigned to particular tasks) and time frames for tests and procedures. It is designed to be used by staff across all professional and administrative groups to organise care, investigation and treatment and to record data on process and outcome. Thus, in theory at least, important elements of care are less likely to be missed and information less likely to be mislaid.

Especially when produced in electronic form and designed across the primary–secondary care interface, ICPs have enormous potential to reduce inefficiency (e.g. double handling, unnecessary paperwork, unnecessary investigations, avoidable time delays, precipitous discharges with subsequent readmission and so on).[37] The structured nature of the ICP allows (indeed, requires) data to be collected in a standardised way, using agreed codes (see Section 5.2); hence facilitating the production of aggregated data for clinical audit and/or epidemiological research. Most ICPs run to several pages (20 is not unusual), so I have not given an example here, but the UK National Electronic Library for Health (http://www.library.nhs.uk/pathways/) provides dozens to download.

It is widely acknowledged that ICPs work only when they are developed collaboratively with input from both primary and secondary care by doctors, nurses, other health professionals, administrators, technical staff and – increasingly – lay experts (patients and carers) and when all players understand that they are not prescriptive – that is, clinical and managerial judgement must also be used. However, in reality, controversy still surrounds the question of 'judgement' when using protocol-based ICPs[38,39] – and probably always will, given the inherent philosophical tensions discussed in Section 5.2 about the nature of disease (and illness). ICPs originated in the acute hospital sector for conditions whose management is likely to follow a defined path (e.g. joint replacement[40,41]) and are considered less suited to conditions that require a high degree of individualization in the course of the episode.[40–48] For patients with comorbidity, special needs and/or uncertain diagnosis, ICPs can still be used to map broad processes and goals, but are less useful when considering the detail of treatment. Increasingly, ICPs span the primary–secondary care interface and cover chronic disease management as well as acute incidents and exacerbations.[49,50] They may be held by patients as they move between community and hospital care, perhaps presenting information in a patient-friendly format and enhancing involvement of patients and carers.

Whilst the reality of ICPs and their centrality in contemporary healthcare is not in doubt, there is no agreement on how to theorise or research them empirically. On the one hand, ICPs sit comfortably in the paradigm of clinical epidemiology (see Section 2.2), since standardised care that incorporates evidence-based guidelines is likely to improve outcome and be more cost-effective. In the UK, the introduction of ICPs was closely linked to the clinical effectiveness, evidence-based practice and quality improvement agendas (see Section 11.2),[51] and there has been a strong professional call to distinguish 'rationalization' of healthcare processes (such as might be achieved via good ICPs) from 'rationing provision' (i.e. cost containment).[51] But in the USA, a more overtly economic model has driven both practice and research. ICPs were developed as an explicit and planned response to the escalating cost of health care.[52] US insurance-based hospitals generally receive a negotiated fee for each patient dependent solely on diagnosis, regardless of the services used or the length of stay. ICPs were introduced as a means of trying to ensure that patients would receive a standard, high-quality but no-frills package for a given diagnosis and that their length of stay would be predefined.

The capacity of ICPs to combine process, practice and audit makes them uniquely able (potentially) to bring together clinical and administrative agendas and meet both quality and business objectives via consistent, cost-effective, integrated care. But this, argue others, is an over-optimistic and theoretically uncritical perspective, which fails to see the care pathway in its social – and micro-political – context. A more sociological perspective sees the ICP as not merely enabling health care but also shaping and constraining its professional roles (and indeed the role of the patient), as well as being efficiently coordinated, formalised and ossified in a pathway development process that is not without political struggles or high-level vested interests. In an excellent article called 'What's in a care pathway?' Ruth Pinder and her colleagues consider the development of care pathways as an exercise in map-making, with all the challenges of 'cultural cartography'.

'[Care pathways] are the geographic maps of managed care. [They] eliminate the boundaries of time and space by removing the walls within a health care setting. [They] rattle our needs for 'turf' and revise our ideas of territory. [They] help us chart the way for truly patient-centred care. (Etheridge, 1986[53]; cited in Pinder[54]).'

This enthusiastic quote from the early days of managed care in the USA suggests (naïvely in retrospect) that the professional relationships and administrative infrastructure would fall into place more easily than actually turned out to be the case. Quoting a contrasting view, Pinder and her colleagues observe that

There is no such thing as a purely objective map, one that reproduces a pre-existing reality. Choices always have to be made about what to represent and how, and what to leave out. To be included on the map is to be granted the status of reality or importance. To be left off is to be denied. (King[55]; cited in Pinder[54]).

In reality, suggest these authors, ICPs explicitly raise – but do not themselves answer – the difficult question of how to work effectively across professional boundaries in the pursuit of seamless care and how to reconcile (or at least, reach a compromise between) different value systems (e.g. care versus cure, evidence-based practice versus cost efficiency, hierarchies versus partnerships).

Even taking account of these caveats, ICPs are not the whole answer to the challenge of coordinating care across professional and organisational boundaries. If, as Charles Handy is often quoted as saying, people are an organisation's most valuable assets (not so much 'human resources' as 'resourceful humans'),[56] then achieving effective and efficient cross-boundary care depends on people at least as much as it depends on systems and protocols. The US Institute of Medicine report 'Crossing the Quality Chasm' identified poor coordination as a key and growing weakness of the current healthcare system, but in my own view, it raised more questions than it answered about how to overcome this problem.[33] I cannot, in this generalist textbook, provide a

---

Box 10.3 Benson's criteria for successful whole systems working.[57]

1 *Ideological consensus* – the extent to which there is agreement on the nature, meaning and value of the task;

2 *Domain consensus* – the extent to which there is agreement about each partner's contribution to the task;

3 *Positive evaluation* – the extent to which those in one part of the partnership have a positive view of the contribution of those in another;

4 *Work coordination* – the extent to which partners are prepared to align work patterns;

5 *Fulfilment of programme requirements* – the degree of compatibility between the goals of the partnership and the goals of the individual stakeholders;

6 *Social importance* – the extent to which there is support for the objectives of the partnership from the range of affected constituencies;

7 *Maintenance of resource flows* – the extent to which there is adequate funding for the objectives of the partnership;

8 *Partnership identity* – the extent to which stakeholders see themselves as working for the partnership rather than representing their constituency.

---

comprehensive overview of the academic literature on coordination in healthcare organisations, but see Section 11.5 where I cover one useful theoretical perspective – organisational sensemaking. Another perspective worth following up further is a seminal paper by J Kenneth Benson on interorganisational networks (from which whole systems theory was subsequently developed by other scholars). Benson proposed that what would now be termed a 'whole systems' perspective on any domain has eight inter-related components (Box 10.3).[57] These components might be applied, for example, when predicting the likely barriers to (and levers for) success in a community development partnership between health and social care organisations (see Section 9.5), or a plan to align the work of primary care diabetes clinics and hospital-based ones. The detailed analysis of healthcare work against Benson's framework is beyond the scope of this book, but if you are interested in the organisational and management dimensions of healthcare from a whole systems perspective, I recommend two recent publications.[58,59]

10.3   The electronic patient record: a road map for seamless care?

No book on contemporary primary health care would be complete without a section on the electronic patient record and a commentary on efforts to date to achieve 'timelessness' and 'spacelessness' in healthcare through a fully networked computer records system, patient-held smart cards and other technology-based innovations. There is no shortage of books, chapters and articles on the EPR and its impact on clinicians and patients, but an alarming proportion of empirical studies on new technologies lack an explicit theoretical perspective (to put it another way, the 'ologies' introduced in Chapter 2 are hard to spot).

The first thing to say about the EPR is that it is not a single, agreed entity. Indeed, 'electronic record' is a highly ambiguous term, relating to both individual (e.g. GP-held) records and a subset of information (either individual or aggregated) that is transferable across sectors. At the time of writing (2007), the strategists and planners in the UK have a particular technology dream for computerised records which includes (in addition to largely paperless GP surgeries and community pharmacies) (a) a live, interactive Internet-based record for every patient, accessible from an Internet-based 'spine'[60]; (b) a technology-supported appointments booking system ('Choose and Book'), in which a patient needing referral can choose a hospital and date, and book an outpatient appointment by phone or Internet[61]; (c) the automatic transfer of prescriptions between GP surgeries and pharmacies[62] and (d) an algorithmic decision support system spanning the primary–secondary care interface (for one example of this, see http://www.medictomedic.com/).

But despite a determined marketing campaign by the UK Department of Health, professionals' resistance to some aspects of the EPR remains strong. The British Medical Association said in 2006 of Choose and Book: *'Many clinicians feel that an electronic referral system which could have improved working practices has been hijacked by a political agenda and this is one of the reasons why the Choose and Book system has not been welcomed'* (www.bma.org.uk; December 2006). Because of what some would see as political dragging of feet (and others as fear of technology or simple lack of engagement), major slippage has plagued the implementation plan for the national IT strategy, at massive cost to the National Health Service (NHS).[63] How might a research dimension help illuminate this uniquely complex and controversial aspect of contemporary primary health care?

The literature on the EPR can be divided into a number of more or less distinct traditions:

1 Descriptive accounts of a particular system, including its technical specifications and instructions for use. One of my lecturers who is undertaking a review of this literature refers this category as 'show and tell' research.

2 Publications on systems of coding, which emphasise the critical importance of the completeness, accuracy and consistency of disease codes (see Section 5.2). Much of this literature comprises detailed definitions of codes according to one or other system (Snomed CT, International Coding System for Primary Care or Read Codes) as well as editorial papers chiding doctors' lukewarm commitment to enforcing these coding standards.[64,65] Others have lamented the loss of the 'story stuff' when the clinical encounter (fundamentally analog in nature – i.e. made up of words and often loaded with ambiguity and uncertainty) is reduced to preordained codes (fundamentally digital – i.e. the person either does or does not count as having a condition represented by a particular code).[66]

3 Research surveys (mostly undertaken by doctors) on the degree of technical success of the EPR, which has documented the proportion of tasks successfully achieved electronically (e.g. compared with a non-computerised system), user satisfaction with the system and impact on clinical outcomes.[62,67–69] Whilst quantitative research is generally highly valued in medical circles, one recent systematic review commented on the limitations of randomized trials for exploring the complexities of EPR implementation and called for a broader methodological approach so that social, cultural and organizational influences on EPR use could be more effectively measured.[68]

4 Qualitative research (mostly undertaken by cognitive and social psychologists) on the impact of the EPR on the clinical encounter and clinical decision making.[69,70] By analysing videoed consultations, psychologists have revealed how the EPR changes the delicate balance between experiential knowledge (subjective, tacit, embodied by individuals, difficult to codify and transmit, particular and specific) and the formal knowledge of evidence-based medicine and clinical coding systems (objective and explicit but too rigid to address the idiosyncrasies of real patients and the complexities of real situations). Some have articulated this as a shift from patient-centred to doctor-centred consulting (see Section 5.4).[71,72]

5 Research into 'change management' (often undertaken by clinicians and informed to a variable extent by sound organisational theory) that has sought to identify key structural, cultural and historical barriers to EPR implementation at organisational level. These studies are mostly based on qualitative interviews with organisational stakeholders, with or without some assessment of implementation success.[62,69,73,74]

6 Socio-technical research (mostly undertaken by sociologists) on the impact of the EPR on work practices, professional identities and organisational routines, studied via in-depth case studies in which detailed observations are made of technology in practice. This relatively sparse literature, whilst often relatively well theorised, has generally been published in journals, which clinicians do not read, and indexed on databases other than Medline.[75–77] A recent scoping review on the EPR, commissioned by the UK Department of Health, did not mention it at all.[69]

It is this final tradition on which I want to expand in this section. Socio-technical systems theory is a specific application of Giddens' structuration theory, which I introduced in Section 9.3. The term 'socio-technical' refers to the essential interdependence between any technical system (such as a networked computer system) and the social system into which it is introduced (such as a GP practice). The term was first coined in the 1960s by researchers at London's Tavistock Institute of Human Relations who were working on the technical changes occurring at the time in the coal mining industry – which had profound knock-on effects on the workers and managers. Since then, a body of theory and practice has developed and is widely used by organisational sociologists (but, I believe, not widely enough by researchers in health services) to study the changes in the organisation of work occurring as information and communication technology systems have become more pervasive and sophisticated.

Applying structuration theory to technologies, there is a reciprocal and very dynamic relationship between any technology and the social system in which it is used.[78] On the one hand, all social systems are technically mediated. Healthcare professionals, managers and patients get an increasing proportion of their information and conduct an increasing proportion of their interactions through technical media: email, the Internet, telephone, management information systems, television and so on. These technologies present, store, index, filter and process information in particular ways – and they require particular practices (such as the use of passwords, the application of technical know-how and helpdesk support) to make them operational. On the other hand, all technical systems are socially mediated. Technology is produced, distributed and managed by people within social structures, for social, economic or political purposes. It is interpreted and used accordingly in particular social situations and with particular social intentions.

A number of concepts underpin the socio-technical perspective. First, that technology *changes the nature of work* and transforms the organisations in which work takes place. As Berg observed back in 1998:

> 'The medical record is a tool . . . it does not 'represent' the work, but it feeds into it, it structures and transforms it in complex ways: it structures communication between healthcare personnel, shapes medical decision making, and frames relations between personnel and patients'.[79]

A common theme in failed initiatives to introduce IT systems in healthcare is failure of designers to take account of how the technology was to be used in practice and how its use might change and threaten established professional identities and work practices.[80]

Second, the socio-technical perspective holds that the acceptability of a technology-based system and the work practices linked to it depends on the *meaning* of the system to individuals and groups. Professionals and managers make sense of new practices in ways that are consistent with their identities, involving such fundamental issues as their mission, roles, status and decision making (as in 'I used to be an independent clinician, now I'm just the guy who puts data in via pull-down menus'). This is why even technologies and practices with a clear 'efficiency advantage' may be resisted. Successful implementation requires changes to both practices and identities, and creation of new organisational routines to legitimate these and give them substance. Typically, clinicians' concerns centre on time-honoured rights and duties such as confidentiality, ownership of data and quality of clinician–patient relationship. Managers' concerns relate to streamlining work flow, automation of care pathways, efficiency of data retrieval, achievement of spacelessness and assurance of accountability, governance, safety and consistent clinical standards.[64,67] Actions in relation to the EPR are susceptible to differing interpretations – for example, 'resisting the new system' versus 'putting patients first'.[81]

The third insight from a (broadly) socio-technical perspective is that there is a political dimension to implementing the EPR, since the new meanings associated with new technologies produce contradictions, generating new tensions and conflicts.* For example, managers have the power to introduce a new technology and provide incentives (e.g. financial); professionals have the power to accept or resist using it and 'work round it'.[73,80,82] Fourth, a socio-technical perspective holds that the messiness and ad hoc nature of clinical work is not a minor issue that will come to be 'tidied up' as clinicians learn to use the EPR more consistently and rationally. Rather, the reality of clinical work – both at the 'micro' level (what clinicians do) and the 'macro' level (organisational routines the social structures that support them) – must be explored and understood as an essential and irreducible dimension of the system as a whole.[73,82,83]

Finally, a socio-technical perspective offers insights into the nature of professional collaboration. Clinical work involving complex technologies is generally done by groups and networks of people. Technology both supports and shapes collaboration and the individual actions that contribute to it (such as a practice nurse undertaking an annual diabetes check or a receptionist booking an appointment). Carsten Østerlund has suggested that the electronic medical record should be thought of not primarily as a 'container' for knowledge about the patient but as an 'itinerary' for work practices relating to the patient.[84] Healthcare staff do not record data merely to describe the patient's problem but to *organise* what they have to do as a team to support the patient in his or her illness journey. What the team is capable of doing is in turn shaped by the capabilities (and the limitations) of the technology.

Here is a controversial suggestion. The high failure rate of so many IT systems in healthcare (such as efforts by GP practices to 'go paperless', government initiatives to produce an electronic 'smart card' patient-held record or Internet-based booking systems for outpatient appointments) is attributable in large part to the fact that such projects have been under-theorised. Specifically, the development of the IT system has been viewed as a technical task that can be separated from the detail of work practices in healthcare organisations and then 'implemented' (with health professionals being 'educated' or 'incentivised' to use particular technologies). Technology developers inevitably simplify the work practices that the information and communication technology system is being designed to support, resulting in a 'clunky' piece of technology that sits oddly (or not at all) in the context of clinical work – which, as Paul Atkinson has so elegantly shown, is complex, subtle, contingent, largely unpredictable and inextricably linked with professional identity.[83]

---

*The purists would probably say that the politics of organisational change is another conceptual category entirely, not part of socio-technical systems research. One could (and my own team often do) spend hours discussing how to classify this complex field of research.

To have even an outside chance of being successfully implemented, information technologies to support health care must be explicitly embedded within, and take full account of, the social relationships, work routines and professional identities which they both support and require. For example, a GP who engages with an electronic ICP that spans the primary–secondary care interface is not merely 'putting data on computer' or 'following the guideline' but is shifting identity from 'individual clinical entrepreneur' to 'member of a care team who are collaborating around the care of the patient'.[82]

In summary, I believe that socio-technical systems theory offers an exciting (and relatively unexplored – at least by health services researchers) approach to the use of technologies in healthcare settings. It re-focuses the analysis from the completion of tasks by individual clinicians to the cooperative work processes that are enacted *between* healthcare staff around the patient's illness trajectory and the wider working relationships and meaning-systems within which particular tasks make sense. Once again, there is huge scope for taking these ideas forward in further research.

10.4 The end of an era?

In this book, and in this chapter in particular, I have deliberately taken a contemporary perspective on primary health care. It is worth reflecting here on the characteristics of 'old-fashioned' general practice on which some traditionalists still look back nostalgically. In the stereotypical GP practice of 40 years ago, the GP (typically male, full-time and in a job for life) worked from owner-occupied premises, perhaps seeing his patients in his own front room, and without the input of nurses or other non-medical clinicians. He may even have mixed and dispensed his own medicines. He worked long hours, did all (or almost all) his own on-call work and employed a minimum of assistants and ancillary staff (perhaps just his own wife to welcome patients into the waiting room and let him know they had arrived). On retirement, he may have passed the practice (along with a tidy guaranteed income) on to his son. The old-fashioned family doctor (as he would have been proud to call himself) had little truck with evidence-based guidelines and was also wary of the creeping bureaucratisation of general practice, preferring to keep paperwork to a minimum and spend his time in direct contact with patients.

The old-fashioned GP's unique selling points (to use an ironically modernist expression) were (a) the intimacy and depth of the doctor–patient relationship, (b) the GP's commitment to the whole patient and (c) the continuity of care that was possible in the world of stable, single-handed street-corner GP practices (see Section 6.3). This GP would have been correct in claiming that most patients would be reluctant to trade depth and continuity of the GP–patient relationship for the bells and whistles of the contemporary health centre (a wide range of specialist clinics, a patient library, nurse practitioners with postgraduate qualifications in health promotion and so on). The UK Small Practices Association (http://www.smallpractices.org.uk/) is a network of GPs who are committed to retaining the service model that they see as encapsulating real 'quality care' (see Chapter 11). It increasingly has to defend its values against onslaughts and jibes from individuals and official bodies who equate 'single-handed practices' with a laggardly approach to technology, indifference to research evidence and an unwillingness to cooperate with cross-boundary care! Rather than taking a side in this particular dispute based on gut reaction or personal memories of good or less good health care experiences with particular GPs, it is worth applying a theoretical perspective to the question of what we have lost (or stand to lose) with the passing of the single-handed, jack-of-all-trades, lives-above-the-shop GP. As with the discussion of the EPR in the previous section, I think that organisational sociology (which considers organisations from perspective of roles, relationships, routines, interactions and professional identities) has the potential to generate light in an area where there is often only heat.

Table 10.2, which is based on some empirical work by my own team as well as independent work by others,[85–87] summarises the characteristics of 'traditional' and 'contemporary' GP practices. My own thinking on the organisational form of the GP practice stemmed from a study on interpreted consultations and the finding that single-handed GPs in London (who at the time of the study were often of South Asian origin) were less likely to use the official interpreting service.[86] This finding was interpreted by primary care trusts (the organisations responsible for primary care standards locally) as 'poor performance' or 'lack of engagement' by these GPs. But an analysis through the lens of organisational sociology reveals a more interesting explanation. To summarise, the traditional GP in an area of high ethnic population, who is usually single-handed (a) often speaks several ethnic languages himself or herself, so sees interpreting as part of his or her own identity rather than something that should be brought in as an add-on; (b) works to a 'family' ethos, and hence is comfortable with multilingual staff whose ad hoc input is recognised and valued (though not generally financially rewarded) and (c) actively encourages family member interpreters and develops routines for using these efficiently. The contemporary GP in a similar area (a) is more often white and monolingual but may have chosen to work in a multicultural area through interest or commitment, (b) adheres to the values of a modern bureaucracy (everyone in the organisation has a job for which they are properly trained and can be trusted to perform), (c) holds a well-differentiated role in a practice with a clear division of labour and active links with external organisations and practitioners and (d) discourages family member interpreters and ad hoc solutions as 'unprofessional'. Such a GP is usually comfortable working with NHS interpreters because the latter represent a 'bureaucratic' solution (i.e. one expressed in terms of a formal role and job description) to an organisational problem.

As Table 10.2 shows, these different organisational forms of GP practice respond very differently to stress (such as an increase in patient numbers without a corresponding increase in resources). The traditional single-handed GP typically responds by restricting his or her remit – by discontinuing all services

Table 10.2 Traditional and contemporary GP practices in the UK.[85,86]

	The traditional GP practice	The contemporary GP practice
Practice	Single-handed or family unit; list size 2000–4000 Offers basic services (General Medical Services) provided by a few core staff	Multipartner; list size 4000–9000 Offers multiple extra clinics and add-on services provided by a wide range of staff and contractors
Premises	Converted house GP usually owner occupier	Purpose-built health centre Owned collaboratively or leased from private funder
Typical history	Established in 1960s or early 1970s following expansion of NHS services with 1964 GP Contract	Established in late 1970s or 1980s, perhaps through merging of several single-handed practices
GP's identity	Family doctor is equal to 'respected pillar of the community', committed to job for life	Member of staff in an efficient and caring organisation, committed as per contract
GP's link to practice	Often lives on site or locally and takes active part in local events, e.g. campaigns, festivals	Often commutes from another area and has no link to the community other than via the list
Practice structure and ethos	Family business with roles and responsibilities defined loosely and informally. Status influenced by kinship and tradition, e.g. senior partner is usually the oldest. Support staff may include doctor's own relatives. Few formal systems, weakly differentiated management roles (GP or spouse may undertake these). Everyone is expected to 'muck in'. Often on call 24 hours for own patients	Bureaucratic organisation with formal and well-differentiated roles and responsibilities and multiple systems and procedures. Status influenced most by qualifications and other external measures of merit. There is often equity of status and parity of pay among all GPs, many of whom work part time and have outside interests. Out of hours care usually contracted out or shared in a cooperative
Values and virtues	Loyalty, thrift, continuity, interpersonal relationships, friendliness, integrity, self-sufficiency	The 'Maxwell six': effectiveness, acceptability, efficiency, accessibility, equity and relevance
Confidentiality defined in terms of	Personal, exclusive and longstanding relationship between patient and a particular GP	Data protection policies and procedures, staff training and supervision
External links	Few and based around GP's social networks	Many and based around collaborative work practices

(Continued)

Table 10.2 (*Continued*)

	The traditional GP practice	The contemporary GP practice
Strategy	Develop and maintain good GP–patient/family relationships Provide a good basic service to the sick Support and care for the family who have chosen you as their GP Don't waste money	Provide comprehensive, up-to-date, evidence-based care for all (including proactive, preventive care) Pay special attention to poor, disempowered and socially excluded patients, whose health problems are often linked to social disadvantage Draw on as many additional services as needed to extend the care package offered to patients
Environmental stress Low	Broad, undifferentiated clinical agenda dealt with by generalist GP GP may pursue a specialism out of personal interest	Economies of scale compared to single-handed practice Professional support and stimulation Weakly developed and voluntary division of labour based on interests of GPs
High	Restriction of remit, e.g. • Limit services to 'core business' (General Medical Services for which GP has contractual obligation) • Limit agenda to biomedical (e.g. refuse to engage with requests to sign housing forms) • Refer complex cases to secondary care • Discourage resource-intensive patients from registering • Close the list	Efficiency measures, e.g. • Limit agenda to biomedical • Strongly developed and enforced division of labour, incorporating 'hierarchy of appropriateness' (see text) • Categorisation and triage of patients according to tasks needed to 'process' them • Extension of opening hours (e.g. evening assistants) to make maximum use of space • Creative use of technology

except core General Medical Services, increasing referrals to secondary care and discouraging resource-intensive patients (such as those who speak languages not offered by practice staff) from registering in the first place. They may also close the list to new patients. Conversely, the contemporary GP practice tends to respond to a similar shock by introducing efficiency measures such as extending and enforcing the interprofessional division of labour, most notably by employing nurses and healthcare assistants to take on some of the GPs' work, triaging patients to the cheapest professional who could complete the tasks needed to 'process' them, increasing throughput (e.g. by extending opening hours) and making creative use of technology.[85,86]

The theoretical distinction between a traditional GP practice run more or less as a 'kinship' organisation and a contemporary practice run as a bureaucratic organisation (in the Weberian sense of roles being defined by job descriptions and person specifications rather than by kinship ties[88]) raises interesting questions about the nature of trust in the doctor, nurse and healthcare system. The family doctor of the 1950s enjoyed an unparalleled degree of trust from his patients – but perhaps this trust was founded on an unequal power relationship and the fact that medical knowledge was a rare commodity, acquired at medical school and carried in the doctor's head, forever inaccessible to the uneducated patient. In the twenty-first-century, equity between clinician and patient is said to be fundamental to a productive relationship, and knowledge (at least in theory) is universally accessible on the Internet. The demise of unquestioning trust in the family doctor is perhaps inevitable, given these critical changes in society.[89]

If trust in clinicians is inexorably being eroded as society changes (and mindful of Onora O'Neill's insightful commentary on the changing nature of trust which I referred to in Section 5.5[89]) what hope is there for clinician–patient trust, and for public confidence in the health professions more generally, as the EPR becomes ubiquitous? In a new book called *The Glass Consumer: Life in a Surveillance Society*, ethicist and lawyer Jonathan Montgomery gives a good description of the changing face of trust and confidentiality in the era of the electronic record:

> 'Health information is particularly personal, and strong commitments to confidentiality have long been seen as an essential prerequisite, giving patients the reassurance that the need before they are comfortable sharing sensitive information with professions. Matters of health are closely connected with self-esteem, reputation and personal identity. Health status can be highly significant in relation to employment prospects, access to insurance (and loans such as mortgages) and, in some contexts, social standing. The increasing sophistication of genetics means that personal health information is increasingly significant in predicting future health, raising the stakes further in respect of potential misuse'.[90,p.188]

Montgomery distinguishes between the traditional confidentiality agreement, which was *'intimate and personal, built on a lifelong relationship of trust'* between patient and GP, and the more contemporary perspective on confidentiality needed now that healthcare is multi-disciplinary, cross-sector and is obtained in a variety of ways from a variety of access points. Because of changes in the nature of illness and how it is managed (see Sections 10.1 and 10.2), assurance of confidentiality *must* shift from being tied to the professionalism of the GP (whose lips are ever sealed to the secrets shared in the consulting room) to being one dimension of data protection in a surveillance society. Of course, professional confidences remain, but there must be trust in the system as well as in the individual clinician. This is a particular example of a wider shift from unquestioning faith in the individual doctor's competence and goodwill to trust in the system-wide culture of accountability and requirement for clinical governance.[91,92]

As Montgomery points out, this fundamental shift in what it means to keep confidentiality raises critical questions about professional (and patient) identity and about the ethics of the new professional–patient relationship (in which, for example, management encroaches more prominently than it did in the past and patients have a right to challenge the professional's account of what is wrong with them). One important part of the solution, he suggests, is to build partnerships between the healthcare system and its users and to ensure that (a) patients understand what 'consent' means in relation to the recording and sharing of information and (b) patients are (with some exceptions) able to access their electronic record and assure themselves of the accuracy and completeness of the information therein. This is the principle behind HealthSpace (https://www.healthspace.nhs.uk/), a development of the electronic patient record in which the patients may access their records, check their accuracy and completeness, and correct errors. At the time of writing, HealthSpace is only available at pilot sites, and its impact on patient care or the illness experience is unknown. Watch this space for research studies on these themes – or, perhaps, think of a research study yourself!

References

1 Pickles W. *Epidemiology in Country Practice*. Bristol: John Wright; 1939.

2 Balint M. *The Doctor, His Patient and the Illness*. London: Routledge; 1956.

3 Fry J. *Common Diseases: Their Nature, Incidence and Care*. 2nd edn. London: Medical & Technical Publishing Co. Ltd.; 1974.

4 Fry J, Sandler G. *Common Diseases: Their Nature, Prevalence and Care*. London: Petroc Press; 1993.

5 Department of Health. *Supporting People with Long Term Conditions: An NHS and Social Care Model to Support Local Innovation and Integration*. London: Department of Health; 2005.

6 Wakely G, Chambers R. *Chronic Disease Management in Primary Care: Quality and Outcomes*. Oxford: Radcliffe; 2005.

7 Hart JT. *A New Kind of Doctor*. London: Merlin Press; 1988.

8 Goldberg RB. Lifestyle interventions to prevent type 2 diabetes. Lancet 2006;368:1634–1636.

9 Department of Health. *National Service Framework for Diabetes*. London: HMSO; 2002.

10 Kvamme OJ, Olesen F, Samuelsson M. Improving the interface between primary and secondary care: a statement from the European Working Party on Quality in Family Practice (EQuiP). Qual Saf Health Care 2001;10:33–39.

11 van den Akker M, Buntinx F, Knottnerus JA. Comorbidity or multimorbidity: what's in a name? A review of the literature. Eur J Gen Pract 1996;2:65–70.

12 Harris MI. Hypercholesterolemia in diabetes and glucose intolerance in the U.S. population. Diabetes Care 1991;14:366–374.

13 Anonymous. Prevalence of overweight and obesity among adults with diagnosed diabetes – United States, 1988–1994 and 1999–2002. MMWR Morb Mortal Wkly Rep 2004;53:1066–1068.

14 Conn JJ, Jacobs HS, Conway GS. The prevalence of polycystic ovaries in women with type 2 diabetes mellitus. Clin Endocrinol (Oxf) 2000;52:81–86.

15 Brown LC, Majumdar SR, Newman SC, Johnson JA. Type 2 diabetes does not increase risk of depression. CMAJ 2006;175:42–46.

16 Hypertension in Diabetes Study (HDS): I. Prevalence of hypertension in newly presenting type 2 diabetic patients and the association with risk factors for cardiovascular and diabetic complications. J Hypertens 1993;11:309–317.

17 Almdal T, Scharling H, Jensen JS, Vestergaard H. The independent effect of type 2 diabetes mellitus on ischemic heart disease, stroke, and death: a population-based study of 13,000 men and women with 20 years of follow-up. Arch Intern Med 2004;164:1422–1426.

18 Musselman DL, Betan E, Larsen H, Phillips LS. Relationship of depression to diabetes types 1 and 2: epidemiology, biology, and treatment. Biol Psychiatry 2003;54(3):317–329.

19 Fortin M, Dionne J, Pinho G, Gignac J, Almirall J, Lapointe L. Randomized controlled trials: do they have external validity for patients with multiple comorbidities? Ann Fam Med 2006;4:104–108.

20 Travers J, Marsh S, Caldwell B, et al. External validity of randomized controlled trials in COPD. Respir Med, epublication ahead of print Nov 2006.

21 McMurdo MET, Witham MD, Gillespie ND. Including older people in clinical research. BMJ 2005;331:1036–1037.

22 van den Akker M, Buntinx F, Metsemakers JF, Roos S, Knottnerus JA. Multimorbidity in general practice: prevalence, incidence, and determinants of co-occurring chronic and recurrent diseases. J Clin Epidemiol 1998;51:367–375.

23 Fortin M, Bravo G, Hudon C, Vanasse A, Lapointe L. Prevalence of multimorbidity among adults seen in family practice. Ann Fam Med 2005;3:223–228.

24 Grumbach K. Chronic illness, comorbidities, and the need for medical generalism. Ann Fam Med 2003;1:4–7.

25 Saltman DC, Sayer GP, Whicker SD. Co morbidity in general practice. Postgrad Med J 2005;81:474–480.

26 Starfield B. William Pickles Lecture. Primary and specialty care interfaces: the imperative of disease continuity. Br J Gen Pract 2003;53:723–729.

27 Fortin M, Lapointe L, Hudon C, Vanasse A. Multimorbidity is common to family practice: is it commonly researched? Can Fam Physician 2005;51:244–245.

28 Gaitatzis A, Carroll K, Majeed A, Sander W. The epidemiology of the comorbidity of epilepsy in the general population. Epilepsia 2004;45:1613–1622.

29 Fortin M, Hudon C, Dubois MF, Almirall J, Lapointe L, Soubhi H. Comparative assessment of three different indices of multimorbidity for studies on health-related quality of life. Health Qual Life Outcomes 2005;3:74.

30 Fortin M, Bravo G, Hudon C, et al. Relationship between multimorbidity and health-related quality of life of patients in primary care. Qual Life Res 2006;15:83–91.

31 Fortin M, Bravo G, Hudon C, Lapointe L, Dubois MF, Almirall J. Psychological distress and multimorbidity in primary care. Ann Fam Med 2006;4:417–422.

32 Starfield B, Lemke KW, Bernhardt T, Foldes SS, Forrest CB, Weiner JP. Comorbidity: implications for the importance of primary care in 'case' management. Ann Fam Med 2003;1:8–14.

33 Institute of Medicine. *Crossing the Quality Chasm: A New Health System for the 21st Century.* Washington, DC: National Academies Press; 2003.

34 Coulter A. What do patients and the public want from primary care? BMJ 2005;331:1199–1201.

35 Wensing M, Jung HP, Mainz J, Olesen F, Grol R. A systematic review of the literature on patient priorities for general practice care. Part 1: Description of the research domain. Soc Sci Med 1998;47:1573–1588.

36 Stange KC. The paradox of the parts and the whole in understanding and improving general practice. Int J Qual Health Care 2002;14:267–268.

37 Renholm M, Leino-Kilpi H, Suominen T. Critical pathways. A systematic review. J Nurs Adm 2002;32(4):196–202.

38 Campbell H, Hotchkiss R, Bradshaw N, Porteous M. Integrated care pathways. BMJ 1998;316(7125):133–137.

39 Harkleroad A, Schirf D, Volpe J, Holm MB. Critical pathway development: an integrative literature review. Am J Occup Ther 2000;54(2):148–154.

40 Pearson SD, Goulart-Fisher D, Lee TH. Critical pathways as a strategy for improving care: problems and potential. Ann Intern Med 1995;123(12):941–948.

41 Benham AJ. Managed care and critical pathway development: the joint replacement experience. Orthop Nurs 1999;18(4):71–75.

42 Brugh LA. Automated clinical pathways in the patient record legal implications. Nurs Case Manag 1998;3(3):131–137.

43 Johnson S, Smith J. Factors influencing the success of ICP projects. Prof Nurse 2000;15(12):776–779.

44 Syed KA, Bogoch ER. Integrated care pathways in hip fracture management: demonstrated benefits are few. J Rheumatol 2000;27(9):2071–2073.

45 Naglie IG, Alibhai SM. Improving outcomes in hip fracture patients: are care pathways the answer? J Rheumatol 2000;27(9):2068–2070.

46 Beavis D, Simpson S, Graham I. A literature review of dementia care mapping: methodological considerations and efficacy. J Psychiatr Ment Health Nurs 2002;9(6):725–736.

47 Kwan J, Sandercock P. In-hospital care pathways for stroke. Cochrane Database Syst Rev 2002;(2):CD002924.

48 Cannon CP, Hand MH, Bahr R, et al. Critical pathways for management of patients with acute coronary syndromes: an assessment by the National Heart Attack Alert Program. Am Heart J 2002;143(5):777–789.

49 Plochg T, Klazinga NS. Community-based integrated care: myth or must? Int J Qual Health Care 2002;14:91–101.

50 Ouwens M, Wollersheim H, Hermens R, Hulscher M, Grol R. Integrated care programmes for chronically ill patients: a review of systematic reviews. Int J Qual Health Care 2005;17:141–146.

51 Oakley P, Greaves E. Process re-engineering: from command to demand. Health Serv J February 23, 1995:32–33.

52 Currie L, Harvey G. Care pathways development and implementation. Nurs Stand 1998;12:35–38.

53 Etheridge ML. Timelines: the maps for managed care. Definition 1986; Fall:1–3.

54 Pinder R, Petchey R, Shaw S, Carter Y. What's in a care pathway? Towards a cultural cartography of the new NHS. Sociol Health Illn 2005;27:759–779.

55 King G. *Mapping Realities: An Exploration of Cultural Cartographies*. London: Macmillan; 1996.

56 Handy C. *Understanding Organisations*. 4th edn. London: Penguin; 1993.

57 Benson JK. The inter-organisational network as a political economy. Adm Sci Q 1975;20:229–249.

58 Hudson B. Whole systems working: a discussion paper for the Integrated Care Network. London: Department of Health; 2004. Available at http://www.integratedcarenetwork.gov.uk.

59 Attwood M, Pedler M, Pritchard S, Wilkinson D. *Leading Change: A Guide to Whole Systems Working*. Bristol: Policy Press; 2003.

60 Granger R. *NHS Connecting for Health Business Plan 2005–6*. London: Department of Health; 2005.

61 Department of Health. *Choose and Book: Patient's Choice of Hospital and Booked Appointment – Policy Framework*. London: Department of Health; 2004.

62 Sugden B. *Electronic Transmission of Prescriptions – Evaluation of Pilots*. University of Newcastle: Sowerby Centre for Health Informatics; 2003.

63 Department of Health. *Information for Health: An Information Strategy for the Modern NHS 1998–2005*. London: NHS Executive; 1998.

64 de Lusignan S, Wells SE, Hague NJ, Thiru K. Managers see the problems associated with coding clinical data as a technical issue whilst clinicians also see cultural barriers. Methods Inf Med 2003;42(4):416–422.

65 de Lusignan S. The barriers to clinical coding in general practice: a literature review. Med Inform Internet Med 2005;30(2):89–97.

66 Kay S, Purves IN. The computerised medical record and the 'story stuff': A narrativistic model. In: Greenhalgh T, Hurwitz B, eds. *Narrative Based Medicine: Dialogue and Discourse in Clinical Practice*. London: BMJ Publications; 1998.

67 Mitchell E, Sullivan F. A descriptive feast but an evaluative famine: systematic review of published articles on primary care computing during 1980–97. BMJ 2001;322(7281):279–282.

68 Delpierre C, Cuzin L, Fillaux J, Alvarez M, Massip P, Lang T. A systematic review of computer-based patient record systems and quality of care: more randomized clinical trials or a broader approach? Int J Qual Health Care 2004;16(5):407–416.

69 Pagliari C. Literature review and conceptual map of the area of E-health. London: NHS SDO Programme; 2005. Available at http://www.sdo.lshtm.ac.uk/ehealth.htm.

70 Booth N, Robinson P, Kohannejad J. Identification of high-quality consultation practice in primary care: the effects of computer use on doctor–patient rapport. Inform Prim Care 2004;12(2):75–83.

71 May C. A rational model for assessing and evaluating complex interventions in health care. BMC Health Serv Res 2006;6:86.

72 Timmermans S, Berg M. *The Gold Standard: The Challenge of Evidence-Based Medicine and Standardization in Health Care*. Philadelphia: Temple University Press; 2003.

73 Heeks R, Mundy D, Salazar A. Why health care information systems succeed or fail. Information Systems for Public Sector Management Working Paper Series. Institute for Development Policy and Management: University of Manchester; 1999. Available at http://www.sed.manchester.ac.uk/idpm/publications/wp/igov/igov_wp09.pdf.

74 Hendy J, Reeves BC, Fulop N, Hutchings A, Masseria C. Challenges to implementing the national programme for information technology (NPfIT): a qualitative study. BMJ 2005;331(7512):331–336.

75 Markus ML, Robey D. Information technology and organizational change: causal structure in theory and research. Manag Sci 1988;34:583–598.

76 Berg M, Bowker G. The multiple bodies of the medical record: toward a sociology of an artefact. Sociol Q 1997;38:513–537.

77 Østerlund C. Documenting practices: the indexical centering of medical records. Outlines Crit Soc Stud 2003;2:43–68.

78 Orlikowski WJ. Using technology and constituting structures: a practice lens for studying technology in organizations. Organ Sci 2000;11:404–428.

79 Berg M. Medical work and the computer-based patient record: a sociological perspective. Methods Inf Med 1998;37(3):294–301.

80 Greenhalgh T, Robert G, Macfarlane F, Bate P, Kyriakidou O. Diffusion of innovations in service organisations: systematic literature review and recommendations for future research. Milbank Q 2004;82:581–629.

81 Walsh SH. The clinician's perspective on electronic health records and how they can affect patient care. BMJ 2004;328(7449):1184–1187.

82 Berg M. Patient care information systems and health care work: a sociotechnical approach. Int J Med Inf 1999;55:87–101.

83 Atkinson P. *Medical Talk and Medical Work*. London: Sage; 1995.

84 Østerlund C. Mapping medical work: documenting practices across multiple medical settings. J Cent Inf Stud 2004;3:35–43.

85 Charles-Jones H, Latimer J, May C. Transforming general practice: the redistribution of medical work in primary care. Sociol Health Illn 2003;25:71–92.

86 Greenhalgh T, Voisey C, Robb N. Interpreted consultations as 'business as usual'? A study of organisational routines in primary care. In: Ethnicity, Health and Health Care: Understanding Diversity, Tackling Disadvantage. Sociology of Health and Illness Monograph 13, in press.

87 Jones L, Green J. Shifting discourses of professionalism: a case study of general practitioners in the United Kingdom. Sociol Health Illn 2006;28:927–950.

88 Weber M. *The Theory of Social and Economic Organisations* (Translated by Henderson AM and Parsons T). Glencoe: Free Press; 1947.

89 O'Neill O. *A Question of Trust: The 2002 Reith Lectures*. Cambridge: Cambridge University Press; 2002.

90 Montgomery J. Personal information in the National Health Service: the demise or rise of patient interests. In: Lace S, ed. *The Glass Consumer: Life in a Surveillance Society*. Bristol: Policy Press; 2005.

91 Halligan A, Donaldson L. Implementing clinical governance: turning vision into reality. BMJ 2001;322:1413–1417.

92 Donaldson LJ. Clinical governance: a mission to improve. Clin Perform Qual Health Care 2000;8:6–8.

93 Bell DSH. Heart failure: a serious and common comorbidity of diabetes. Clin Diabetes 2004;22(2):61–65.

94 Herpertz S, Albus C, Wagener R, et al. Comorbidity of diabetes and eating disorders. Does diabetes control reflect disturbed eating behavior? Diabetes Care 1998;21:1110–1116.

CHAPTER 11

Quality

Summary points

1 Quality means different things to different people, and any primary care quality initiative must be addressed from multiple perspectives. It has different dimensions (e.g. the 'Maxwell six': effectiveness, efficiency, acceptability, access, equity, relevance). Indicators used to assess progress in any quality initiative may be more or less valid and more or less susceptible to 'gaming'.

2 A rational biomedical approach to quality improvement is to set evidence-based standards of care, create incentives for clinicians to meet those standards and use criterion-based audit to monitor progress towards the standards. This has formed the basis of the UK Quality and Outcomes Framework for general practice, which early reports suggest has been successful in improving outcomes for patients. But this approach has been criticised for being resource-intensive, inherently dull (hence demotivating) and linked politically to the new public management with its emphasis on standardisation, centralised control and accountability to the state.

3 Significant event audit uses case stories as the basis for reflection and action. It may be used in both research and (as a relatively rapid and resource-light approach) service improvement. Story-based approaches may engage and motivate staff and promote reflection on ethical issues.

4 Informal peer discussion groups have a long and honourable history in UK general practice. They use social learning and social influence methods to raise motivation, promote reflective learning and initiate action to improve practice. They may be particularly effective when linked with audit or other quality improvement techniques.

5 A 'mystery shopper' is an individual who poses as a patient in order to experience a service and provide unique feedback based on 'living through' the healthcare system. Mystery shopper techniques are especially useful when seeking to improve services for stigmatising conditions. Such approaches might be fruitfully studied through the lens of phenomenology.

6 Many determinants of quality in health care have been shown to lie at organisational rather than individual level. Organisational level interventions aimed at wholescale transformation of a general practitioner (GP) practice or equivalent should be analysed using theoretical models that address the level of the organisation. One such model is Weick's notion of organisational

(Continued)

(Summary points continued)

> sensemaking – a theoretical perspective which helps explain why team-focused, locally owned, locally adapted, interprofessional and formative quality initiatives tend to be considerably more successful than individually focused, top-down, one-size-fits-all, uniprofessional and summative ones.

11.1   Defining and measuring quality

Quality has been a hot topic in healthcare for around 10 years (see, for example, the US Institute of Healthcare Improvement; http://www.ihi.org/ihi and the International Forum on Quality and Safety in Healthcare; http://www.quality.bmjpg.com/). Books on quality in healthcare are ubiquitous – see the individual sections below for some examples; I must confess to having written a book on quality myself a few years ago,[1] though the field has moved on considerably since then.

Despite widespread interest, there are relatively few analyses of quality in healthcare that take what I would call an academic perspective (see Section 1.4). This seems a shame, but perhaps it is for good reason. The main character in Robert Pirsig's *Zen and the Art of Motorcycle Maintenance* is a philosophy teacher who sets his students an essay with the title 'What is quality?'[2] The question, which seems so simple and straightforward, eventually sends the teacher crazy. Intuitively, and at a pragmatic, seat-of-the-pants level, we know what quality is, but when we try to nail it to a definition, especially one that all players agree on, the concept becomes slippery. Indeed, an important characteristic of 'quality' is that both the definition of the term and its different dimensions, and the appropriate way to measure it vary with whose perspective you take (Figure 11.1 and Box 11.1).

Perhaps we should be content to see quality work as more practical than intellectual, needing little more than a few checklists such as 'six simple steps to improving patient satisfaction' or 'ten tips for achieving organisational change'. I'm not sure. There is nothing so practical as a good theory, and theoretical insights will not only inform the design of quality initiatives that are likely to work, but may also help explain our failures and partial successes. In the remaining sections in this chapter, I have not attempted a comprehensive coverage of all the possible approaches to assuring and improving quality in primary care. Instead, I have given what I hope will prove to be a range of contrasting examples of quality initiatives, each of which is underpinned by a different theoretical model. None of these approaches is necessarily better than the others – but one of them (or some other that I have not covered here) may well prove more fit for purpose in any given situation and context. The choice of the 'best' approach to quality in your own practice (or, perhaps, your own MSc or PhD project) must be made on a combination of theoretical and practical grounds.

Before we move on to specific examples, let me first offer some definitions of quality terms, for which I have my colleague Jill Russell to thank. *Quality*

The senior GP's perspective
The senior partner is an old-fashioned GP who has lived and worked in the area for many years. He sees quality mainly in terms of the Prentice family's ongoing relationship with their family doctor, which will be built through years of continuity of care and mutual trust. He defines quality failures in terms of mutual misunderstandings and 'hidden agendas' not raised.

The pharmacist's perspective
The community pharmacist sees quality in terms of the timely and cost-efficient supply of medication to the Prentices, perhaps supported by shared electronic records and automatic transfer of prescriptions. She defines quality failures in terms of breaks in the supply chain for long-term medication, adverse reactions to medication and poor compliance (perhaps due to patients' limited understanding of medicine-related issues).

The practice manager's perspective
The manager sees quality in terms of the smooth running of the practice, generation of adequate income and efficient human resource practices (including appraisal and training). He or she defines quality failures primarily in terms of administrative complaints (e.g. length of time to see a doctor), failure to meet income targets and disaffection or poor performance in staff.

The Prentice family have recently moved into the area and are looking for a GP practice to register with. Mrs Prentice is 44; she has heavy periods and may need a hysterectomy in the future. Mr Prentice, 47, is diabetic and has high blood pressure. Florence Prentice is 17; she sees the nurse for contraception and had a (secret) termination of pregnancy recently. Mrs Prentice's mother, Ruby Brown, 79, lives with the family and has memory problems.

Mr Prentice's perspective
Mr Prentice sees quality in terms of good diabetes and blood pressure control, absence of complications and living a 'normal life.' He would see a missed recall for retinal screening as a quality failure.

Florence Prentice's perspective
Florence sees quality in terms of accessible, free contraception and prompt, discreet management of personal health problems. Quality failure would be if her medical record were seen by her parents or a future partner.

The nurse's perspective
The practice nurse, who runs the clinics for chronic disease management, sees quality in terms of completeness of patient registration and recall, evidence-based protocols followed, and clinical targets achieved. She defines quality failures mainly in terms of losses to follow-up, delayed diagnoses and ineffective treatments.

Ruby Brown's perspective
Mrs Brown sees quality in terms of living in her own home. She would see the need to go into residential care as a quality failure.

Figure 11.1 Different perspectives on quality in primary care.

assurance means maintaining or enhancing service quality using systematic assessment of performance against predetermined standards. *Quality improvement* generally refers to approaches that seek to improve care, and prevent poor care, on a continuous basis as part of an everyday routine. Such approaches are generally developmental, whereas with quality assurance the emphasis is more on monitoring. *Quality control* is a mechanism for ensuring that an output (product or service) conforms to a predetermined specification. A *quality indicator* is something that can be measured (usually but not always quantitatively) to assess progress towards a particular quality goal or alert people to a fall (or impending fall) in quality. The selection of valid and appropriate quality indicators is fraught with controversy, mainly because when financial

> **Box 11.1 Some frameworks for considering different dimensions of quality.**
>
> The Donabedian Three[3]
> - Structure (the design and organisation of the service)
> - Process (what is done, e.g. in terms of procedures, protocols, etc.)
> - Outcome (what happens as a result)
>
> The Maxwell Six[4]
> - Effectiveness
> - Efficiency
> - Acceptability
> - Equity
> - Access
> - Relevance
>
> The framework for organisational learning (Argyris and Schon)[5]
> - Effectiveness
> - Efficiency
> - Respect and caring
> - Safety
> - Timeliness
>
> *Note:* 'Effectiveness' is generally defined as 'doing the right things'; 'efficiency' is 'doing things right'. See the third footnote in Chapter 1, page 14.

rewards are attached to particular indicators, gaming quickly results and if the indicator is not robust, poor practice will be rewarded as generously as good practice. Box 11.2 shows the features of an ideal quality indicator.

One aspect of quality that is increasingly recognised as important in both research and policymaking is the subjective experience of illness and the impact of health interventions on this.[7,8] The UK Medical Research Council warns grant applicants that without a robust measure of health-related quality of life, their trial is unlikely to be funded (see www.mrc.ac.uk/). The National Institute for Clinical Excellence makes extensive use of quality of life data when judging whether a drug or procedure should be made available on the National Health Service (see www.nice.org.uk/). Researchers' desire to compare the subjective impact of treatments across clinical trials[9] has spawned a growth industry of 'standardised' health-related quality of life scales – both generic (such as the SF-36, the Nottingham Health Profile or the EuroQol[10–12]) and disease-specific (for use in people with diabetes, HIV, respiratory disease or heart disease, for example[13–16]), and instruments specifically designed to measure the impact of comorbidity (discussed in Section 10.1).[17,18] Box 11.3 lists some examples of questions from one widely used quality of life instrument.

Countless studies have been published demonstrating that particular quality of life instruments have robust psychometric properties – for example, that

---

Box 11.2 Features of the ideal quality indicator.[1,6]

A quality indicator:
- Should measure an important and relevant aspect of the illness experience or healthcare;
- Should be reliable, reproducible, easily quantifiable using readily available information, affordable and should exhibit a 'dose-response' effect (i.e. increases in the level of the indicator should indicate better quality);
- Should be a true predictor of quality and not merely express exposure to a covariable (see Section 8.2);
- Should be sensitive, that is a high score on the indicator should indicate quality in a particular aspect of care, and specific, that is a low score should indicate that the quality of this aspect of care is inadequate. These characteristics will make the indicator less vulnerable to gaming, – that is unscrupulous individuals bypassing the quality work and going merely for the incentive points;
- Should be amenable to quality control monitoring designed to distinguish gaming from genuine improvements;
- Should be aggregable (i.e. individual data may be summed to produce comparative data within and across practices);
- Changes in the levels of the indicator should rapidly and accurately reflect the success of attempts to improve quality of care.

---

they give similar results on repeated testing of the same individual (reliability), that the scores on a random sample of respondents are normally distributed and that scores show a similar distribution pattern in two different populations (equivalence). But this is not the same as demonstrating that the instrument is actually measuring all the aspects of quality of life that are meaningful and important to all individuals studied, nor that these aspects have been appropriately weighted in the scoring system (validity).

Several reviews have argued convincingly that statistical manipulation alone can never demonstrate the validity of quality of life scales and that more extensive *qualitative* studies of the experience of illness and disability should be undertaken before tick-box instruments are developed.[12,21–24] For people whose language is not English, it is standard practice to translate an established English (or American) instrument and 'validate' it by back-translation followed by factor analysis of a pilot data set,[8] though this approach has been rightly challenged for assuming that if a questionnaire can be *reliably* translated and back-translated into language X, and if response patterns of population samples are statistically comparable, the instrument is necessarily *valid* in that language and culture.[25–28] Paterson has developed a 'customisable' instrument for measuring quality of life, the Measure Yourself Medical Outcomes Profile (MYMOP), in which each respondent first identifies the three most important dimensions of their own quality of life and then scores each of these on a scale

Box 11.3 Examples of generic, disease-specific and patient-specific quality of life questions.

Generic questions (from the SF-36[19])

   1 In general, would you say your health is
     □ Excellent
     □ Very good
     □ Good
     □ Fair
     □ Poor
   2 Compared to 3 months ago, how would you rate your health in general now?
     □ Much better than 3 months ago
     □ Somewhat better than 3 months ago
     □ About the same as 3 months ago
     □ Somewhat worse than 3 months ago
     □ Much worse than 3 months ago

Disease-specific questions (from the St George's respiratory questionnaire[16])

   1 Over the last 3 months, I had shortness of breath
     □ Most days
     □ Several days per week
     □ A few days per month
     □ Only when I had a respiratory infection
     □ Never
   2 My cough or shortness of breath embarrasses me in public
     □ Agree
     □ Disagree
   3 I feel that my respiratory disease is out of my control
     □ Agree
     □ Disagree

Patient-specific questions (from a 'MYMOP' scale,[20] completed by a patient)
Choose one or two symptoms (physical or mental) that bother you the most.
Now, consider how bad each symptom is, over the last week, and score it by
   circling your chosen number.
SYMPTOM 1 = *Can't get upstairs*
As bad as it could be 0 1 2 ③ 4 5 6 As good as it could be
SYMPTOM 2 = *Afraid to go out of the house*
As bad as it could be 0 ① 2 3 4 5 6 As good as it could be

of 1–5.[20,29,30] This (in theory at least) gets around the problem that different individuals value different aspects of their lives and lifestyles differently, and hence 'standardisation' (though crucial for comparing findings across different trials[31]) is an over-rated virtue in quality of life instruments. One of my students is currently using the MYMOP instrument to evaluate a yoga course for people with diabetes, and is finding that different people want (and get) different things out of joining the course.

The use of health-related quality of life instruments is illustrated in Section 4.4 where I describe trials of self-management programmes for chronic illness. If you plan to develop such an instrument yourself (or choose and use an off-the-peg one), note that this is an especially tricky area for the novice. Make sure you read Section 3.4 on questionnaire research and pursue relevant references from that section and that you find yourself a supervisor who has worked with these instruments before, otherwise you will waste a lot of time on research that could prove unpublishable.

11.2   A rational biomedical perspective: evidence-based targets, planned change and criterion-based audit

A good introductory article on quality in primary care, which takes what is very much the current 'mainstream' perspective on the topic, is Campbell and colleagues' 'Defining quality of care'.[32] They argue that the starting point for both defining and measuring quality is the individual patient and that two principal dimensions of quality should be considered: access to care and effectiveness of care. Effectiveness has two key components – clinical and interpersonal. These individual, patient-focused dimensions of quality, they argue, should inform system-level aspects such as the structure of the health care system, key processes of care and chosen outcome measures. But because one person's quality care is another's lengthy waiting list or blacklisted procedure, care for individuals (at least in publicly funded healthcare systems) must be balanced against the needs of the entire population. These considerations require additional dimensions of quality, including equity (everyone matters equally; hence queue-jumping and 'postcode lotteries' should be avoided) and efficiency (there is a limited pot for all, so waste should be avoided).

Campbell et al.'s article (from the National Primary Care Research and Development Centre in Manchester) has been followed by numerous further studies by the same team and has set the foundations for a national system of quality targets and financial rewards for UK GPs, known as the Quality and Outcomes Framework or QOF (Box 11.4; see http://www.ic.nhs.uk/services/qof).[33] I had a walk-on part in the development of this framework some years ago, when I was invited to sit on a panel of experts that set the standards by which access and effectiveness would be defined for one particular clinical condition (diabetes).[6] We (the panel members) were all sent a set of reprints containing the best and most up-to-date research evidence on diabetes care, and we spent a couple of days in heated discussion around a large table considering the implications of the research for the design and delivery of services. We continued

> **Box 11.4 The UK Quality and Outcomes Framework (based on 2006–2007 figures).**
>
> The QOF is a voluntary reward and incentive programme for UK GP practices that began in 2004. Achievement points are available in four domains:
> • *Clinical care*, which covers the major chronic diseases such as asthma, cancer, coronary heart disease and diabetes – up to 550 QOF points;
> • *Good organisation*, which covers the quality of medical records, patient communications, education and training, practice management and medicines management – up to 184 QOF points;
> • *Positive patient experience*, which covers how well practices manage patient surveys and consultation length – up to 100 QOF points;
> • *Extra services*, for practices that provide cervical screening, child health surveillance, maternity services and contraceptive services – up to 36 QOF points.
> There are further bonus QOF points for overall clinical achievement (up to 100 points), overall achievement in the organisation (up to 30 points) and access standards (up to 50 points).

our deliberations by email and eventually came up with a set of standards for diabetes care that satisfied most if not all the people on the panel. A few years later (and suitably updated), these standards formed the benchmarks against which GPs' performance in diabetes care was measured, incentivised and financially rewarded.

At the time of writing, articles and commentaries are only beginning to appear on the impact of the QOF on quality of primary care in the UK. See, for example, Colin Kenny's upbeat assessment of the impact of the QOF on diabetes care, in which he claims evidence for substantial improvements in patient-relevant outcomes,[34] and the companion articles by consultant diabetologists[35] and the ensuing online correspondence (http://www.bmj.com) which suggests that (a) the QOF indicators measured some but not all of the key dimensions of diabetes care – in particular they omitted the knock-on effect on secondary care services and GPs' non-diabetic patients; (b) gaming may have occurred to a significant degree in some practices, allowing GPs to reap financial rewards without actually improving care (see Box 11.2) and (c) many of the improvements attributed to the QOF were merely continuation of a general trend and not the result of the QOF (i.e. they would have happened anyway).

The purpose of this section is not to judge the impact of the UK QOF or comparable initiatives in other countries, but to consider where its protagonists are coming from and the assumptions on which their work is based. Initiatives such as the QOF take a strong rationalist perspective – that is, they are based on the assumption that quality initiatives can (and should) be planned and implemented according to a structured sequence, more or less as follows: Set

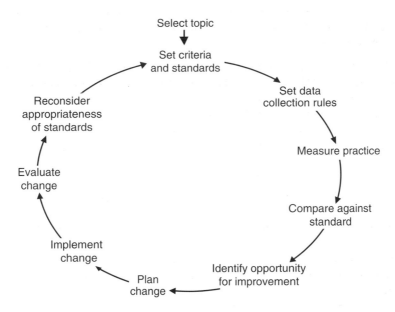

Figure 11.2 Criterion-based audit.

a standard for clinical care (ideally, evidence-based); plan specific changes (guidelines, training programmes, financial incentives and so on) to achieve that standard; put resources behind the plans; monitor progress and tweak input accordingly. This is the basic model of criterion-based audit (the standard 'audit cycle') in which a quality goal is pursued – at least in theory – by making changes in structure and process of care (Figure 11.2).

The formal planning of care and the use of criterion-based audit to monitor progress is a model with much going for it, combining as it does evidence-based medicine (see Section 2.2) and conventional management theory (i.e. change is seen as a rational, planned process requiring clear vision, firm leadership and close monitoring against predefined targets). Without doubt, health care can often be significantly improved using this model. Martin Roland, who was the academic lead on the development of the QOF, has summarised the evidence for different approaches to quality assurance within this model.[36] In short, effective strategies tend to be multifaceted, adequately resourced, driven by clear leadership, linked to structural or financial incentives and accompanied by a cultural ('hearts and minds') change in attitudes and priorities.

But the rationalist theoretical lens, with its emphasis on standard-setting, targets, monitoring, and the 'milestones' of the quality initiative may prove more illuminating in some circumstances than others. In some situations, the presumed 'clockwork universe' that can be adjusted here or there to improve an output further down the clinical production line fails to match the experience on the ground. In an important study of the limitations of criterion-based audit as perceived by clinicians, Johnston found that they had five main bug-bears: lack of resources, lack of expertise or advice in project design and analysis, problems between groups and group members, lack of an overall plan for audit and organisational impediments.[37] Whilst Johnston's own analysis is largely from within the rationalist frame of reference (he talks of 'barriers' that should be 'overcome' so that audit-driven quality initiatives can enjoy greater success), 'problems in the team' and 'organisational impediments' might be more productively analysed through alternative theoretical lenses such as social learning (described in Section 2.8 and 11.4) or organisational sensemaking (Section 11.6).

It is also worth noting the historical (and political) context within which the rationalistic perspective on quality has risen to prominence. Arguably, this particular take on quality is a product of its time, closely aligned as it is with the new public management, whose emphasis is 'finding out what works and implementing it' and whose discourse links economic efficiency with accountability and performance management.[38,39] Both Ian Sanderson (a political scientist) and Andrew Van de Ven (a sociologist who studies innovation in hospitals) as well as my own team have argued that the evidence-based case for 'what works' can be constructed rhetorically to support particular political positions and marginalise others.[40-42] That is not to suggest that the QOF has been 'spun' to serve particular political ends, but it is worth bearing in mind that the standards which are set and pursued in the audit cycle are to some extent socially constructed. It is also worth noting an alternative perspective on the extent to which any organisational change can be 'planned' and 'implemented', as depicted in Figure 11.2. Paul Bate (an organisational ethnographer) and his colleagues have recently argued (based on an extensive literature review) that many change efforts in the National Health Service have the characteristics of social movements – that is, they occur organically in an emergent rather than programmable way, and whilst much good can come of them, their unfolding cannot be predicted or controlled with any accuracy.[43] Whist planned and programmed change against evidence-based standards has its place in quality improvement, it is not a panacea.

11.3   A narrative perspective: significant event audit

I used to run a module on change management in the MSc in Primary Health Care at University College London, in which I required students to report on a standard criterion-based audit (see previous section). Whilst some students completed the assignment as intended, others used it as an opportunity for describing how they had begun their audit with high hopes but abandoned it when participating staff either lost momentum or became distracted by competing demands. There is no doubt that whilst such projects are often very worthy, maintaining motivation and finding time to see the project through is often a major challenge.

An alternative approach, significant event audit, uses the inherent attraction of the story form (see Box 11.4). Significant event audit is defined as the study of

'individual cases in which there has been a significant occurrence (not necessarily involving an undesirable outcome for the patient) are analysed in a systematic and detailed way to ascertain what can be learnt about the overall quality of care and to indicate changes that might lead to future improvements'.[44]

It is also known as critical event audit, critical incident analysis, structured case analysis and facilitated case discussion. There are subtle semantic differences between these different terms (such as the balance between patient and professional focus), but in practice they are often used synonymously. All of them are based on a careful and structured dissection of a single case, and all ask the crucial question, 'How could things have been different, what can we learn from what happened, and what needs to change?'

The technique was originally developed during World War II by an aviation psychologist called Flanaghan.[45] At that time, there was an urgent need to train flight crews in a very short time and to understand the specific behaviours that led to the success or failure of a mission. Flanaghan defined an incident as *'any observable human activity that is sufficiently complete in itself to permit inferences and predictions about the person performing the action'.* His painstaking work on the critical incident technique (which he extended after the war to other areas of individual and organisational behaviour) laid the foundations for its widespread use in business, health care, organisational psychology and education. Flanaghan believed that critical incident analysis was different from other forms of qualitative research in that it was particularly focused on providing quick solutions to challenging practical problems. Furthermore, he argued, greater emphasis should be placed on collecting as many independent, dispassionate observations as possible rather than focusing on the subjective experience of a single individual. Data may be collected by face-to-face individual interviews, group interviews, self-administered questionnaires or direct observation, though individual and group interviews are most commonly used. Participants should be encouraged to report the incident in as much detail as they can remember, since (as Flanaghan said in his original paper) if people can only produce vague impressions, this suggests that the incident is not well remembered and may be inaccurate.

For a critical incident technique to be a useful learning experience or trigger for change, three pieces of information must be included as well as the incident itself: a description of the situation that led to the incident, the actions or behaviours of the focal person in the incident and the results or outcomes of the behavioural actions.[46] These key elements bear a close resemblance to Aristotle's essential features of a story (see Section 2.6): chronology, characters, context, emplotment and trouble (in this case, the critical incident). Whilst critical incident narratives in healthcare are rarely examined as literature (but watch this space – one of my PhD students is doing just this),

---

Box 11.5 Ten unique selling points of stories in the context of quality improvement.[47]

1 Stories are *perspectival*. They are told subjectively from the viewpoint of the narrator, drawing attention to the individual rather than the institution and thus highlighting the view of particular patients or staff.

2 Stories *make sense of experience*. The structuring devices of time and plot retrospectively align events and actions so as to modify mental schemas.

3 Stories are *non-linear*. They convey multiple and complex truths, depicting events as emerging from the interplay of actions, relationships and environments.

4 Stories are *embedded in a context*. A particular story about what went on in an organisation is nested within an over-arching meta-narrative of 'what tends to go on around here'.

5 Stories have an *ethical dimension*. They depict both acts and omissions, reflecting society's expectations about what a 'good doctor' or 'good daughter' should have done in such circumstances.

6 Stories *bridge the gap* between the formal, codified space of an organisation (roles, job descriptions and lines of accountability) and informal, uncodified space (relationships, feelings, 'unwritten rules' and subcultures).

7 Stories offer insights into what *might have been* (what Bruner calls 'subjuncivization'[48]). The imaginative reconstruction of the end of a story allows us to consider different options for change.

8 Stories are *action-oriented*, depicting what people did (and what happened to them) and also igniting and shaping their future action.

9 Stories are *inherently subversive*, since (in Bruner's terminology) they embrace the tension between the canonical (i.e. an organisation's standard routines and procedures) and the unexpected (i.e. new ways of thinking and working).

10 Leadership is related to storytelling. *'Leaders are people who tell good stories, and about whom good stories are told'.*[49]

---

the story form has a number of inherent advantages in quality improvement efforts (Box 11.5).

In an excellent overview, Kemppainen gave examples of the use of critical incident technique in determining patients' perceptions of quality in health services. The informant was asked to 'think back to your last encounter with a doctor/nurse. Describe something that you found particularly memorable'.[50] The person was then prompted to describe the situation in detail, focusing on the actions and behaviours of the health professional(s) and the outcome of those actions. A minority of incidents in Kemppainen's overview related to perceptions of excellence and were particularly attributed to 'nurturing' behaviour on the part of a health professional. Most negative incidents identified by patients were characterised by perceived failure of communication or poor personal care. My own team used a significant event prompt in our qualitative study of interpreted consultations (see Section 6.5) in which we asked both patients and health professionals to 'describe a recent interpreted consultation that went particularly well' and also 'tell us about an interpreted consultation that didn't go so well'.[51]

Whilst the analysis of stories by or about patients is increasingly used in research (and in that context the stories usually require extensive analysis), storytelling can be a quick and effective form of audit in a service context, as described in a short article by Robinson and colleagues[52] and in more detail by Mike Pringle's team.[44] Using a semi-formal group discussion led by a trained facilitator, participants are asked to recall situations that they think are examples of good or bad practice in the particular setting being studied. The participants describe what first occurred, the subsequent events and why they perceived the incident to be an example of effective or ineffective practice (Box 11.6).

Kemppainnen's qualitative study explored the practical barriers to effective significant event audit in general practice.[50] These included:
• Practical problems such as lack of space and lack of privacy
• Lack of trust – especially when junior members of staff were required to work in groups with the most senior members
• Insufficient protected time available for discussion of sensitive cases
• The risk of making things worse rather than better
• Poor facilitation skills of the person leading the discussion
• Role conflict when junior staff are asked to adopt 'egalitarian' ethos in group meetings
• Concern from non-doctors that the doctors' agenda tends to dominate the meetings

In addition to these practical issues, there are some important theoretical and methodological bugbears to address if you plan to use significant event audit in a piece of academic work (such as a research study or evaluation of a quality improvement project). On the one hand, the significant event in a facilitated discussion potentially exposes and illuminates 'system errors' in a 'blame free' forum, and the use of multiple narrators (it is generally assumed) will lend objectivity to the technique. The narratives are used merely as a means to an end: Find out where the problem exists in the system with a view to fixing it. But stories, as I explained briefly in Section 2.6, are never a quick way to objective truth, since narrative truth and scientific truth are different epistemological forms. The best we can ever expect from a collection of stories about a particular incident is an illumination of how the events and actions were differently constructed and emplotted by different actors and observers. We will be able to determine, for example, who is constructed as the hero and the villain of the scenario and how events are rhetorically described in particular (implicitly causal) sequences. But if we accept that narrative has the properties listed in Box 11.5, we must be careful not to confuse it with scientific 'fact'.

Box 11.6 Stages in significant event audit in a GP practice setting.[52]

1 Decide who will be included in the group (ideally 8–10 participants).
2 Either appoint a facilitator from within the group or bring in an external person. The facilitator's role is to

Explain the aims and process of the discussion

Structure the discussion – that is, keep to time, encourage contributions from all participants and clarify and summarise frequently

Apply the basic ground rules of group discussion and maintain confidentiality

Facilitate the suggestions for improvement when areas of concern arise

Encourage participants to accept responsibility for initiating change

Recognise emotion within the discussion and allow appropriate expression within the group

Remain 'external' to the group

3 Allocate a defined time for the meeting. Use a comfortable, quiet room and ensure that routine business (e.g. answering the phone) will be dealt with by someone outside the group. More junior staff (e.g. receptionists) might like to have an informal preparatory meeting in which they plan what they will say.
4 Choose a case or cases. Cases may be chosen at random or, alternatively, those of particular concern or interest may be selected. Ideally, the facilitator, or by agreement a member of the group, should prepare a brief, written summary of the case and circulate this to all participants, preferably before the meeting.
5 At the meeting, the participant who has been most involved in the case should open the discussion by summarising his or her recollections outlining good aspects of care first, and then suggesting areas of concern. Other members are then invited by the facilitator to add their observations until everyone, as appropriate, has participated.
6 At this point, the facilitator should summarise the discussion, helping the team to identify the good aspects of care and highlighting the areas of concern, encouraging the group members to suggest improvements. The facilitator should end the discussion by requesting final comments and summarising the improvements to be implemented.
7 The facilitator should provide written feedback as soon as possible after the discussion. Ideally, regular review sessions should also be held to check that the suggested improvements have been implemented, and if not, to explore the reasons for this.
8 Confidentiality should be maintained by providing clear explanation to all staff of the importance of this dimension and by ensuring that the patient's name and other identifying details are not included on the written record of the discussion.

In summary, significant event audit has many theoretical advantages and draws on the inherent attraction of the story form to overcome motivational barriers to quality improvement. It is potentially a powerful technique for learning and change, but it must be used sensitively in the service context and not taken at face value in the academic context. If you are interested in exploring the theoretical dimension of significant event audit, try Rick Iedema's clever paper on critical incident analysis in the Australian flying doctor service.[53] Incidentally, this approach to audit is increasingly used in patient safety research – an important topic that I have omitted from this textbook purely due to lack of space.[54]

11.4 A social learning perspective: peer review groups and quality circles

Since the time of Balint (see Section 6.3), and probably for many years before him, GPs have met together on a regular and semi-formal basis to discuss their practice with a view to improving it. A recent survey of 26 European countries found that some form of peer review groups or quality circles was widespread in ten of these (The Netherlands, the UK, Denmark, Belgium, Ireland, Sweden, Norway, Germany, Switzerland and Austria).[55] Participation in these groups was as high as 86% in some countries (and as low as 2% in others). The world-renowned primary care quality guru, Richard Grol, has identified reflective practice (via quality circles or otherwise) and peer review as two key approaches for improving quality in primary care.[56] Whilst Balint's disciples took an explicitly psychoanalytic theoretical perspective to their group work, modern-day groups often nail their colours to a different mast – such as evidence-based practice, reflective practice or simply 'professional development'. Let's take a look at these approaches and consider how they work.

Peer review groups and quality circles are somewhat different in design and purpose, and take different formats in different countries.[55,57,58] The former tend to be more informal and driven by friendly group discussion, whereas the latter tend to be part of a wider, more formal quality improvement programme such as the European Foundation for Quality Management which includes checklists for self-assessment and guidance for formal practice audit, and which may include external inspection by doctors of one another's practices.[59,60] But even in very formal, structured peer review initiatives (and in no small part due to Grol's influence on the design of programmes throughout Europe), there is now strong emphasis on self-assessment and reflection by the 'inspected' practice with the external 'inspectors' providing formative feedback rather than summative judgement.

Typically, a peer review group meets fortnightly or monthly and covers a pre-agreed topic such as antibiotic prescribing or dealing with difficult patients. Participants may or may not undertake audits (see Section 11.2) on the topic area and bring data to the meeting. They may or may not look up relevant research evidence. The focus of the meeting is informal discussion and learning from one another. In their recent review, Contencin et al. capture both the diversity and the underlying common spirit of these meetings well:

> *The mainspring of peer-review groups tends to be personal motivation – a desire to learn and share. A group provides interaction between practices, a sense of cohesion and the support afforded by group policies. In Germany, group meetings are attended mostly by single-handed GPs seeking an exchange of views and constructive criticism. In the UK, the peer-review element was a particularly valued facet in a team based, multi-professional and formative quality initiative. To motivate participants, most peer group meetings are run by trained moderators. In Denmark, psychologists teach 'moderator-GPs' problem-solving techniques, communication skills and how to prevent burn-out. In Switzerland, hundreds of volunteer tutors (doctors or allied health professionals) have been trained. They chair groups of doctors and encourage them to improve their performance. An important factor is maintaining early enthusiasm and quality of assessment. Cyclic quality improvement procedures are useful in this regard.*[57]

If all this sounds somewhat ad hoc and a little too jolly to count as a quality initiative, let us consider the nature of learning and personal development. In Section 2.8, I introduced three theories of learning: experiential learning theory (Lewin, Kolb and Dewey), social learning theory (Bandura) and social development theory (Vygotsky). Whilst these theories have important differences, they have much in common with one another – especially the central importance placed by all of them on social discourse as a means of promoting reflection and consolidating or changing understanding. As Paulo Friere said: *'Knowledge emerges only through invention and reinvention, through the restless, impatient, continuing, hopeful inquiry men pursue in the world, with the world, and with each other'.*[61] The link between experiential learning, social interaction and quality improvement in organisations has been eloquently made by Donald Schon in his excellent book *The Reflective Practitioner*, which I strongly recommend.[62] If this topic interests you, see also the recent paper by Stark et al. on 'guided reflection'.[63]

In other words, informal chit-chat is no bad thing. The experiential learning cycle (Figure 2.2, page 51) does not progress solely by individual accumulation of new facts and experiences but by the construction of these facts and experiences into meaningful stories and the sharing of these stories with other individuals who are seen as homophilous (i.e. 'someone like me, facing the same problems as me') and hence worth listening to. In a learning group – either formally established (as in a peer review group) or informally gathered (as in a café or coffee queue) – learners' stories are the vehicle through which the meaning of a shared or common experience is negotiated and re framed. Individual experiences (usually told in the form of stories), ideas and observations are placed into a 'rummage-bin' which can be drawn upon in discussion.

An interesting example of social learning (and, arguably, of the Vygotskian notion that learning is often social *before* it becomes internalised) is John Gabbay and Andrée le May's ethnographic study of how GPs and nurses introduce improvements to their clinical practice. After several months' ethnographic work in a single GP practice, and extensive analysis of qualitative data (observations and interviews), these researchers concluded that the traditional 'evidence into practice' sequence (identify clinical problem → look up research evidence [e.g. in a guideline] → apply evidence) never actually occurred! Rather, these clinicians relied on 'mindlines', defined as 'collectively reinforced, internalised, tacit guidelines', which developed iteratively through browsing journals (often infrequently), informal chats with colleagues, experience from individual patients and discussions with pharmaceutical representatives.[64] It is worth quoting directly from the researchers' discussion:

> *'When describing what we call mindlines, clinicians told us, for example, that they were grown from experience and from people who are trusted; they were 'stored in my head' but could be shared and tested and then internalised through discussion, while leaving room for individual flexibility. Once compiled, each individual practitioner's mindlines were adjusted by checking them out against what was learnt from brief reading or from discussions with colleagues, either within or outside the practice. The mindline might well be modified when applied to an individual patient after discussion and negotiation during the consultation; at this stage patients' ideas of what is the appropriate evidence about their particular case (their own personal history, what their family has experienced, what they have read in the media, and so on) could influence the application or even the continuing development of the mindline. Further adjustment might subsequently happen during swapping stories with colleagues or in audit or 'critical incident meetings'.'*

This is not to say that evidence-based guidelines are unimportant or that they have no influence on the practice of GPs. Some years ago, my colleague Hannah-Rose Douglas and I studied the attitudes of doctors and nurses to training courses in evidence-based medicine and found that most of them did not want to be trained in the evaluation of research evidence![65] They valued the principles of evidence-based medicine and wanted to learn and apply them, but they believed that this would happen mostly by talking to experts and colleagues whom they trusted as 'knowing the evidence'. Gabbay and le May's research suggests that these clinicians understood better than we ourselves did at the time how learning occurs in primary care.

As someone who qualified as a doctor almost 25 years ago, and who has since spent many fruitful evenings in informal discussions with peers about how to improve our practice, I am largely reassured that there is a theoretical basis for the 'informal' end of the spectrum of quality improvement methods. Although I have presented criterion-based audit, significant event audit and peer review groups as separate approaches to quality improvement, in reality these approaches are often applied in combination and fed into one another.

11.5   A phenomenological perspective: the patient as mystery shopper

I was introduced to the concept of 'mystery shopping' in quality improvement initiatives by Dr Paula Baraitser, a sexual health specialist in south London who has used this approach particularly creatively. I am grateful to Paula for illuminating the concept to me. In this section, I first summarise the literature on mystery shopping before adding my own commentary – a suggestion that the mystery shopper approach might be analysed and refined using insights from phenomenology (See Section 2.7.1).

We all know from our own experience as patients how important it is to be treated with respect, retain our dignity and have confidence in our clinician. In Section 10.2, I briefly discussed Wensing's research, which identified 'humaneness' as patients' top priority for their clinician.[66] I have heard countless stories from my women friends of doctors failing to introduce themselves, making sexist comments while examining them or leaving the curtains open while doing an intimate procedure. Whilst respect and dignity are important issues in any area of health care, they are perhaps especially crucial to optimising outcome in sensitive and potentially embarrassing areas such as gynaecology or sexual health.

Research has shown that the patient satisfaction survey (a widely used tool for evaluating services) consistently underestimates the level of dissatisfaction and unease with services dealing with stigmatising conditions and intimate examinations.[67–70] Patients who gave qualitative interviews as well as filling in closed-item questionnaires described the detail of their personal experiences and disclosed their fears only in the former. It is worth speculating on why this is so. Patients may be reluctant to criticise a local service in a box-ticking format or they may attribute their experience (such as a long waiting time) to circumstance, luck or their own fault rather than to a problem with the service itself.[68] They may be unwilling to comment on 'technical' aspects of the service – or perhaps, their comments in this area may be dismissed by experts as ill-informed.[71]

The use of mystery shoppers (also known as simulated patients or clients, pseudo-patients and undercover careseekers) has a long history in educating medical students,[72,73] assuring quality in telephone advice lines[74] and evaluating services in general practice,[75–79] community pharmacy,[80–83] mental health[84] and sexual health.[82,85–88] The quality agenda in sexual health services is especially challenging, since few patients attending this service would want to define themselves in terms of their links to the clinic (contrast this with patients who have chronic, relatively non-stigmatising illnesses such as diabetes or kidney disease, who are often quite happy to join self-help groups and accept invitations to be the service user on a quality improvement steering group). Many sexual health problems (e.g. sexually transmitted infections, teenage pregnancy) are closely linked to social inequality, especially the triple jeopardy of being young, poor and lacking social capital (see Section 9.2), and are much commoner in certain minority ethnic groups. The target population for sexual health services includes a highly mobile, hard-to-reach and sometimes overtly disaffected sector of the population. For all these reasons, capturing the patient experience in a way that is meaningful and representative is no easy task.

Against this background, Paula and her team were delighted when they heard that a group of middle-aged white women had begun to sample the local gynaecology services incognito and provide feedback to the clinics. They asked the women to join forces and help develop the local Mystery Shopper Project, in which participants from a broad range of social and ethnic groups and sexual orientations were recruited and taught how to present with one of several standardised stories to different parts of the sexual health services. After each encounter, the mystery shopper filled out a questionnaire containing both open- and closed-item questions (see Section 3.4) which covered perceptions of confidentiality and staff attitudes at reception, length of time spent waiting at each stage (including time to book an appointment), quality of the waiting room environment, staff attitudes and manner during the clinical consultation, and their information needs at all stages of the visit. The data were analysed thematically to identify patients' chief concerns, and these were fed back to the staff in each clinic with a view to triggering action for quality improvement (this part of the work is ongoing). In this particular study, more than half the mystery shoppers had a positive experience but almost all identified important quality issues. The most common ones raised were difficulty booking an appointment, lack of confidentiality in the waiting area, rudeness and perceived judgemental attitudes by receptionists, and an offhand manner by clinicians.

In their paper on the Mystery Shopper Project, Paula and her team emphasise the importance of initial training and ongoing support (e.g. by telephone) for people who work as mystery shoppers.[86] Even though these individuals had no current sexual health problem (though some had been recruited after a previous clinic encounter), living through the experience of a long wait in an uncomfortable waiting room with a receptionist peering over her spectacles at you can be potentially traumatising. When a member of my own team visited a family planning clinic in Lambeth to discuss research, people at a nearby bus stop shouted offence ('dirty slag') as she queued outside the door! Add to this the stress of the undercover agent: One study in the USA reported that 13% of mystery shoppers were 'exposed' during the encounter.[89]

There is something underhand and perhaps frankly dishonest in the idea of the mystery shopper, and there is no doubt that some clinicians are resistant to this approach to quality improvement.[80,90] It could be argued that the exposure of poor practice justifies the deception that is integral to the mystery shopper model, but in the UK, research ethics committees have required informed consent from all potential participating clinicians before such projects can go ahead. These and other issues are discussed extensively in a recent review by Herrera.[91] In the remainder of this section I want to offer a philosophical slant on the question: What is the justification for placing the personal experience of the mystery shopper so centrally in a quality improvement project?

In some respects, mystery shopper initiatives can be thought of as an example of ethnographic method applied in clinical services. Ethnography, more usually applied by anthropologists visiting far-flung tribes, requires the researcher not merely to observe but to participate in all aspects of the alien culture and (thereby) reach a true understanding of why things occur as they do.[92] Ethnographic work is written up (to a greater or lesser extent) as personal story, and particularly powerful are the 'confessional' and 'impressionist' tales that place experiences within the identity and lifeworld of the researcher rather than offering a third-person 'view from nowhere'.[93] Mystery shopper projects rest, therefore, on the authenticity of the participants' experience: If the shopper is too nervous about the context or the procedure to take note of his or her perceptions or if he or she becomes over-familiar (so that, for example, anxiety-provoking experiences cease to provoke anxiety), relatively weak data will be generated.

Is it really necessary to experience a cervical smear in order to assess quality in a smear clinic? Phenomenologists (see Section 2.7.1) would argue that it is, since perceptions are necessarily embodied – that is, the experience is brought about by and through an individual.[94] All experiences are structured through what phenomenologists call intentionality, which is a particular property of consciousness. A person cannot merely be conscious; he or she must be conscious in relation to *something*. The directing of consciousness towards that something – with the assignment of meaning and significance through particular concepts, thoughts, ideas and images – comprises intentionality. When a mystery shopper attends for a cervical smear and subsequently reports in a free text response or a telephone interview that she perceived the nurse as 'brusque' and 'dismissive', she has generated data that could not have been obtained from more conventional research techniques. Of course, terms like 'brusque' and 'dismissive' are open to multiple interpretations and cannot be objectively verified. Indeed, nothing in phenomenology can be objectively verified – it is an inherently subjective branch of philosophy. This privileging and celebration of the subjective tends to make rationalist researchers very uneasy, but provided that the mystery shopper presents her experience honestly, subjective data can have real value. Moran defined phenomenology as 'the unprejudiced, descriptive study of whatever appears to consciousness, precisely in the manner in which it so appears'.[95] If the mystery shopper *experiences* the nurse as brusque and dismissive, that is important data!

The use of a phenomenological theoretical lens to inform research design and help interpret data in healthcare has been very much led by nursing academics, who have emphasised the critical need to capture *subjective* experience using careful qualitative methods and appropriate analytic techniques (see Section 3.2).[96–99] But to date, published mystery shopper studies have been led by doctors (and occasionally pharmacists), who have generally emphasised the use of 'objective' research tools such as closed questionnaires and precise measurement of waiting times and who tend to express findings in terms such as '35% of clinicians refused to....', using qualitative data only as illustrative quotes to spice up an essentially quantitative study. In other words, whilst (in my view) the theoretical value of the mystery shopper approach is its potential for rich phenomenological insights that could capture the meaning that particular experiences have for individual patients, I cannot find a single example of such an analysis in the literature, and nor did a systematic review of over 300 empirical studies of user involvement in healthcare planning.[100]

An overview by Angela Coulter from the influential Picker Institute (see http://www.pickereurope.org/) argues that whilst questionnaire surveys have their place, the time is ripe for research on the patient experience to go beyond box-ticking and include a wide range of qualitative and quantitative approaches.[101] Wensing and Elwyn recently argued even more forcefully in favour of a shift towards open-ended qualitative studies of the patient experience. One area that is wide open for further theoretical and methodological work is the work of the mystery shopper![102]

11.6 A sociological perspective: Quality Team Development as organisational sensemaking

Many determinants of quality in health care have been shown to lie at organisational rather than individual level.[103–105] This finding has led to a growing emphasis on the team or organisation as the unit of analysis in quality improvement initiatives – especially the notion of the 'learning organisation' (one in which the acquisition, processing and sharing of knowledge is actively supported and rewarded).[56,105–109] There are numerous examples of organisational approaches to quality improvement in the literature. In this section I have chosen to describe one particular initiative – the UK Royal College of General Practitioners' (RCGP) Quality Team Development (QTD) programme (http://www.rcgp.org.uk/quality_/quality_home.aspx; Box 11.7).

A few years ago, I was part of a team led by Dr Fraser Macfarlane to evaluate QTD.[113] We found that this approach had been introduced by the RCGP following a literature review of research on previous organisational-level quality initiatives in primary care, which had revealed eight factors that appeared critical to success:

a The initiative should be locally owned and delivered rather than imposed.
b Targets and standards should be locally adaptable to take account of local circumstances and priorities.
c The initiative should be professionally rather than managerially led.
d There should be a focus on the team rather than the individual GP.
e The initiative should be explicitly interprofessional rather than doctor-led.
f The initiative should draw on interpersonal influence and other informal change mechanisms.
g The initiative should be developmental and formative rather than (or as well as) summative.
h There should be interorganisational collaboration and learning.

> ### Box 11.7 The RCGP QTD programme.
>
> The QTD programme was developed by the UK RCGP in partnership with other professional bodies, including the Institute of Healthcare Management and the Royal College of Nursing, and with input from patient organisations. An expert multi-professional group drew on an extensive review of the literature on quality in general practice, and also on the College's 20 years' experience of developing and evaluating peer-review-based methods of assessing performance in practice, including 'What Sort of Doctor?'[110] approval for practices that train new GPs[111] and Practice Team Accreditation.[112]
>
> QTD aims to support quality improvement through a process of practice team development, education and service planning. The programme requires teams to set and work towards their own development targets. It includes a team self-assessment exercise, a patient survey and a multi-disciplinary peer review visit by a team of three independent assessors. Assessors (GPs, nurses and managers) are volunteers who are recruited from participating local practices; they receive 1 day's compulsory training by the RCGP. At an initial meeting, the assessors review the practice's self-assessment report and plan the practice visit. At the visit, they provide immediate verbal feedback to the practice; structured written feedback is expected within 6 weeks. The lead assessor (usually but not always a GP) has responsibility for planning, coordinating and writing up the assessment.

According to the official evaluation, the RCGP QTD programme, which was the first UK programme to meet all the above criteria, appeared to be highly successful and greatly valued in the small number of practices that signed up to it.[113] In this section, I do not want to address the detail of the QTD programme, but to consider the theoretical basis for the critical success factors listed above. These factors are not, of course, a formula for achieving quality, nor does every factor need to be present to assure quality, but they are nevertheless worth analysing from an academic perspective.

One theoretical perspective that, I believe, provides useful insights here is Karl Weick's notion of organisational sensemaking.[114] I recommend his book *Sensemaking in Organizations* as one of the most readable and coherent management texts on the bookshelves. Box 11.8 lists the seven characteristics that Weick believed marked out the sensemaking organisation. Let's see how far they help us analyse the provisional critical success factors that were built into QTD.

The first thing to note is that quality initiatives take place in a social context. As Weick perceptively observed, these initiatives are tied to people, to people's working relationships with each other and to their sense of participation (or not) in organisational life. Secondly, a quality initiative is crucially linked to the identity of the individuals involved. Professional staff are not cogs in the organisation's machinery but more or less free agents who must choose to

> **Box 11.8 Weick's seven characteristics of sensemaking in organisations.**[114]
>
> **1** *Social context.* Action in an organisation requires, and gains energy from, the actual, implied or imagined presence of others.
>
> **2** *Personal identity.* Organisational initiatives are closely tied up with each person's sense of who he or she is in a particular setting, together with any threats that exist to this sense of self and what is available to enhance the sense of self.
>
> **3** *Retrospect.* The world perceived by the members of the organisation is actually a past world in the sense that we look back at our own actions and those of others and thereby make sense of where we are now.
>
> **4** *Salient clues.* People involved in an organisational effort use initiative and resourcefulness to elaborate tiny indicators into full-blown stories of 'success', 'failure', 'pulling together' and so on, creating what may amount to self-fulfilling prophecies (hence, perhaps, the widely recognised importance of 'early wins').
>
> **5** *Ongoing projects.* Sensemaking is constrained by the speed with which events flow into the past and become outdated.
>
> **6** *Plausibility.* Sensemaking requires that stories about events and collective achievements hang together coherently and authentically.
>
> **7** *Enactment.* Sensemaking is active, not passive. It depends on more or less continuous action by individuals to gain some sense of what they are up against (e.g. by asking questions, making declarations, probing to see how something or someone reacts and so on).

get involved in an improvement initiative or not, and will do so on terms that make sense locally and contingently. In a systematic review of complex service innovations in healthcare, my team studied the role of individuals in the assimilation of such innovations and concluded:

> *'People are not passive recipients of innovations. Rather (and to a greater or lesser extent in different individuals), they seek innovations out, experiment with them, evaluate them, find (or fail to find) meaning in them, develop feelings (positive or negative) about them, challenge them, worry about them, complain about them, 'work round' them, develop know-how about them, modify them to fit particular tasks, and try to improve or redesign them – often through dialogue with other users'.*[115]

Epstein has coined the term 'mindfulness' to describe professionals' awareness of, and commitment to, the quality agenda in their individual practice and in organisational improvement initiatives.[116] Any organisational-level quality initiative gains its energy and retains its focus by becoming part of people's raison d'etre. Conversely, if the initiative fails to be taken up by 'hearts and minds', it will quickly lose momentum. Different organisational forms (the 'traditional' versus the 'contemporary' GP practice as described in Section 10.4) are associated with radically different GP identities (see Table 10.2, page 265), and more generally, the identity of a member of the primary health care team profoundly affects how (and with what degree of mindfulness) they enact each aspect of their role.[117,118] Others have shown that tensions arise in organisations when what people are expected to *do* conflicts with who they *are*.[119] I like to think of 'local ownership' of a quality initiative as shorthand for the process by which it becomes appropriated in the identity of the individuals who must see it through.

To illustrate this principle using a counter-example, let me tell you an anecdote about a 'top-down' improvement initiative that was doomed to failure. My neighbour (let's call him Bruno), who is a fellow academic, recently received an email from the Provost of his university requiring staff to dress more smartly when teaching students. He was henceforth required to wear a shirt, tie and jacket so as to convey the high professional standards expected at this top-class university. Bruno's response to this missive was to deliberately 'dress down', not only refusing to wear a tie but selecting his scruffiest pair of jeans whenever he was down to lecture his students. Why did this senior professional behave so petulantly when asked to pull together for a quality initiative? Because, I think, Bruno defined 'professionalism' very differently from his boss. For him, professionalism was about the intellectual content of his lectures, not the clothes he wore when he delivered them. The Provost's instruction conveyed the message that Bruno (who did not own a jacket or tie) was 'unprofessional' and delivering 'poor quality' lectures. He felt (perhaps rightly) insulted and undervalued. The so-called quality initiative cut to the core of his identity. It is likely, even, that dressing casually to give lectures was not incidental to Bruno's professional identity but was actually an enactment of aspects of it – his desire to appear approachable to his students, his rejection of the material over the intellectual, his identification with the 'academic' rather than the 'management' community and so on. Had the Provost of this particular university engaged the lecturers in his quality initiative, a compromise might have been possible in which lecturers were somehow able to construct 'smartening up' as aligned with, rather than conflicting with, the people they saw themselves as. This seemingly trivial example illustrates a more general point made powerfully by Weick in his book – that everything we ask the members of an organisation to do has a symbolic meaning, and Bruno's conflict highlights that one person's 'smart dress' is another's 'style over substance'.

Three more critical success factors that informed the design of the RCGP QTD initiative were a focus on the team, interprofessional involvement and the use of informal interpersonal influence. All this is very politically correct, but what is its theoretical justification? Again, Weick offers some explanatory clues. He argues that organisational members are active 'framers', cognitively making sense of the events, processes, objects and issues that comprise (say) a complex quality initiative. A schema of a person's construction of reality provides the frame though which he or she recalls prior knowledge and interprets new information. Eveland, writing in the 1980s, uses the example of the personal computer – described variously as a 'typewriter', 'calculator' and 'terminal' by members of one organisation – to show how different linguistic metaphors construct a different reality around an innovation and both create and block opportunities for its use:

> 'Seeing PCs as typewriters implies one-to-one access, usually by secretaries, on desks or in typing pools with relatively little consultation by system engineers with those who use them except about aesthetics or ergonomics. The 'calculator' metaphor implies that the tools will be used one-on-one in professional offices, with choices about both equipment and usage left largely to the individuals. Others see PCs as 'terminals' – an approach that implies they should be scattered around, spaced roughly equally apart, for open use by anyone who wanders by. None of these metaphors is precisely wrong – but each tends to limit the choices of users in critical ways . . .'. [120]

This historical example offers us some interesting intellectual tools with which to study resistance to change, in terms of meanings and metaphors based on particular cognitive schemas. With the wisdom of hindsight, and knowing how networked computer systems transformed organisations in the 1990s, we can see how inappropriate the 'calculator' and 'typewriter' metaphors were, but this was not, of course, clear at the time. A generation later, there is a similar degree of confusion about the Internet-based electronic patient record: what does this innovation *mean* ('universally accessible summary of key health problems' or 'loss of the personal GP–patient relationship and a threat to confidentiality')? Depending on whether clinicians take the former or the latter view, the introduction of Internet-based records will meet with different degrees of resistance.

To return to QTD, the basis of success in this and comparable organisation-wide change efforts is ensuring that all members share a frame of reference (or at least, that they hold frames that are compatible with one another) on the nature of the change and why it is needed. Good leadership is about telling the story that sets this shared framing, and about introducing the opportunities for discussion that allow people to negotiate and challenge meanings so that common understandings can emerge. This, I believe, is the reason why a team focus and interprofessional involvement and dialogue are so essential. An initiative that means one thing to the doctors in a GP practice, another thing to the nurses and another to managers will not get beyond first base. As well as promoting social learning (see Section 11.4), the use of informal interpersonal influence is likely (though by no means guaranteed) to accelerate the development of such shared frames.

The next critical success factor that informed QTD was a developmental and formative rather than judgmental and summative approach. This aligns with another of Weick's characteristics of sensemaking: retrospect. By this, he meant that people in organisations first engage in a continuous stream of action, which inevitably generates equivocal situations (especially when change is afoot), and then retrospectively impose a structure or schema on the situations they have faced in order to make them sensible. New knowledge can be thought of as a retrospectively imposed interpretation of our organisational stream of experience. Formative quality initiatives create space for retrospective sensemaking; those that are purely summative stifle this crucial emergent element of the change process.

The final critical success factor identified by the RCGP when they designed the QTD initiative was interorganisational collaboration and learning. Whilst this is by no means incompatible with Weick's sensemaking framework, it fits more closely with Abrahamson's notion of interorganisational macrocultures and the 'fads and fashions' that these macrocultures support.[121,122] The use of interorganisational learning collaboratives to drive quality improvement initiatives is currently very popular in both the UK and the USA, and whist such collaboratives demand much from their members, the impact on practice can be profound.[108,109,123,124]

In conclusion, I have offered a unique (and, some would argue, idiosyncratic) theoretical perspective on what many experts currently see as the 'gold standard' quality initiative in UK general practice. Weick's theory of organisational sensemaking offers one unifying explanation (though it is not the only compatible explanation) for most of the critical success factors underpinning the design of QTD. Furthermore, like all good theories, this rich framework offers interesting hypotheses for refining the QTD model – for example, the introduction of clearer and more explicit mechanisms for staff to negotiate the meaning of suggested changes and fit them into their cognitive schemas. Once again, there is considerable scope for further research.

References

1 Greenhalgh T, Eversley J. *Quality in General Practice: Towards a Holistic Approach*. London: Kings Fund; 1998.
2 Pirsig R. *Zen and the Art of Motorcycle Maintenance*. London: Bodley Head; 1974.
3 Donabedian A. Evaluating the quality of medical care. Milbank Mem Fund Q 1966;44:166–206.
4 Maxwell R. Dimensions of quality revisited: from thought to action. Qual Health Care 1992;1:171–177.
5 Argyris C, Schon D. *Organizational Learning: A Theory of Action Perspective*. London: Addison-Wesley; 1978.
6 Campbell SM, Hann M, Hacker J, Durie A, Thapar A, Roland MO. Quality assessment for three common conditions in primary care: validity and reliability of review criteria developed by expert panels for angina, asthma and type 2 diabetes. Qual Saf Health Care 2002;11:125–130.
7 Wilson IB, Cleary PD. Linking clinical variables with health-related quality of life. A conceptual model of patient outcomes. JAMA 1995;273:59–65.
8 Scientific Advisory Committee of the Medical Outcomes Trust. Assessing health status and quality-of-life instruments: attributes and review criteria. Qual Life Res 2002;11:193–205.

9 Garratt AM, Schmidt L, Fitzpatrick R. Patient-assessed health outcome measures for diabetes: a structured review. Diabet Med 2002;19:1–11.

10 Kind P, Dolan P, Gudex C, Williams A. Variations in population health status: results from a United Kingdom national questionnaire survey. BMJ 1998;316:736–741.

11 Coons SJ, Rao S, Keininger DL, Hays RD. A comparative review of generic quality-of-life instruments. Pharmacoeconomics 2000;17:13–35.

12 Ravens-Sieberer U, Erhart M, Wille N, Wetzel R, Nickel J, Bullinger M. Generic health-related quality-of-life assessment in children and adolescents: methodological considerations. Pharmacoeconomics 2006;24:1199–1220.

13 Bradley C, Speight J. Patient perceptions of diabetes and diabetes therapy: assessing quality of life. Diabetes Metab Res Rev 2002;18(suppl 3):S64–S69.

14 Clayson DJ, Wild DJ, Quarterman P, Duprat-Lomon I, Kubin M, Coons SJ. A comparative review of health-related quality-of-life measures for use in HIV/AIDS clinical trials. Pharmacoeconomics 2006;24(8):751–765.

15 Oldridge N, Saner H, McGee HM. The Euro Cardio-QoL Project. An international study to develop a core heart disease health-related quality of life questionnaire, the HeartQoL. Eur J Cardiovasc Prev Rehabil 2005;12(2):87–94.

16 Ferrer M, Villasante C, Alonso J, et al. Interpretation of quality of life scores from the St George's Respiratory Questionnaire. Eur Respir J 2002;19:405–413.

17 Fortin M, Lapointe L, Hudon C, Vanasse A, Ntetu AL, Maltais D. Multimorbidity and quality of life in primary care: a systematic review. Health Qual Life Outcomes 2004; 2:51.

18 Fortin M, Hudon C, Dubois MF, Almirall J, Lapointe L, Soubhi H. Comparative assessment of three different indices of multimorbidity for studies on health-related quality of life. Health Qual Life Outcomes 2005;3:74.

19 McHorney CA, Ware JE, Jr, Raczek AE. The MOS 36-item short-form health survey (SF-36): II. Psychometric and clinical tests of validity in measuring physical and mental health constructs. Med Care 1993;31:247–263.

20 Paterson C. Measuring outcomes in primary care: a patient generated measure, MYMOP, compared with the SF-36 health survey. BMJ 1996;312(7037):1016–1020.

21 Muldoon MF, Barger SD, Flory JD, Manuck SB. What are quality of life measurements measuring? BMJ 1998;316:542–545.

22 Bernheim JL. How to get serious answers to the serious question: 'How have you been?': subjective quality of life (QOL) as an individual experiential emergent construct. Bioethics 1999;13:272–287.

23 Wade DT. Outcome measures for clinical rehabilitation trials: impairment, function, quality of life, or value? Am J Phys Med Rehabil 2003;82(suppl 10):S26–S31.

24 Hickey A, Barker M, McGee H, O'Boyle C. Measuring health-related quality of life in older patient populations: a review of current approaches. Pharmacoeconomics 2005;23(10):971–993.

25 Hendrickson SG. Beyond translation . . . cultural fit. West J Nurs Res 2003;25:593–608.

26 Bowden A, Fox-Rushby JA. A systematic and critical review of the process of translation and adaptation of generic health-related quality of life measures in Africa, Asia, Eastern Europe, the Middle East, South America. Soc Sci Med 2003;57:1289–1306.

27 Herdman M, Fox-Rushby JA, Badia X. 'Equivalence' and the translation and adaptation of health-related quality of life questionnaires. Qual Life Res 1997;9:316–322.

28 Boynton PM, Wood GW, Greenhalgh T. A hands-on guide to questionnaire research part three: reaching beyond the white middle classes. BMJ 2004;328:1433–1436.

29 Paterson C. Seeking the patient's perspective: a qualitative assessment of EuroQol, COOP-WONCA charts and MYMOP. Qual Life Res 2004;13(5):871–881.

30 Paterson C, Britten N. In pursuit of patient-centred outcomes: a qualitative evaluation of the 'Measure Yourself Medical Outcome Profile'. J Health Serv Res Policy 2000;5(1): 27–36.

31 Garratt A, Schmidt L, Mackintosh A, Fitzpatrick R. Quality of life measurement: bibliographic study of patient assessed health outcome measures. BMJ 2002;324:1417.

32 Campbell SM, Roland MO, Buetow SA. Defining quality of care. Soc Sci Med 2000;51: 1611–1625.

33 Marshall M, Roland M, Campbell SM, et al. *Measuring General Practice: A Demonstration Project to Develop and Test a Set of Primary Care Clinical Quality Indicators.* London: Nuffield Trust; 2003.

34 Kenny C. Diabetes and the quality and outcomes framework. BMJ 2005;331:1097–1098.

35 Greenwood R, Shaw K, Winocour P. Diabetes and the quality and outcomes framework: integrated care is best model for diabetes. BMJ 2005;331:1340.

36 Roland M. Choosing effective strategies for quality improvement. Qual Health Care 2001;10:66–67.

37 Johnston G, Crombie IK, Davies HT, Alder EM, Millard A. Reviewing audit: barriers and facilitating factors for effective clinical audit. Qual Health Care 2000;9:23–36.

38 Pope C. Resisting evidence: the study of evidence-based medicine as a contemporary social movement. Health 2003;7:267–282.

39 Harrison S. The politics of evidence-based medicine in the United Kingdom. Policy Polit 1998;26:15–31.

40 Sanderson I. Getting evidence into practice; perspectives on rationality. Evaluation 2004;10:366–379.

41 Van de Ven AH. The rhetoric of evidence-based medicine. Health Care Manage Rev 2006;27:89–91.

42 Russell J, Greenhalgh T, Byrne E, McDonnell J. The argumentative turn in healthcare policy analysis: an agenda for research. J Health Serv Res Policy, submitted.

43 Bate P, Robert G, Bevan H. The next phase of healthcare improvement: what can we learn from social movements? Qual Saf Health Care 2004;13:62–66.

44 Pringle M, Bradley CP, Carmichael CM, Wallis H, Moore A. Significant event auditing. A study of the feasibility and potential of case-based auditing in primary medical care. Occasional Paper 70. London: Royal College of General Practitioners; 1995.

45 Flanaghan J. The critical incident technique. Psychol Bull 1954;51:327–358.

46 Anderson L, Wilson S. Critical incident technique. In: Whetzel DL, Wheaton GR, eds. *Applied Measurement Methods in Industrial Psychology.* Palo Alto, CA: Davies-Black Publishing; 1997.

47 Greenhalgh T, Russell J, Swinglehurst D. Narrative methods in quality improvement research. Qual Saf Health Care 2005;14:443–449.

48 Bruner J. *Acts of Meaning.* Cambridge, MA: Harvard University Press; 1990.

49 Gardner H. *Leading Minds: An Anatomy of Leadership.* London: Harper Collins; 1995.

50 Kemppainen JK. The critical incident technique and nursing care quality research. J Adv Nurs 2000;32:1264–1271.

51 Greenhalgh T, Robb N, Scambler G. Communicative and strategic action in interpreted consultations in primary health care: a Habermasian perspective. Soc Sci Med 2006;63:1170–1187.

52 Robinson LA, Stacy R, Spencer JA, Bhopal RS. Use facilitated case discussions for significant event auditing. BMJ 1995;311:315–318.

53 Iedema R, Flabouris A, Grant S, Jorn C. Narrativizing errors of care: critical incident reporting in clinical practice. Soc Sci Med 2006;62:133–144.

54 Vincent CA. Analysis of clinical incidents: a window on the system not a search for root causes. Qual Saf Health Care 2004;13:242–243.

55 Beyer M, Gerlach FM, Flies U, et al. The development of quality circles/peer review groups as a method of quality improvement in Europe: results of a survey in 26 European countries. Fam Pract 2003;20:443–451.

56 Grol R. Improving the quality of medical care: building bridges among professional pride, payer profit, and patient satisfaction. JAMA 2001;286:2578–2585.

57 Contencin P, Falcoff H, Doumenc M. Review of performance assessment and improvement in ambulatory medical care. Health Policy 2006;77:64–75.

58 Rhydderch M, Edwards A, Elwyn G, et al. Organizational assessment in general practice: a systematic review and implications for quality improvement. J Eval Clin Pract 2005;11:366–378.

59 Nabitz U, Klazinga N, Walburg J. The EFQM excellence model: European and Dutch experiences with the EFQM approach in health care. European Foundation for Quality Management. Int J Qual Health Care 2000;12:191–201.

60 Heaton C. External peer review in Europe: an overview from the ExPeRT Project. External Peer Review Techniques. Int J Qual Health Care 2000;12:177–182.

61 Friere P. *Education for Critical Consciousness*. New York: Continuum; 1974.

62 Schon D. *The Reflective Practitioner*. New York: Basic Books; 1983.

63 Stark P, Roberts C, Newble D, Bax N. Discovering professionalism through guided reflection. Med Teach 2006;28:e25–e31.

64 Gabbay J, le May A. Evidence based guidelines or collectively constructed 'mindlines?' Ethnographic study of knowledge management in primary care. BMJ 2004;329:1013–1017.

65 Greenhalgh T, Douglas H-R. Experiences of general practitioners and practice nurses of training courses in evidence-based health care: a qualitative study. Br J Gen Pract 1999;49:536–540.

66 Wensing M, Elwyn G. Research on patients' views in the evaluation and improvement of quality of care. Qual Saf Health Care 2002;11:153–157.

67 Sitzia J, Wood N. Patient satisfaction: a review of issues and concepts. Soc Sci Med 1997;45:1829–1843.

68 Dougall A, Russell A, Rubin G, Ling J. Rethinking patient satisfaction: patient experiences of an open access flexible sigmoidoscopy service. Soc Sci Med 2000;50:53–62.

69 Avis M, Bond M, Arthur A. Satisfying solutions? A review of some unresolved issues in the measurement of patient satisfaction. J Adv Nurs 1995;22:316–322.

70 Avis M, Bond M, Arthur A. Exploring patient satisfaction with out-patient services. J Nurs Manag 1995;3:59–65.

71 Calnan M. Towards a conceptual framework of lay evaluation of health care. Soc Sci Med 1988;27:927–933.

72 McAvoy BR. Teaching clinical skills to medical students: the use of simulated patients and videotaping in general practice. Med Educ 1988;22:193–199.

73 Pickard S, Baraitser P, Rymer J, Piper J. Can gynaecology teaching associates provide high quality effective training for medical students in the United Kingdom? Comparative study. BMJ 2003;327:1389–1392.

74 Moriarty H, McLeod D, Dowell A. Mystery shopping in health service evaluation. Br J Gen Pract 2003;53:942–946.

75 Owen A, Winkler R. General practitioners and psychosocial problems: an evaluation using pseudopatients. Med J Aust 1974;2:393–398.

76 Rethans JJ, Sturmans F, Drop R, Van Der. Assessment of the performance of general practitioners by the use of standardized (simulated) patients. Br J Gen Pract 1991;41:97–99.

77 Rethans JJ, Drop R, Sturmans F, Vleuten C. A method for introducing standardized (simulated) patients into general practice consultations. Br J Gen Pract 1991;41:94–96.

78 Renaud M, Beauchemin J, Lalonde C, Poirier H, Berthiaume S. Practice settings and prescribing profiles: the simulation of tension headaches to general practitioners working in different practice settings in the Montreal area. Am J Public Health 1980;70:1068–1073.

79 Kinnersley P, Pill R. Potential of using simulated patients to study the performance of general practitioners. Br J Gen Pract 1993;43:297–300.

80 Norris PT. Purchasing restricted medicines in New Zealand pharmacies: results from a 'mystery shopper' study. Pharm World Sci 2002;24:149–153.

81 Greenhalgh T. Drug prescription and self-medication in India: an exploratory survey. Soc Sci Med 1987;25:307–318.

82 Madden JM, Quick JD, Ross-Degnan D, Kafle KK. Undercover careseekers: simulated clients in the study of health provider behavior in developing countries. Soc Sci Med 1997;45:1465–1482.

83 Bennett W, Petraitis C, D'Anella A, Marcella S. Pharmacists' knowledge and the difficulty of obtaining emergency contraception. Contraception 2003;68:261–267.

84 Winkler RC. Research into mental health practice using pseudopatients. Med J Aust 1974;2:399–403.

85 Sykes S, O'Sullivan K. A 'mystery shopper' project to evaluate sexual health and contraceptive services for young people in Croydon. J Fam Plann Reprod Health Care 2006;32: 25–26.

86 Baraitser P, Pearce V, Horne N, Boynton PM. Mystery shoppers: a tool for sexual health service evaluation. Qual Saf Health Care, submitted.

87 Huntington D, Schuler SR. The simulated client method: evaluating client-provider interactions in family planning clinics. Stud Fam Plann 1993;24:187–193.

88 Huntington D, Lettenmaier C, Obeng-Quaidoo I. User's perspective of counseling training in Ghana: the 'mystery client' trial. Stud Fam Plann 1990;21:171–177.

89 Woodward CA, McConvey GA, Neufeld V, Norman GR, Walsh A. Measurement of physician performance by standardized patients. Refining techniques for undetected entry in physicians' offices. Med Care 1985;23:1019–1027.

90 Borfitz D. Is a 'mystery shopper' lurking in your waiting room? Med Econ 2001;78:63–70.

91 Herrera CD. Reconsidering the pseudo-patient study. Camb Q Healthc Ethics 2001;10: 325–332.

92 Geertz C. *The Interpretation of Cultures.* New York: Basic Books; 1973.

93 Van Maanen J. *Tales of the Field: On Writing Ethnography.* Chicago, IL: University of Chicago Press; 1986.

94 Merleau-Ponty M. *The Primacy of Perception* (Translated by Edie J). Evanston, IL: North Western University Press; 1964.

95 Moran D. *Introduction to Phenomenology.* London: Routledge; 2000.

96 Crotty M. *Phenomenonlogy and Qualitative Nursing Research.* London: Churchill Livingstone; 1995.

97 Benner P. *Interpretive Phenomenology: Embodiment, Caring and Ethics in Health and Illness.* London: Sage; 1994.

98 Edward KL. A theoretical discussion about the clinical value of phenomenology for nurses. Holist Nurs Pract 2006;20:235–238.

99 Davis LA. A phenomenological study of patient expectations concerning nursing care. Holist Nurs Pract 2005;19:126–133.

100 Crawford MJ, Rutter D, Manley C, et al. Systematic review of involving patients in the planning and development of health care. BMJ 2002;325:1263–1267.

101 Coulter A, Fitzpatrick R. The patient's perspective regarding appropriate health care. In: Albrecht G, Fitzpatrick R, Scrimshaw S, eds. *The Handbook of Social Studies in Health and Medicine*. London: Sage; 2003.

102 Wensing M, Elwyn G. Methods for incorporating patients' views in health care. BMJ 2003;326:877–879.

103 Berwick DM. A primer on leading the improvement of systems. BMJ 1996;312:619–622.

104 Carroll JS, Edmondson AC. Leading organisational learning in health care. Qual Saf Health Care 2002;11:51–56.

105 Davies HTO, Nutley SM. Developing learning organisations in the new NHS. BMJ 2000;320:998–1001.

106 Koeck C. Time for organisational development in healthcare organisations. BMJ 1998;317:1267–1268.

107 Moss M, Garside P, Dawson S. Organisational change: the key to quality improvement. Qual Health Care 1998;7(suppl):S1–S2.

108 Bate SP, Robert G. Report on the 'Breakthrough' collaborative approach to quality and service improvement in four regions of the NHS. A research based evaluation of the Orthopaedic Services Collaborative within the Eastern, South and West, South East, and Trent regions. Birmingham: Health Services Management Centre, University of Birmingham; 2002.

109 Wilson T, Plsek P, Berwick D. *Learning from Around the World: Experiences and Thoughts of Collaborative Improvement From Seven Countries*. Boston: Institute for Healthcare Improvement; 2001.

110 Royal College of General Practitioners. What Sort of Doctor? J R Coll Gen Pract 1981;31:698–702.

111 Schofield T, Hasler J. Approval of trainers and training practices in the Oxford Region. BMJ 1984;288:538–540.

112 Schofield T, Blakeway-Phillips C. Practice Team Accreditation. In: Walshe K, Walsh N, Schofield T, Blakeway-Phillips C, eds. *Accreditation in Primary Care: An Approach to Clinical Governance*. Abingdon, VA: Radcliffe Press; 1999.

113 Macfarlane F, Greenhalgh T, Schofield T, Desombre T. RCGP Quality Team Development programme: an illuminative evaluation. Qual Saf Health Care 2004;13:356–362.

114 Weick KE. *Sensemaking in Organizations*. Thousand Oaks, CA: Sage; 1995.

115 Greenhalgh T, Robert G, Macfarlane F, Bate P, Kyriakidou O. Diffusion of innovations in service organisations: systematic literature review and recommendations for future research. Milbank Q 2004;82:581–629.

116 Epstein RM. Mindful practice. JAMA 1999;282:833–839.

117 Charles-Jones H, Latimer J, May C. Transforming general practice: the redistribution of medical work in primary care. Sociol Health Illn 2003;25:71–92.

118 Greenhalgh T, Voisey C, Robb N. Interpreted consultations as 'business as usual'? A study of organisational routines in primary care. In: Ethnicity, Health and Health Care: Understanding Diversity, Tackling Disadvantage. Sociology of Health and Illness Monograph 13, in press.

119 Pratt MG, Rockmann KW, Kaufmann JB. Constructing professional identity: the role of work and identity learning cycles in the customization of identity among medical residents. Acad Manag J 2006;49:235–262.

120 Eveland JD. Diffusion, technology transfer and implementation. Knowledge Creation Diffusion Util 1986;8:303–322.

121 Abrahamson E. Managerial fads and fashions: the diffusion and rejection of innovation. Calif Manag Rev 1991;16:586–612.

122 Abrahamson E, Fombrun CJ. Macrocultures: determinants and consequences. Acad Manag Rev 1994;19:728–755.

123 Ovretveit J, Bate P, Cleary P, et al. Quality collaboratives: lessons from research. Qual Saf Health Care 2002;11:345–351.

124 Leatherman S. Optimizing quality collaboratives. Qual Saf Health Care 2002;11:307.

Index